Comprehensive Care Coordination for Chronically Ill Adults

Comprehensive Care Coordination for Chronically Ill Adults

Editors

Cheryl Schraeder, RN, PhD, FAAN

Director of Policy and Practice Initiatives
Institute for Healthcare Innovation
UIC College of Nursing
Chicago, IL, USA

Paul Shelton, EdD

Senior Research Specialist
Institute for Healthcare Innovation
UIC College of Nursing
Chicago, IL, USA

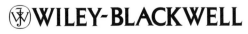

WILEY-BLACKWELL

A John Wiley & Sons, Ltd., Publication

This edition first published 2011 © 2011 by John Wiley & Sons, Inc.

Wiley-Blackwell is an imprint of John Wiley & Sons, formed by the merger of Wiley's global Scientific, Technical and Medical business with Blackwell Publishing.

Registered office: John Wiley & Sons Ltd, The Atrium, Southern Gate, Chichester,
West Sussex, PO19 8SQ, UK

Editorial offices: 2121 State Avenue, Ames, Iowa 50014-8300, USA
The Atrium, Southern Gate, Chichester, West Sussex, PO19 8SQ, UK
9600 Garsington Road, Oxford, OX4 2DQ, UK

For details of our global editorial offices, for customer services, and for information about how to apply for permission to reuse the copyright material in this book please see our website at www.wiley.com/wiley-blackwell.

Library of Congress Cataloging-in-Publication Data

Comprehensive care coordination for chronically ill adults / editors, Cheryl Schraeder, Paul Shelton.
       p. ; cm.
   Includes bibliographical references and index.
   ISBN-13: 978-0-8138-1194-9 (pbk. : alk. paper)
   ISBN-10: 0-8138-1194-5
   1. Chronically ill–United States.   2. Chronic diseases–United States.   3. Integrated delivery of health care–United States.   I. Schraeder, Cheryl.   II. Shelton, Paul.
   [DNLM: 1. Chronic Disease–United States.   2. Comprehensive Health Care–United States.   3. Delivery of Health Care, Integrated–United States.   4. Health Services Needs and Demand–economics–United States.   5. Socioeconomic Factors–United States.   WT 30]
   RC108.C647 2011
   616.02′8–dc23
                                                                         2011018145

A catalogue record for this book is available from the British Library.

This book is published in the following electronic formats: ePDF 9780470960868; ePub 9780470960875; Mobi 9780470960882

Set in 10/12.5 pt Times by Aptara® Inc., New Delhi, India
Printed and bound in Singapore by Fabulous Printers Pte Ltd

1   2011

Contents

SECTION 4 MEDICAID MODELS

SECTION 5 PRACTICE CHANGE

Editors and Contributors

Editors

Cheryl Schraeder, RN, PhD, FAAN
Clinical Associate Professor
College of Nursing
University of Illinois at Chicago
Chicago, IL
USA

Paul Shelton, EdD
College of Nursing
University of Illinois at Chicago
Chicago, IL
USA

Contributors

Kyle R. Allen, DO, AGFS
Professor of Internal and Family Medicine
Northeastern Ohio Universities Colleges
of Medicine & Pharmacy
Medical Director, Post Acute & Senior
Services
Chief, Division of Geriatric Medicine
Summa Health System
Akron, OH
USA

Robert M. Atkins, MD, MPH
Senior Medical Director-Integration
Aetna-Schaller Anderson
Indianapolis, IN
USA

Emma Barker, MSW
Associate Program Officer
New York Academy of Medicine
New York, NY
USA

Robert Berenson, MD
Institute Fellow
The Urban Institute
Washington, DC
USA

Carrie Berger, BA, MSW Candidate
College of Nursing
University of Illinois at Chicago
Chicago, IL
USA

**Michael K. Berkes, BS, MSW
Candidate**
Visiting Research Specialist
College of Nursing
University of Illinois at Chicago
Chicago, IL
USA

Chad Boult, MD, MPH, MBA
Professor and Director
The Lipitz Center for Integrated Health
Care
Department of Health Policy and
Management
Bloomberg School of Public Health
Johns Hopkins University
Baltimore, MD
USA

Randall S. Brown, PhD
Mathematica Policy Research
Princeton, NJ
USA

Cherie P. Brunker, MD
Associate Professor
Division of Geriatric Medicine
University of Utah
Chief of Geriatrics
Intermountain Healthcare
Salt Lake City, UT
USA

Eric A. Coleman, MD, MPH
Professor of Medicine
Division of Health Care Policy and
Research
Department of Medicine
University of Colorado
Denver, CO
USA

Beverly J. Court, MHA, PhD
Research Manager
Washington State Medicaid Purchasing
Administration
Olympia, WA
USA

Meg Cristofalo, MSW, MPA
University of Washington
Seattle, WA
USA

L. Gail Dobell, PhD
Measurement and Evaluation Specialist
Residents First - Advancing Quality in
Ontario Long-Term Care Homes
Ontario Health Quality Council
Toronto, ON
Canada

David A. Dorr, MD, MS
Associate Professor
Primary: Department of Medical
Informatics & Clinical Epidemiology
Joint: Department of Internal Medicine &
Geriatrics
Oregon Health & Science University
Portland, OR
USA

Mark E. Douglas, JD, MSN, RN
Director of Clinical Project Coordination
Aetna-Schaller Anderson
Indianapolis, IN
USA

Linda Fahey, RN, MSN
Decatur Memorial Hospital
Decatur, IL
USA

**Sandee Ferguson, RN, BBA,
MS, Fellow**
Manager, Long Term Care Access &
Integration
Community Long Term Care Division
Ohio Department of Aging
Columbus, Ohio
USA

**Angela M. Gerolamo, PhD,
APRN, BC**
Nurse Researcher
Mathematica Policy Research
Princeton, NJ
USA

Arkadipta Ghosh, PhD
Researcher
Mathematica Policy Research
Princeton, NJ
USA

Robyn L. Golden, LCSW
Director of Older Adult Programs
Rush University Medical Center
Chicago, IL
USA

Lee Greer, MD, MBA
Chief Quality and Safety Officer
North Mississippi Health Services
Tupelo, MS
USA

Carol Groves, RN, MPA
Senior Director of Continuing Care
Kaiser Foundation Health Plan of the
Mid-Atlantic States, Inc.
Rockville, MD
USA

Beth A. Hale, PhD, RN
Director of Admissions
Hospice of the Valley
Phoenix, AZ
USA

Allison Hamblin, MSPH
Center for Health Care Strategies
Hamilton, NJ
USA

Susan Hazelett, RN, MS
Manager HSREI
Summa Health System
Akron, OH
USA

Lynda Hedstrom, MSN, APRN, NP-C
Senior Director Professional Practice and
Clinical Training

UnitedHealthcare Medicare and
Retirement

Mike Herndon, DO
Medical Director
Health Care Management
Oklahoma Health Care Authority
Oklahoma City, OK
USA

Ida Hess, MSN, FNP-BC
Visiting Nurse Practice Specialist
Institute for Healthcare Innovation
College of Nursing
University of Illinois at Chicago
Mahomet, IL
USA

Carolyn Holder, MSN, RN, GCNS-BC
Manager, Transitional Care
Post Acute and Senior Services
Summa Health System
Akron, OH
USA
Adjunct Faculty, College of Nursing
Kent State University
Kent, OH
USA

Julianne R. Howell, PhD
Independent Technical Consultant
Centers for Medicare & Medicaid Services
Baltimore, MD
USA

Krista L. Jones, DNP, MSN, ACHN, RN
Clinical Instructor
College of Nursing
University of Illinois
Urbana, IL
USA

Molly M. King, BA
Research Assistant II
Oregon Health & Science University
Portland, OR
USA

Antoinette Krupski, PhD
Associate Director, CHAMMP
Research Associate Professor
Department of Psychiatry and Behavioral
Sciences
University of Washington at Harborview
Medical Center
Seattle, WA
USA

Daniel S. Lessler, MD, MHA
Professor of Medicine
School of Medicine, University of
Washington
Associate Medical Director, Harborview
Medical Center
Seattle, WA
USA

David Mancuso, PhD
Senior Research Supervisor
Washington State Department of Social
and Health Services
Research and Data Analysis Division
Olympia, Washington
USA

Eran D. Metzger, MD
Assistant Professor of Psychiatry
Harvard Medical School
Associate Director of Psychiatry at
Hebrew SeniorLife
Boston, MA
USA

Robert Newcomer, PhD
Professor
Institute for Health & Aging
University of California
San Francisco, CA
USA

Tracy Novak, MHS
Associate Director
Director of Communications

The Lipitz Center for Integrated Health
Care
Department of Health Policy and
Management
Bloomberg School of Public Health
Johns Hopkins University
Baltimore, MD
USA

**Joo-bong Park Oh, MN, MS,
PsyD, RN**
Supervisor
LAC USC Medical Center
Los Angeles, CA
USA

Anthony J. Perry, MD
Director, Johnston R. Bowman Health
Center
Associate Professor of Internal Medicine
Rush University Medical Center
Chicago, IL
USA

Maria C. Raven, MD, MPH, MSc
Assistant Professor
Department of Emergency Medicine
Division of General Internal Medicine
New York University School of Medicine
Bellevue Hospital Center
New York, NY
USA

**Carolyn J. Reconnu, RN,
BSN, CCM**
Manager
Health Management Program
Oklahoma Health Care Authority
Oklahoma City, OK
USA

Daniel A. Reece, MSW, LCSW
PeaceHealth Oregon Region
Strategy, Innovation and Development
Eugene, OR
USA

Karyn Rizzo, RN, CHPN, GCNS
Executive Director
Notre Dame Hospice
Worcester, MA

Benjamin Ronk, BA
Visiting Research Specialist
College of Nursing
University of Illinois at Chicago
Chicago, IL
USA

Madeleine Rooney, MSW, LCSW
Program Coordinator, Transitional Care
Older Adult Programs
Rush University Medical Center
Chicago, IL
USA

Susan Rosenbek, RN, MS
Division of Health Care Policy and
Research
Department of Medicine
University of Colorado
Denver, CO
USA

Joseph L. Ruby, BA, MA
President & CEO
Area Agency on Aging
Uniontown, OH
USA

Jennifer Schore, MSW, MS
Mathematica Policy Research
Princeton, NJ
USA

Gayle E. Shier, MSW
Program Coordinator
Rush University Medical Center
Chicago, IL
USA

Stephen A. Somers, PhD
Center for Health Care Strategies
Hamilton, NJ
USA

Brenda Sulick, PhD
Vice President
Congressional Affairs & Advocacy
National PACE Association
Alexandria, VA
USA

Chandra L. Torgerson, RN, BSN, MS
SVP Quality Management and Chief
Nursing Officer
UnitedHealthcare Medicare & Retirement

Christine van Reenen, PhD
Senior Vice President for Public Policy
National PACE Association
Alexandria, VA
USA

Patricia J. Volland, MSW, MBA
The New York Academy of Medicine
Senior Vice President, Strategy and
Business Development
Director, Social Work Leadership Institute
New York, NY
USA

Valerie Waldschmidt, BSE
Visiting Research Coordinator
College of Nursing
Institute for Healthcare Innovation
University of Illinois at Chicago
Chicago, IL
USA

Nancy Whitelaw, PhD
Senior Vice President
Healthy Aging
National Council on Aging
Washington, DC
USA

Adam B. Wilcox, PhD
Assistant Professor
Department of Biomedical Informatics
College of Physicians and Surgeons
Columbia University
New York, NY
USA

Mary E. Wright
Program Associate, Social Work
Leadership Institute, and Executive
Assistant
New York Academy of Medicine
New York, NY
USA

Phyllis Yoders, RN, BSN
Long Term Care Nursing Consultant
Area Agency on Aging
Uniontown, OH
USA

Weon-seob Yoo, PhD, MPH, MD
Assistant Professor
College of Medicine
Eulji University
Joong-Gu, Daejeon
Republic of Korea

Chad Zhu, MS
Research and Data Analysis Division
Washington State Department of Social
and Health Services

Acknowledgments

There are a number of people we would like to thank that have contributed to and helped shape our thinking and understanding of coordinated health care for adults with chronic illnesses. We thank Sandra Reifsteck, at the time an administrator with the Carle Clinic Association, Urbana, IL, who fostered a vision that primary care desperately needed to be improved for patients with chronic illness and provided opportunities for moving that vision forward. We thank Anna Bergstrom, when she was with the Medical Group Management Association, for her help and guidance with a case management project within multispecialty group practices that targeted chronically ill adults. We thank Donna Regenstrief and Christopher Langston, with the John A. Hartford Foundation, who provided the opportunity to expand a collaborative coordinated care intervention in primary care, and Dennis Nugent and Cindy Mason, with the Centers for Medicare & Medicaid Services, who worked with us for a number of years on different demonstrations to improve the health management of chronically ill Medicare beneficiaries. We thank Kelly Cunningham and Jean Summerfield of Healthcare and Family Services for the opportunity to improve the management of Medicaid beneficiaries transitioning from nursing facilities to the community. We thank Patricia Volland and Robyn Golden, at the New York Academy of Medicine Social Work Leadership Institute, for their continuing efforts to improve the care coordination for chronically ill older adults. We thank Eric Coleman, MD, Mark Sager, MD, and David Dorr, MD, for sharing their vast clinical insights and research experiences accumulated from working in the health management of chronically ill adults within primary care, and to Robert Newcomer of the University of California at San Francisco and Randall Brown of Mathematica Policy Research for sharing their unique perspectives and viewpoints on different aspects to consider when evaluating chronic care delivery models. We thank Ida Hess and Donna Dworak for their commitments to help define and advance nursing roles in a collaborative practice with physicians, patients, and their families, and to Robert Kirby, Robert Parker, Curtis Krock, Paul Schaap, and John Stoll, primary care physicians at the Carle healthcare system, Urbana, IL, who had the foresight and interest to work in collaborative care teams with nurses and who contributed to quality efforts to improve the care of their chronically ill patients. Our heartfelt thanks goes out to Cynthia Fraser, director of our coordinated care programs; she is a unique individual with exceptional organizational and interpersonal skills that were integral to providing necessary and needed services to chronically ill adults. A big debt of gratitude is owed to Senator Richard Durbin from the state of Illinois and his legislative director, Dena Morris, for the commitment, time, and insight they shared in advocating for and advancing the care of the chronically ill at the federal level. And most importantly, this book would not have been possible if not for the thousands of patients and their caregivers who have participated in the coordinated care programs that we have conducted over the past 20 plus years. It is because of their interest and commitment in helping others through sharing their stories, their insights concerning the frustrations and successes of managing their illnesses, and their experiences in navigating the fragmented health care system that makes the effort that much more worth while. Also, a special thanks goes to our spouses, Claire and Thomas, and our children for their endless encouragement and support.

Introduction

Cheryl Schraeder and Paul Shelton

One of the most frequently noted criticisms of the U.S. health care industry is the fragmented nature of its delivery system and payment structure. This fragmented disconnect has resulted in excessive duplication and overuse of medical services, a lack of access to essential services, and patients who are not fully engaged in their care. Our health care industry is especially deficient in providing high quality, coordinated, and cost effective care to adults with multiple chronic health conditions.

Despite these limitations of the current health care system, a number of policymakers, health care professionals, and researchers are engaged in developing and testing new models of care for patients with co-morbidities. Many of these models involve physicians, nurses, and other professionals working in collaborative relationships with patients and their caregivers, implementing evidence-based best practices and comprehensive coordinated care. The primary goals of these programs are to reduce unnecessary emergency department visits and avoidable hospital admissions, and to improve patients' quality of life and satisfaction with care.

These program results to date have demonstrated success in improving processes of care, quality of life, and satisfaction with care for multi-morbid patients, but have produced limited success in reducing their use and cost of health services. However, the results suggest that certain components are integral to and have the potential to be cost effective when included in comprehensive efforts to manage the health care needs of adults with multiple chronic illnesses.

This book is intended for medical, nursing, allied health, and social service professionals, and students who are interested in and/or involved in providing care and the coordination of health and community services for chronically ill adults. It presents concise information drawn from a number of disciplines and sources that has been learned over the past two plus decades from pilot studies, randomized clinical trials, and federal demonstrations that can be used as a resource and starting point for improvements in the delivery of chronic care.

These lessons learned are presented in two major sections. The first section presents background on the theoretical concepts of comprehensive care coordination, including: the demographic and health characteristics of chronically ill adults; relevant coordinated care practices in the acute, primary, and community setting; intervention components that have been successful and are essential in reducing hospital readmissions; different aspects and approaches to program evaluation; essential elements of health information technology systems; alternative payment methods for supporting chronic care management; and approaches to educating interdisciplinary team members. The second section uses a case study format to present a number of nationally recognized best practices that use different approaches in providing comprehensive care coordination, including: community-based primary care; transitional care; acute care discharge planning; and managed care and integrated health care systems. Programs are also described that provide services to Medicaid and Medicare populations, services for patients with specific chronic conditions, telemedicine services, and an example of a population-based approach to chronic illness in the Republic of Korea.

In the pages that follow we have tried to present a picture of some notions of what evidence-based, best practice comprehensive coordinated care might look like, as well as different ways it is currently provided and could be delivered in the future. Although the quest for the best pathway to high quality, cost effective chronic illness care remains elusive, the search will likely gain momentum, especially in an electrically charged atmosphere of health care reform, and the rapidly aging of America. It is our hope that the information contained in the following chapters makes some contribution to the development of innovative models that improve the quality of life and medical care of chronically ill adults.

Part 1

Theoretical concepts

Chapter 1

Chronic illness

Paul Shelton, Cheryl Schraeder, Michael Berkes,
and Benjamin Ronk

Introduction

The demographic landscape of the United States has changed significantly. Americans are living longer than ever before. The average life span has increased from 47 years for individuals born in 1900 to 78 years for those born in 2006 (National Center for Health Statistics [NCHS] 2010). The result has been an exponential growth in the number and percentage of older Americans, which is unique to our nation's history. This longevity is primarily due to advances in modern medical science that have produced new screening and diagnostic technologies, pharmaceuticals, and medical procedures, as well as comprehensive initiatives that have greatly diminished or eliminated infectious diseases and improved public health problems. Americans living in the twenty-first century can expect to live longer than any previous generation. Longer life expectancy combined with the baby-boom generation, individuals born after World War II from 1946 through 1964, will double the number of individuals who are 65 years and older during the next 25 years.

This aging of America has created problems and challenges for our health care system. As longevity has increased so have the numbers of Americans living with chronic illnesses. Chronic illnesses afflict people of all ages, and although a majority of individuals living with chronic illnesses are not elderly, the likelihood of having a chronic illness increases dramatically with advancing age. Current projections estimate that approximately 66% of Americans 18 years of age and older suffer from at least one chronic illness, and as much as 80% of individuals 50 years of age and older suffer from at least one chronic illness (Machlin *et al.* 2008). These individuals seek and receive health care in a system that is designed, structured, and financed for treating acute episodes of care. The current system has been extensively criticized for being overly deficient in providing coordinated care for individuals with chronic illnesses who are primarily insured through Medicare and Medicaid (Institute of Medicine [IOM] 2001), and who are not receiving optimum chronic illness care (McGlynn *et al.* 2003).

The new generation of older Americans, the baby boomers, will be distinctly different from previous generations. They will be more educated, have more discretionary income, be more racially diverse, have fewer children, and have less disability compared

Comprehensive Care Coordination for Chronically Ill Adults, First Edition. Edited by Cheryl Schraeder and Paul Shelton.
© 2011 John Wiley & Sons, Inc. Published 2011 by John Wiley & Sons, Inc.

to their parent's generation (Federal Interagency Forum on Aging-Related Statistics 2008; IOM 2008). Their sheer numbers alone will dramatically affect the future of our health care system. During the next two decades the number of older adults will double, from approximately 37 million to over 70 million, accounting for an 8% overall increase within the total population, currently from 12% to 20% (IOM 2008). While this approaching demographic shift has been anticipated for over 50 years, our health care system is not prepared for its arrival. More providers with specialized training and resources, and new approaches to delivering chronic care are needed to meet the aging population's health care needs (Bodenheimer *et al.* 2009; IOM 2008). Presenting a stark reality, the IOM (2008) asserted that providers are inadequately prepared in general knowledge of geriatrics, the health care workforce is not large enough to meet older patients' needs, and the scarcity of workers currently specializing in geriatrics is even more pronounced. These shortages will become more pronounced in the future.

According to the IOM (2001), improving care for the chronically ill is one of the most important health care challenges facing our nation today. The IOM report makes clear that there are no easy means or readily available answers to improving this care. Despite some consensus regarding what optimum chronic care should resemble, its delivery remains elusive (Wolff & Boult 2005). Research has demonstrated that achieving and sustaining improvements in the care coordination and medical management of these chronically ill adults is extremely difficult and is hindered by a general lack of knowledge, experience, and financial mechanisms necessary for the optimal care for this large and ever expanding segment of the population (Norris *et al.* 2008; Wallace 2005). Dysfunctional incentives have created fragmentation within our current system which fails to address the underlying causes of disease, and far too many care decisions are not under the control of clinicians and patients.

In this chapter we (1) define chronic illness, its general prevalence, and the main causes for its dramatic increase; (2) present a demographic profile of the adult population 55 years of age and older, (3) present a demographic profile for adults 65 years of age or older, with additional characteristics related to Medicare beneficiaries; and (4) present specific characteristics of chronically ill adults. A basic understanding of the scope and magnitude of chronic illness is necessary in order to begin to design, implement, and evaluate effective comprehensive care coordination programs for the tidal wave of chronically ill adults who will hit the health care system, especially Medicare, with brute force in the very near future.

What is a chronic illness?

Chronic illness is a general term that refers to a diagnosed illness, functional limitation, or cognitive impairment that lasts at least a year, places limits on a person's daily activities, and often requires regular attention and medical care (Hwang *et al.* 2001; Anderson 2010). Chronic illnesses are often preventable, usually develop in later adulthood, and last for years. They are typically managed with proper care from clinicians, self-care activities, and often with help from family members acting as informal caregivers. Some of the most prevalent chronic illnesses include arthritis, asthma/bronchitis, cancer, cardiovascular disease, depression, and diabetes (American Association of Retired Persons [AARP] 2009a; Center for Disease Control and Prevention [CDCP] 2009).

Having a chronic illness affects people in multiple ways. Many chronic illnesses reduce a person's quality of life and/or limits their performance of normal activities without some form of assistance. Approximately 20% of people who have a chronic illness also have one or more limitations in activities of daily living (ADLs) or instrumental activities of daily living (IADLs; Agency for Healthcare Research and Quality [AHRQ] 2006). Typically, people with multiple chronic illnesses have significantly higher rates of hospital admissions and emergency room (ER) visits, and experience higher medical expenses compared to people without a chronic illness. Chronic illnesses account for 70% of annual mortality rates; heart disease, cancer, and stroke are the causes of 50% of all deaths each year (CDCP 2009).

The prevalence of chronic illness is steadily on the rise, and will increase exponentially in the future. In 1995 there were approximately 118 million individuals living with a chronic illness. This number is projected to increase 45% by 2030 to 171 million (NCHS 2010). In 2006, over 20% of all individuals had at least one chronic illness, and 28% had two or more (Anderson 2010). Hypertension was the most common chronic illness (33%), followed by lipid disorders (22%), upper respiratory diseases (19%), non-traumatic joint disorders (17%), heart disease (14%), diabetes mellitus (13%), eye disorders (11%), asthma (10%), and chronic respiratory infections (10%; Anderson 2010).

There are several factors that contribute to the increase of these illnesses. An aging population is a prominent factor, as the proportion of individuals with chronic illnesses increases dramatically with age. For example, one in fifteen children has multiple chronic illnesses (7%) compared to three out of four elderly individuals (75%). National statistics highlight these differences for distinct age groups (AHRQ 2006): 27% of children from birth to age 19 have one chronic illness, 7% have two or more; 40% of adults aged 20 to 44 have one chronic illness, 17% have two or more; 68% of adults aged 45 to 64 have one chronic illness, 43% have two or more; and 91% of the elderly have one chronic illness while 73% have two or more. In comparison, respiratory disease (36%) and asthma (30%) are the most prominent pediatric chronic illnesses, while hypertension (60%), cholesterol disorders (41%), arthritis (28%), heart disease (25%), and eye disorders (23%) are the most common in adulthood (Anderson 2010).

The increased use of evidence-based clinical guidelines have broadened the definitions of disease, and advances in treatment modalities have led to more people being screened and subsequently diagnosed with chronic illnesses. Treatment advances have allowed providers to diagnose chronic illnesses and identify people who might benefit from medications or therapies at an earlier age, while public awareness of certain chronic illnesses has led to more people requesting testing and treatment (AARP 2009a). Two examples that highlight these advances are the increased percentage of adults that are either under surveillance or are being actively treated for hypertension (Ostchega *et al.* 2007) and/or high cholesterol (Hyre *et al.* 2007), with the intent of preventing or delaying the onset of heart disease or stroke. As a result, the most prominent form of chronic illness treatment with adults is hypertension and elevated cholesterol.

Several behaviors identified with the American lifestyle are also responsible for the increase in chronic illnesses. Three modifiable health risk behaviors, lack of physical activity, tobacco use, and poor nutrition (CDCP 2009), are linked to several chronic illnesses, including chronic obstructive pulmonary disease (COPD), diabetes, and cancer (AARP 2009a). Less than half of all adults (48.8%) meet Healthy People 2010 minimum recommendations for physical activity, and 23% report no leisure-time physical activity at all during the month (Carlson *et al.* 2008). Approximately 20% of adults (NCHS 2010) and 23% of high school students are cigarette smokers (CDCP 2008).

Obesity has reached epidemic proportions in America and is one of the biggest public health challenges the country has ever faced (U.S. Department of Health and Human Services 2001). An estimated 34% of adults aged 20 years and over are overweight, 34% are obese, and 6% are extremely obese (Flegal *et al.* 2010), while over 20% of children and teens between the ages of 6 and 19 are obese (Ogden *et al.* 2008). Body Mass Index (BMI), calculated as weight in kilograms divided by height in meters squared (kg/m^2), is commonly used to classify people as overweight (BMI 25.0-29.9), obese (BMI equal to or greater than 30.0), and extremely obese (BMI equal to or greater than 40.0). Researchers at RAND Health (2002) estimated that obese individuals have 67% more chronic illnesses than normal-weight individuals, and long-term smokers have 25% more chronic illnesses compared to individuals who have never smoked.

A profile of adults aged 55 years and over

In this section we present selected sociodemographic characteristics of the adult population aged 55 and over. This age cohort was selected because they will constitute nearly one-third (31%) of the total population by 2030 (U.S. Census Bureau 2008), and it is during the ages of 55 to 64 that some adults begin to experience chronic illnesses typical of older adults (Paez *et al.* 2009). Most of the information presented in this section is based on data from the U.S. Census Bureau (2008) and the 2004-2007 National Health Interview Survey (Schoenborn & Heymen 2009). This overview incorporates the latest data available and covers demographics, health status and specific chronic illnesses, specific health behaviors, and health service utilization. Comparisons are made between the following age groups: 55 to 64 (near elderly); 65 to 74 (elderly); 75 to 84 (old); and 85 and over (very old). The data are summarized in Table 1.1.

Demographics

In 2007, adults aged 55 and over accounted for approximately 24% of the population (U.S Census Bureau 2008). When examined by age category, 11% represented the near elderly, 7% elderly, 5% old and 1% very old. Approximately 55% were female, a percentage that increased with older age: 52% of the near elderly; 56% of the elderly; 59% of the old; and 66% of the very old. Minorities comprised 20% of the total population as well as the four age groups.

Marital status followed a similar pattern: 62% were married, but this figure decreased to 50% of the old and 28% of the very old. Widowhood reflected a mirror image: 18% were widowed, but this figure increased to 39% of the old and 63% of the very old

(U.S. Census Bureau 2008). Educational attainment was quite high; 83% graduated from high school, and 26% were college graduates (15% with an undergraduate degree and 11% with an advanced degree).

Household income primarily reflected differences in employment and retirement status. The median household income in 2008 for adults 55 to 64 years of age was about $57,000, and $30,000 for individuals 65 years and older (DeNavas-Walt *et al.* 2009); 54% of the total population had household income of $35,000 or more (U.S. Census Bureau 2008). About 13% of very old individuals (85 years of age and older), compared to 9% of the total population, lived below the poverty level (poor). Health insurance coverage was also governed by employment and age. Approximately 88% of individuals aged 55 to 64 had some form of health insurance, either through employment-based health benefits/individually purchased coverage (68%) or public coverage (20%), which includes the disabled (10%) and those covered by Medicaid (7%; DeNavas-Walt *et al.* 2009). Almost all individuals aged 65 and over were covered by Medicare (93%), with 10% covered by both Medicare and Medicaid (U.S. Census Bureau 2008). About 59% of the 65 and older age group had some type of private health insurance, and a little over 7% had military-based health insurance, Tricare (Administration on Aging [AoA] 2009).

Health status

Overall, about 23% of adults aged 55 and over rated their health as fair or poor (Schoenborn & Heymen 2009), ranging from 20% in the near elderly to 32% in the very old. There were no differences in health status by gender, except males in the very old age group were more likely than women to rate their health as fair or poor. Individuals whose household income was below the poverty level, who were not married, and who had Medicaid health insurance coverage were more likely to be in fair or poor health.

Total chronic conditions varied accordingly with age. A little over 20% of adults 55 to 64 years had one chronic condition in 2005, and 57% had two or more. This prevalence was in sharp contrast to older adults. Almost 15% of elderly adults had one chronic condition, and 77% had two or more (Machlin *et al.* 2008). About 50% of adults aged 55 and over had hypertension, ranging from 41% in the near elderly group to 56% in the old age group (Schoenborn & Heymen 2009). Between the ages of 55 and 64 men were more likely than women to have hypertension, but the difference was just the opposite for those 65 years and older; women were more likely than men to have hypertension. African American adults and those with Medicaid coverage had the highest rates of hypertension compared to all adults 55 years of age and older.

Heart disease increased with age; 25% of adults aged 55 and over had the disease, but rates more than doubled when comparing the near elderly (17%) with the very old (40%; Schoenborn & Heymen 2009). Compared to all adults 55 years and older, men were more likely than women to have heart disease, and so were men or women who lived in poverty. The prevalence of diabetes did not consistently increase with age. About 16% of the total population had diabetes, with a high of 19% in the elderly group compared to a low of 13% in the very old. Individuals who were poor or had Medicaid coverage were more likely to be diagnosed with diabetes.

Overall, 32% of adults aged 55 and over had some form of hearing impairment and 14% had vision problems, even when wearing glasses (Schoenborn & Heymen 2009). These incidences increased substantially with age; approximately 62% of the very old had hearing difficulties and 27% had vision impairments. The highest rates of vision impairments were again associated with poverty and Medicaid coverage.

Aging takes its toll on performing everyday activities (Schoenborn & Heymen 2009). The percentage of adults 55 years and older who had difficulty performing physical and social activities increased with age. At least 20% to 25% had some limitations in walking any distance, walking up steps, or standing for any length of time. Researchers have suggested that these disability rates among the near elderly will rise over 40% in the future if depression, diabetes, and nervous system conditions continue to be diagnosed in record numbers (Martin *et al.* 2010). These limitation rates more than doubled for old and very old individuals. About 10% of all adults had difficulties shopping or socializing, and once again these numbers doubled with the old and very old age groups. Arthritis and other musculoskeletal conditions and heart or circulatory problems were the primary causes of their physical limitations (NCHS 2010). As a general trend, women were more likely than men to have limitations performing physical or social activities with prominent differences emerging among the elderly. Adults with Medicaid coverage and who lived in poverty had higher rates of difficulty, and individuals who were married had lower rates of difficulty compared to individuals who were not married.

Health behaviors

About half of adults aged 55 and over (52%) participated in some type of leisure-time physical activity in the past year (Schoenborn & Heymen 2009). The prevalence decreased to less than 30% in the very old. There was little variation in physical activity between men and women. The percentage of adults who did some type of leisure-time physical activity on a regular basis plummeted to 24%. Individuals who were living in poverty, were covered by Medicaid, or were not married were less likely to engage in any type of physical activity.

This cohort of adults contributed to the nation's obesity epidemic. About 23% were considered obese in 2002 (Rhoades 2005). The old and very old age groups were the least likely to be obese (14%). African American and Hispanic adults (34%) were more likely to be obese compared to Caucasian or Asian individuals (12%). Only 34% of all adults were at a healthy weight, ranging from 30% for the near elderly to 53% for the very old (Schoenborn & Heymen 2009). Typically, women were more likely to be at a healthy weight than men. Half of adults aged 55 and older had never smoked cigarettes (50%) and another 27% were former smokers (Schoenborn & Heymen 2009). These percentages increased with age, and women usually were more likely than men to have never smoked.

Health service utilization

The use of almost all types of health care services increased with advancing age (Schoenborn & Heymen 2009). Most adults 55 years of age and older had a regular source of care (94%). Uninsured adults were less likely to have a regular source of care than any other group (65%). A majority of these adults visited their doctors at least yearly (88%); almost all adults 65 years and older (over 95%) visited a doctor at least once in the past year.

Approximately one-fifth (22%) of adults aged 55 and over had at least one ER visit in the past 12 months, ranging from 19% in the near elderly age group to 33% in the very old age group. Poor adults and those with Medicaid coverage were more likely than other adults to have an ER visit regardless of age. ER visit rates were also higher for unmarried individuals compared to those who were married, regardless of age. In 2007, approximately 13% of adults 55 to 64 years of age were hospitalized at least once in the previous year compared to 33% of adults 65 years of age and older (NCHS 2010). The primary reasons for these admissions were either cardiac or respiratory related and were similar between age groups (Russo *et al.* 2009). The primary reasons for hospitalization among near elderly adults were (1) coronary arteriosclerosis, (2) osteoarthritis, (3) nonspecific chest pain, (4) pneumonia, and (5) congestive heart failure (CHF)/acute myocardial infarction. For adults 65 to 74 years of age reasons included (1) coronary arteriosclerosis, (2) osteoarthritis, (3) CHF, (4) pneumonia, and (5) COPD/cardiac dysrhythmias. For adults 80 years of age and older reasons in 2002 included (1) CHF, (2) pneumonia, and (3) cardiac dysrhythmias (NCHS 2010).

People who receive their health insurance coverage from Medicaid present a different picture of chronicity compared to the general population of adults 55 years of age and older. The Medicaid program is the largest single purchaser of nursing home and long-term care services in the country, and in 2006 Medicaid spending accounted for approximately one in six health care dollars. It accounted for 7% of all federal outlays and consistently averages at least 20% of state budgets, placing substantial pressure on public resources (Kronick *et al.* 2007). Adults comprised approximately 27% of the total Medicaid population, the disabled accounted for 16%, and the elderly accounted for 9% (Williams 2004). More than 60% of adult Medicaid enrollees had a chronic or disabling illness, primarily diabetes, hypertension, asthma, psychoses, or chronic depression.

Nearly half (48%) of adult Medicaid enrollees also had at least one physical or cognitive limitation, and almost half of these individuals (46%) had a mental health problem. People with physical or cognitive disabilities were more likely to have three or more chronic illnesses (35%) compared to non-disabled adults (10%). The most common occurring chronic illnesses for disabled beneficiaries were hypertension (23%), diabetes (14%), and behavioral health disorders, such as affective psychoses (9%) and schizophrenia (9%; Kronick *et al.* 2007).

Medicaid beneficiaries with disabilities and the elderly had different types of chronic illnesses (Kronick *et al.* 2007). The elderly were more likely to have cardiovascular disease (52%) compared to people with disabilities (32%), while individuals with disabilities were more likely to have a psychiatric diagnosis (29%) than the elderly.

Medicaid enrollees with multiple chronic illnesses and disabilities had complex health problems that resulted in more intensive health care use and subsequently much higher expenditures. For example, the elderly and disabled account for only 25% of the total Medicaid population, yet they consume 70% of Medicaid's resources (Williams 2004). Average annual expenses for these beneficiaries were more than 15 times compared to beneficiaries without these conditions.

Table 1.1   Selected Characteristics of Adults 55 Years of Age and Older

Characteristic	Percent of Population
Total population	24
Total population by age category	
55–64 years	11
65–74 years	7
75–84 years	5
85+ years	1
Female	55
55–64 years	52
65–74 years	56
75–84 years	59
85+ years	66
Minority race	20
Not Married	48
Education	
Less than high school	17
College degree (bachelor's or above)	26
Household income below poverty level	9
Health insurance coverage	
55–64 years	88
Employer/private	68
Disabled	10
Medicaid	7
65+ years	
Medicare	93
Medicare and Medicaid	10
Medigap	59
Military-based	7
Health rated fair/poor	23
Chronic Illnesses	
55–64 years	
1 chronic condition	20
2+ chronic conditions	57
65+ years	
1 chronic condition	15
2+ chronic conditions	77
Hypertension	55
Heart disease	25
Diabetes	16
Hearing problems	32
Vision problems	14
Obesity	23
Any difficulty with physical activities	25
Any difficulty with social activities	10
Health Behaviors	
Leisure-time physical activity	52
Current smoker	23
Prior healthcare use	
Regular source of care	94
Any ER visit	22
Any hospital admission	
55 to 64 years	13
65+ years	33

Sources: DeNavas-Walt *et al.* 2009; Machlin *et al.* 2008, NCHS 2010; Schoenborn & Haymen 2009; U.S. Census Bureau 2008.

A profile of older adults aged 65 years of age and older

The increasing number of Americans 65 years of age and older, coupled with their complex health needs, is one of the leading causes of escalating costs of health care. The 65-and-over age group has grown twice as fast as the rest of the U.S. population in the past 20 years. One out of eight Americans is now 65 or older (AoA 2009). These growing numbers of older Americans, especially those 75 years of age and over, will present the greatest challenge from economic and human service perspectives because age 75 appears to be the point in the lifespan when disability, morbidity, and mortality rates begin to rapidly increase.

The Medicare program enables older Americans to obtain health care services. However, in its current form, Medicare lacks many of the essential components of a high-quality, efficient health system (Medicare Payment Advisory Commission [MedPAC] 2010a). Program spending and utilization have increased substantially over the last three decades, primarily because for Medicare beneficiaries chronic illness is the norm rather than the exception (Wolff & Boult 2005). It is estimated that if current spending and utilization trends continue, the long-term viability and sustainability of Medicare is in jeopardy (MedPAC 2010a).

Despite the increased prevalence of chronic illness, generalizations about health concerning the elderly are difficult because they are not a homogeneous group. Many people remain relatively healthy and vigorous into their 70s and beyond, while others develop serious illnesses and functional impairment in their 50s and 60s. Chronic illnesses are associated with varying levels of severity (Anderson 2010). Some chronic illnesses are extremely debilitating and others produce effects that are hardly noticeable on an individual's health. Some chronic illnesses are not disabling when diagnosed, but may lead to poorer health later on in life if not treated early and effectively. Some people with chronic illnesses live full, productive lives even with limitations; others experience depression, isolation, and a reduced quality of life.

In this section, we present a summary of demographic and health-related characteristics of adults 65 years of age and older and also specific characteristics of Medicare beneficiaries. The principal sources of data for this section are from the U.S. Bureau of the Census, the NCHS, the Bureau of Labor Statistics, and the Centers for Medicare & Medicaid Services (CMS) Medicare Current Beneficiary Survey. All summary statistics are based on the latest published data available. Selected characteristics are summarized in Table 1.2.

Demographics

Adults 65 years and older represented 13% of the total population in 2008, and are estimated to be over 19% by 2030 (AoA 2009). Females outnumbered males at a 1.36 to 1.0 ratio (136 women for every 100 men). Minorities comprised 19% of the population but are projected to account for 38% of the population by 2050 (Federal Interagency Forum on Aging-Related Statistics 2008). Older men were more likely to be married than older women (72% versus 42%), and widowhood was more common among older women than men (AoA 2009). Marital status had a direct relationship with living arrangements; 19% of older men lived alone compared to 39% of older women. Approximately 78% of both women and men were high school graduates, and about 20% were college graduates.

Older men had higher rates of college graduation than women (25% versus 20%; AoA 2009; Federal Interagency Forum on Aging-Related Statistics 2008). Median household income was $44,000 and 10% had incomes below the poverty level (AoA 2009). A greater percentage of minorities lived in poverty than Caucasians. These low-income elderly represent a diverse and complex group that frequently has socioeconomic stressors, limited or low health literacy, and limited access to health care (Counsel *et al.* 2007).

About half of the total population of individuals aged 65 or older (51%) lived in nine states: California, Florida, New York, Texas, Pennsylvania, Illinois, Ohio, Michigan, and New Jersey. In 11 states they comprised 14% or more of the state population: Florida (17%); West Virginia (16%); Pennsylvania, Maine, Iowa, Hawaii, and North Dakota (each 15%); South Dakota and Arkansas (each 14%), and Rhode Island (14%).

Health status

Only 39% of adults 65 and older rated their current health as excellent or very good (AoA 2009). Racial minorities were less likely to rate their health as excellent or very good compared to Caucasians. Over 50% of adults had at least one chronic illness and many had multiple illnesses. The most frequently occurring chronic illnesses were hypertension (53%), arthritis (46%), heart disease (30%), COPD (22%), any cancer (21%), diabetes (18%), and stroke (9%; Federal Interagency Forum on Aging-Related Statistics 2008). Women reported higher rates of arthritis than men (54% versus 43%); men reported higher levels of heart disease (37% versus 26%) and cancer (24% versus 19%) than women. African Americans reported higher levels of hypertension and diabetes than other racial groups. Almost half of men (48%) and approximately one-third of women (35%) reported trouble hearing. Vision trouble affected about 17% of both men and women. Older adults who lived in poverty consistently had higher rates of kidney disease, CHF, heart disease, mental illness, and diabetes, compared to middle or upper-income older adults (AHRQ 2006).

Some form of disability (difficulty with memory, walking, self-care, or independent living) was reported by 38% of older adults, and 16% needed some type of assistance as a result (AoA 2009). There was a strong correlation between disability status and health status. Among those with a severe disability, 64% were in fair or poor health. Based on 2005 data, 42% had at least one ADL or IADL limitation, and women had higher levels of functional limitations than men (Federal Interagency Forum on Aging-Related Statistics 2008).

Health habits

The percentage of older adults who engaged in regular leisure-time physical activity is somewhat small; only about 26% of adults aged 65 to 74 engaged in regular physical activity, and only 19% of persons 75 years of age or older did so (AoA 2009). Based on height and weight combinations 31% were obese; there were no significant differences in obesity based on gender. Only about 9% were still smokers. Poverty was associated with higher levels of inactivity and cigarette smoking but not obesity (NCHS 2010).

Health service utilization

Almost one in every four adults 65 years of age or older had an ER encounter at least once in the previous year (23%) and 9% had two or more visits (NCHS 2010). Poverty and Medicaid coverage increased the likelihood of ER usage. It has been estimated that ER visit rates will steadily increase among the elderly in coming decades (Wilber *et al.* 2006) which will place more strain on health care resources. The emergency care of older adults is often time and resource intensive, and complicated by underlying chronic illnesses. This increase in future utilization is especially noteworthy since about 33% of elderly patients discharged from the ER are prone to experience an adverse event within 90 days of the index visit, returning to the ER for another visit with or without a hospital admission, nursing home admission, or death (Hastings *et al.* 2008).

About 33% of adults were hospitalized at least once during the past 12 months (Levit *et al.* 2009), and 6% experienced two or more hospital admissions during the same time period (NCHS 2010). Rehospitalization rates among Medicare beneficiaries are high. In 2004, almost one fifth (19.6%) of beneficiaries who had been discharged from a hospital were rehospitalized within 30 days, and 34% were rehospitalized within 90 days; 67% of patients who had been discharged with medical conditions and 52% with surgical procedures were rehospitalized or died within 12 months after discharge (Jenks *et al.* 2009). Among patients rehospitalized within 30 days after a surgical procedure, about 70% were rehospitalized with a medical condition. The most frequent medical reasons for rehospitalization included CHF, pneumonia, COPD, psychoses, and GI problems. The most frequent surgical reasons for rehospitalization included cardiac stent replacement, major hip/knee surgery, other vascular surgery, major bowel surgery, and other hip or femur surgery.

In 2006, the median annual health care cost for these adults was approximately $4,000 per person; about 25% had no expenses or expenses under $1,750; and 25% had expenses over $9,300 (Machlin 2009). Over 50% of individual out-of-pocket spending, excluding health care coverage, was for prescription medications (NCHS 2010). Viewed from another perspective, in 2002 the elderly accounted for 36% of all health care expenses (Cohen & Yu 2006).

Medicare beneficiaries

The Medicare program provides health insurance coverage to Americans who are age 65 or older, under age 65 with certain disabilities, and individuals of all ages diagnosed with End-Stage Renal Disease (ESRD). Medicare Part A, the Hospital Insurance Program, assists in the coverage of inpatient hospital care, inpatient care in a skilled nursing facility, hospice services, and some home health care services. Beneficiaries are automatically enrolled and do not pay a monthly premium for Part A. Medicare Part B, the Medical Insurance Program, helps pay for physician services, outpatient care, some preventive services, and some services not covered under Part A, such as home health care and physical and occupational therapy. Beneficiaries are automatically enrolled unless they opt out, and they must pay a monthly premium for Part B that is deducted from their monthly Social Security benefits. Medicare Part D is a prescription drug benefit provided by private insurance companies. Part D may help lower prescription drug costs for some beneficiaries, and premiums must be paid for by the beneficiary. Below we present a snapshot of the Medicare fee-for-service (FFS) population, with an emphasis on health care utilization and expenditures.

The Medicare population in 2006 was composed of the elderly (84%), the disabled (16%), and individuals with ESRD (less than 1%; MedPAC 2010b). The typical Medicare beneficiary was a Caucasian female (56%) between 65 and 74 years of age (42%), who lived with her spouse (49%), attended some college or was a college graduate (41%), and rated her health as good or fair (51%). Most beneficiaries lived in urban areas (76%), had annual household incomes between $15,000 and $25,000 (22%; CMS 2002), and had some form of supplemental insurance coverage (90%). Their chronic illnesses were arthritis (55%) and hypertension (55%), and they had no ADL or IADL limitations (CMS 2002). Medicare spent an average of $8,865 in 2006 for their health care services (MedPAC 2010b). For more characteristics of the Medicare population see Table 1.2.

Table 1.2   Selected Characteristics of the Medicare Population

Characteristic	Percent of Population
Gender	
Male	44
Female	56
Race	
Caucasian	78
African American	9
Hispanic	8
Other	5
Age Categories	
< 65 years	15
65–74 years	42
75–84 years	31
85+ years	13
Not Married	44
Less than high school	27
Household income below poverty level	15
Medicaid eligible	16
Lives alone	28
Lives in rural area	24
Health rated fair/poor	30
Chronic Illnesses	
Hypertension	55
Arthritis	55
Obesity	31
Heart disease	30
Pulmonary disease	22
Cancer (any)	21
Diabetes	18
Osteoporosis	15
Stroke	11
Alzheimer's disease	4
Prior healthcare use	
Any ER visit	23
2+ ER visits	9
Any hospital admission	33
2+ hospital admissions	6

Sources: CMS 2002; Federal Interagency Forum on Aging-Related Statistics 2008; NCHS 2010; MedPAC 2010b.

Dual-eligible beneficiaries, those who qualify for both Medicare and Medicaid, accounted for 16% of the total Medicare population in 2006 (MedPAC 2010b). They were eligible for Medicaid because of low household income: 51% lived below the poverty level. They were more likely to be female, African American or Hispanic American; they lacked a high school education, had more ADL and/or IADL limitations, lived in rural areas, and lived either in an institution, alone, or with persons other than a spouse. They were more likely to be under 65 years of age (41%), have higher rates of poor health (20%), diabetes, COPD, stroke, and Alzheimer's disease compared to non-dual-eligibles. They accounted for 27% of total Medicare expenditures and averaged per capita expenses of $15,384, which is more than twice that for non-dual-eligible beneficiaries.

In 2008, health care spending was approximately $1.95 trillion (MedPAC 2010b), and accounted for 16% of the gross domestic product (Stanton & Rutherford 2006). Medicare is the largest single purchaser of health care in the United States, and accounted for 23% of total spending in 2006 (MedPAC 2010b). The rest of health care spending came from private insurance payers (35%) and from out-of-pocket spending. All public programs, including Medicare, Medicaid, the State Children's Health Insurance Program, and other programs, accounted for 47% of total spending.

Medicare spending presents a more complex picture than beneficiary demographics and their health status. In 2008 Medicare accounted for 29% of all national spending on hospital care, 21% of physician and clinical services, 41% of home care services, 19% of nursing home care, 30% of durable medical equipment, and 22% of prescription drugs (MedPAC 2010b). According to 2009 data, inpatient hospital services accounted for 27% of Medicare expenditures, 13% for physician services, and 12% for prescription drugs under Part D. Total Medicare expenditures in any given calendar year are spent among a very small number of beneficiaries. In 2006, the costliest 5% of beneficiaries accounted for 39% of total Medicare spending. In contrast, 50% of beneficiaries accounted for only 4% of total program expenses. The costliest beneficiaries tended to be the chronically ill, who experienced multiple hospital admissions, were covered by both Medicare and Medicaid (dual-eligibles), and were within in the last year of their lives.

The burden of chronic illness

Over half of Americans suffer from at least one chronic illness. Despite tremendous advances in treatment, chronic illness rates have risen dramatically. Diabetes has become a "new" national epidemic, and escalating rates of obesity and cardiovascular disease threaten to derail previous advances made in reducing these disease rates (DeVol & Bedroussian 2007). It has been estimated that without significant change in chronic illness care and lifestyle, the incidence of cancer, mental disorders, and diabetes will increase by 50% in the next two decades, and heart disease will increase by more than 40% (Partnership to Fight Chronic Disease 2009).

Chronic illnesses are having an enormous impact on human and economic aspects of society. It has been suggested that the health of Americans and the economy depend on our ability to focus efforts on reducing the burden of chronic illness, because if not, the socioeconomic consequences will be staggering and could negatively impact the lifestyles of all Americans (DeVol & Bedroussian 2007). In this section we present a snapshot of the burdens caused by chronic illnesses.

Chronic illness prevalence

Today, 50% of Americans suffer from at least one chronic illness (Partnership to Fight Chronic Disease 2009), and four out of five older adults, aged 50 and older, suffer from at least one chronic illness (AARP 2009a). This prevalence differs by race: 77% of African Americans have at least one chronic illness, as do 68% of Hispanic Americans; 64% of Caucasians; and 42% of Asian Americans (Collins *et al.* 2002). A quarter of Americans (28%) have multiple chronic illnesses (Anderson 2010).

Additionally, some chronic illnesses are associated with higher risk of co-morbidity than others. For example, people with CHF, kidney disease, or stroke are more likely to have five or more other chronic illnesses than people with arthritis, mental disorders, or cancer (AARP 2009a). Similarly, the relationship of select chronic illness and co-morbidity-risk are associated with age and gender. Using an algorithm developed by Weiss and colleagues (2007), it is possible to estimate major chronic illness co-occurrence in older adults. For example, following their formula, approximately 14% of elderly women with chronic lower respiratory tract illness (emphysema, chronic bronchitis, or asthma) will also have both diabetes and severe arthritis compared to 20% of elderly men. However, few researchers have studied the clustering of chronic illnesses, which has a direct impact on how care is provided to these individuals and ultimately on clinical outcomes (Vogeli *et al.* 2007).

Chronic illnesses' impacts on health service use

Individuals with chronic illnesses, typically adults 55 years of age or older and those with multiple chronic illnesses, are the heaviest users of health care services. They are the highest users in all major health service areas including hospitalizations, physician visits, home health care, and prescription medications (Anderson 2010). They account for a majority of annual health care expenditures. Based on recent 2006 data, individuals with one or more chronic illnesses accounted for: 79% of physician visits, 97% of home health visits, 79% of hospital admissions, and 93% of individuals filling prescription medications (Anderson 2010).

Both home health care and physician visits have increased significantly alongside the number of chronic illnesses (Anderson 2010). Physician visits increased from an annual average of three visits for one chronic illness, to twelve visits for someone with five or more chronic illnesses (or four times as many annual visits). Home health visits showed a similar trajectory; visits for one chronic illness averaged one annual visit versus eleven visits for someone with five or more chronic illnesses. Additionally, the same pattern of chronic illnesses, combined with ADL or IADL limitations, impacted these visits. Physician visits increased from five annual visits for an individual with one chronic illness and any ADL/IADL limitation compared to fourteen visits for someone with five or more chronic illnesses, or three times as many annual visits. Individuals with one chronic illness and any ADL/IADL averaged six annual home health visits compared to seventeen for someone with five or more chronic illnesses.

A different pattern emerged when physician visits for elderly adults were examined, regarding those 65 years of age or older and covered by Medicare. The burden placed on health care providers was magnified radically (Berenson 2007). Medicare beneficiaries with one chronic illness averaged 8 annual visits with 4 different physicians. These numbers increased noticeably based on the number of chronic illnesses. Medicare beneficiaries with two chronic illnesses averaged 11 visits with 5 different physicians; beneficiaries with three chronic illnesses averaged 15 visits with 7 different physicians; beneficiaries with four chronic illnesses averaged 20 visits with 8 different physicians; and beneficiaries with five or more chronic illnesses averaged 37 visits with 14 different physicians.

Individuals with chronic illness were more likely to be hospitalized (Anderson 2010). About 4% of individuals with no chronic illnesses were hospitalized in a 12-month period; however, the incidence increased to 6% with one chronic illness, 10% for two, 14% for three, 19% for four, and 27% for five or more. A similar pattern emerged when comparing any ADL/IADLs limitation with the number of chronic illnesses. Individuals with a chronic illness and any ADL/IADL limitation had a hospitalization rate of 13%, and increased to 17% for two chronic illnesses, 23% for three chronic illnesses, 26% for four chronic illnesses, and 31% for five or more chronic illnesses.

Individuals with chronic illnesses accounted for the majority of prescription medications (Anderson 2010). On average, individuals with one chronic condition filled 7 prescriptions annually, which increased to 16 prescriptions for two chronic illnesses, 27 for three chronic illnesses, 36 for four chronic illnesses and 57 for five or more. This same pattern was visible when comparing the likelihood of filled prescription medications and number of chronic illnesses. Approximately 13% of individuals with one chronic illness and any ADL/IADL limitation filled a prescription in a 12-month period compared to 22% for individuals with two chronic illnesses, 35% for individuals with three chronic illnesses, 42% for individuals with four chronic illnesses, and 65% for individuals with five or more chronic illnesses.

Chronic illness impact on health care costs

In 2006, 50% of individuals diagnosed with one or more chronic illness accounted for 84% of all health care spending (Anderson 2010). These expenditures were disproportional compared to the percentage of individuals with no chronic illnesses and their insurance coverage: 78% of private health-insurance spending was on the 48% of individuals with chronic illnesses; 79% of Medicaid spending was on the 40% of non-institutional individuals with chronic illnesses; and 98% of Medicare spending was on beneficiaries with chronic illnesses. The number of chronic illnesses accelerated health care spending. Compared to individuals with no chronic illnesses, annual expenditures are almost three times greater for someone with one chronic illness, over seven times greater for someone with three chronic illnesses, and almost 15 times greater for someone with five or more chronic illnesses (Anderson 2010). There was also a significant difference in health care spending on chronically ill individuals with ADL or IADL limitations. Individuals with one or more ADL/IADL limitations and five or more chronic illnesses had average annual health expenditures that were more than double compared to individuals with one or more ADL/IADL limitations and only one chronic illness (approximately $17,000 versus $6,000).

Ultimately, how much a particular chronic illness contributes to health care spending is a product of the total cost of treatment and the impact the disease has on life expectancy (AARP 2009a). For example, a 65-year-old adult with a serious chronic illness will cost Medicare an additional $1,000 to $2,000 per year until death, compared to a similar aged adult without the condition (Joyce *et al.* 2005). Over an adult's remaining life expectancy from age 65, diabetes is estimated to be more costly than cancer ($15,000 in additional spending versus $13,500), and hypertension more costly than stroke ($11,000 versus $4,000), despite differences in shorter life expectancy associated with the chronic illnesses. Lifetime Medicare spending on elderly individuals who are obese is estimated to be $25,000 to $37,000 more compared to beneficiaries of normal weight (Thorpe & Ogden 2010). From age 70 until death, Medicare spends approximately 35% more on obese beneficiaries compared to those of normal weight, primarily because of higher co-morbidity among very old obese beneficiaries (Yang & Hall 2008).

Although inpatient care is the largest category of Medicare expenditures, in recent years the prevalence and changing mix of treatment locations for chronic illnesses have had noticeable effects on the rise in Medicare spending (Thorpe *et al.* 2010; Decker *et al.* 2009). Increases in the rates of diabetes, kidney disease, hypertension, hyperlipidemia, mental disorders, and arthritis among Medicare beneficiaries have reduced spending growth for inpatient hospital services. At the same time, because these illnesses are primarily treated in the outpatient setting and at home by prescription drugs, the growth of Medicare spending has largely been attributable to increases in physician visits, prescription medications, and home health care services.

Chronic illness impact on patient care and caregivers

An older America, coupled with advances in medical technology and treatment, has resulted in a substantial reported increase in chronic illnesses. We have seen that this phenomenon has resulted in significantly higher health care utilization and spending, but how have these trends impacted chronically ill adults, their families, and caregivers? Two surveys have highlighted that unfortunately, these individuals and their caregivers have often experienced shortcomings in chronic illness care that they have received (Harris Interactive 2001; AARP 2009b). These surveys found that chronically ill adults experienced numerous quality of care problems, including issues with timely access to care when sick, a lack of care coordination and adequate information, major medical errors, unnecessary medical tests, potentially unnecessary hospital readmissions, and inadequate follow-up care after hospital discharge.

Ongoing challenges for chronically ill adults in receiving care included not being able to see a physician when they felt it was necessary, concerns that their insurance did not cover all types of care needed, and that the costs of care were a financial burden (Harris Interactive 2001; AARP 2009b). Chronically ill adults with three or more chronic illnesses experienced consistently high out-of-pocket expenses compared to those with no chronic illnesses, especially the near elderly (Cunningham 2009; Paez *et al.* 2009). Chronically ill adults also experienced different diagnoses for the same symptoms from

Table 1.3 A Synopsis of Chronic Illness

Chronically Ill Adults
- The number of individuals with chronic illness is increasing substantially and rapidly.
- The type and number of chronic illnesses varies by race and socioeconomic status.
- Hypertension is the most common chronic illness in adults, followed by lipid disorders, arthritis, heart disease, and eye disorders.
- Approximately 50% of individuals with a chronic illness have multiple chronic illnesses.
- Elderly adults, 65 years of age and older, have a higher likelihood of having multiple chronic illnesses.
- Elderly women are more likely to have chronic illnesses than men.
- Approximately 25% of individuals with chronic illnesses have some type of physical or social activity limitation.

Chronic Illness and Health Care Utilization
- Individuals with chronic illnesses are the largest consumers of health care services.
- Individuals with multiple chronic illnesses have the highest likelihood of hospitalization.
- Outpatient health care utilization, especially physician visits and home health care visits, increase substantially with the number of chronic illnesses an individual has.
- Over 60% of annual health care spending is for individuals with multiple chronic illnesses.
- 98% of annual Medicare expenditures are for individuals with chronic illnesses and over 66% of expenditures are for those with five or more chronic illnesses.

Chronic Illness' Impact on Individuals and Their Caregivers
- Quality of care for individuals with chronic illnesses varies by race.
- Over 50% of individuals with chronic illnesses have more than three different physicians.
- Individuals with chronic illnesses report not receiving adequate information from clinicians and health care providers.
- Out-of-pocket expenses increase substantially with the number of chronic illnesses an individual has.
- Caregiving children and spouses are more likely to suffer from depression.
- Family caregivers provide a majority of all long-term care services to the chronically ill.

different physicians, and some were warned by a pharmacist about a potentially harmful interaction between medications prescribed for them by one or more of their physicians.

Poor communication patterns were prominent among providers and chronically ill adults and their caregivers (AARP 2009b). Common problems included that the provider did not have all the needed information when the patient arrived for the visit, the patient and/or caregiver did not understand what they had been told by the provider, and they were not told the purpose of or how to take a newly prescribed medication.

Chronically ill adults were reluctant to ask for help, and few of them ever asked for assistance from outside the immediate family (Harris Interactive 2001). On average, family caregivers had provided care for a loved one for about four and a half years. When these caregivers needed help, they more often sought assistance from local religious and/or community organizations they were familiar with. Like the chronically ill adult they cared for, caregivers were not likely to ask for assistance, even from other relatives or close friends.

Family caregivers are a critical support structure for individuals with chronic illnesses. In any given year, over 50 million Americans find themselves in a caregiving role (Partnership to Fight Chronic Disease 2008). Almost one in five (17%) family caregivers provide 40 hours of care a week or more, and provide a majority (80%) of all long-term care services for those with a chronic illness or disability. Family caregivers who experience extreme stress while caring for their loved one with chronic illness or disability have been shown to be more prone to chronic diseases themselves and they age prematurely. Children of aging parents are twice as likely as non-caregivers to suffer from depression, and spouses are six times as likely to suffer from depression (Partnership to Fight Chronic Disease 2008). Caregiving families tend to have incomes that are $15,000 less than non-caregiving families, yet they spend 2.5 times more on out-of-pocket expenses.

Summary

As Americans have become increasingly older, so have the number living with chronic illnesses. Our current health care system was not designed to provide coordinated care for these individuals who are primarily insured by the Medicare and Medicaid programs. As a result, these individuals are not receiving optimum quality of care for many of their chronic illnesses. As the "baby boom generation" gets ready to become Medicare beneficiaries, more providers with specialized training, resources, and new approaches to delivering care for chronic illnesses will be needed to meet their health care needs.

Improving care for the chronically ill is one of the most important challenges facing our health care system. Research has consistently demonstrated that maintaining and sustaining improvements in care management and coordination for chronically ill adults is extremely difficult. Additionally, dysfunctional incentives have contributed to a fragmented system that has failed to address the fundamental causes of chronic illness, and too many care decisions have been removed from the control of clinicians and patients.

The prevalence of chronic illness is steadily increasing, and by 2030 it is estimated that the number of adults with at least one chronic illness will be in excess of 171 million. Besides longevity, lack of physical activity, tobacco use, and poor nutrition habits are directly responsible for increased rates of chronic illnesses, including cancer, COPD, diabetes, and heart disease. The chronically ill have significantly higher rates of disability, mortality, health care utilization, and medical expenses compared to people without chronic illnesses.

Rates of chronic illness are correlated with socioeconomic status and ethnicity. Adults who live near or below the poverty level and are racial minorities experience significantly higher levels of chronic illnesses and disability. Projections indicate that these incidences will only get worse in the future.

The data indicate that the current care provided to chronically ill adults and their caregivers often leads to poor outcomes. In clinical practice, chronic illness management typically falls short of effective communication and coordination across different care settings and providers. As a result, patients and their families/caregivers experience the brunt of the chronic illness burden.

It has been acknowledged and acclaimed by medical experts and policy makers that our health care system is dysfunctional and for all purposes, broken. Almost all agree that changes are necessary, especially when it comes to financing and delivering medical care for individuals with chronic illnesses. In the proceeding chapters we present information that addresses the current state of chronic illness care, and we offer evidence-based suggestions that have the potential to positively impact care management and address the issues of fragmentation and care coordination for the chronically ill.

References

Administration on Aging. (2009) *A Profile of Older Americans: 2009*. U.S. Department of Health and Human Services, Washington, DC.

Agency for Healthcare Research and Quality. (2006) *Medical Expenditure Panel Survey Household Component*. Agency for Healthcare Research and Quality and National Center for Health Statistics, Rockville, MD.

American Association of Retired Persons. (2009a) *Chronic Care: A Call to Action for Health Reform*. American Association of Retired Persons Public Policy Institute, Washington, DC.

American Association of Retired Persons. (2009b) *Beyond 50.09 Survey Report*. American Association of Retired Persons, Washington, DC.

Anderson, A. (2010) *Chronic Care: Making the Case for Ongoing Care*. Robert Wood Johnson Foundation, Princeton, NJ.

Berenson, R.A. (2007) *The Emerging Challenge of Chronic Care*. The Urban Institute, Washington, DC.

Bodenheimer, T., Chen, E., & Bennett H.D., (2009) Confronting the growing burden of chronic disease: can the U.S. workforce do the job? *Health Affairs*, 28(1), 64–74.

Carlson, S.A., Fulton, J.E., Galuska, D.A., *et al.* (2008) Prevalence of self-reported physically active adults – United States, 2007. *Morbidity and Mortality Weekly Report*, 57, 1297–1300.

Centers for Disease Control and Prevention. (2008) Cigarette use among high school students – United States, 1991–2007. *Morbidity and Mortality Weekly Report*, 57, 689–691.

Centers for Disease Control and Prevention. (2009) *Chronic Disease Overview*. Centers for Disease Control, Atlanta, GA. Available at: http://www.cdc.gov/chronicdisease/overview/index.htm.

Centers for Medicare & Medicaid Services. (2002) *Program Information on Medicare, Medicaid, SCHIP, and Other Programs*. U.S. Government Printing Office, Washington, DC.

Cohen, S., & Yu, W. (2006) *The Persistence in the Level of Health Care Expenditures Over Time: Estimates for the U.S. Population, 2002–2003*. Statistical Brief #124. Agency for Healthcare Research and Quality, Rockville, MD.

Collins, K.S., Hughes, D.L., Doty, M.M., *et al.* (2002) *Diverse Communities, Common Concerns: Assessing Health Care Quality for Minority Americans*. Commonwealth Foundation, New York, NY.

Counsel, S.R., Callahan, C.M., Clark, D.O., *et al.* (2007) Geriatric care management for low-income seniors. *Journal of the American Medical Association*, 298, 2623–2633.

Cunningham, P.J. (2009) *Chronic Burdens: The Persistently High Out-of-Pocket Health Care Expenses Faced by Many Americans with Chronic Conditions*. The Commonwealth Fund, New York, NY.

DeNavas-Walt, C., Proctor, B.D., & Smith, J.C. (2009) *Income, Poverty, and Health Insurance Coverage in the United States: 2008*. U.S. Census Bureau, Current Population Reports. U.S Government Printing Office, Washing, DC.

Decker, S.L., Schappert, S.M., & Sisk, J.E. (2009) Use of medical care for chronic conditions. *Health Affairs*, 28(1), 26–35.

DeVol, R., & Bedroussian, A. (2007) *An Unhealthy America: The Economic Burden of Chronic Disease*. The Milken Institute, Santa Monica, CA.

Federal Interagency Forum on Aging-Related Statistics. (2008) *Older Americans 2008: Key Indicators of Well-Being*. U.S. Government Printing Office, Washington, DC.

Flegal, K.M., Carrol, M.D., Ogden, C.L., *et al.* (2010) Prevalence and trends in obesity among U.S. adults, 1999–2008. *Journal of the American Medical Association*, 303, 235–241.

Harris Interactive. (2001) *Chronic Illness and Caregiving: Survey of the General Public, Adults with Chronic Conditions and Caregivers*. Harris Interactive, New York, NY.

Hastings, S.N., Oddone, E.Z., Fillenbaum G., *et al.* (2008) Frequency and predictors of adverse health outcomes in older Medicare beneficiaries discharged from the emergency department. *Medical Care*, 46, 771–777.

Hyre, A.D., Munter, P., Menke, A., *et al.* (2007) Trends in ATP-III defined high blood cholesterol prevalence, awareness, treatment and control among U.S. adults. *Annals of Epidemiology*, 17, 548–555.

Hwang, W., Weller, W., Ireys, H., *et al.* (2001) Out-of-pocket medical spending for care of chronic conditions. *Health Affairs*, 20, 267–278.

Institute of Medicine. (2001) *Crossing the Quality Chasm: A New Health System for the Twenty-first Century*. National Academies Press, Washington, DC.

Institute of Medicine Committee on the Future of Health Care Workforce for Older Americans. (2008) *Retooling for an Aging America: Building the Health Care Workforce*. National Academies Press, Washington, DC.

Jenks, S.F., Williams, M.V., & Coleman, E.A. (2009) Rehospitalizations among patients in the Medicare fee-for-service program. *New England Journal of Medicine*, 360, 1418–1428.

Joyce, G.F., Keeler, E.B., Shang, B., *et al.* (2005) The lifetime burden of chronic disease among the elderly. Web exclusive. Health Affairs, W5-R18-W5-R29, 26 September. Available at: http://content.healthaffairs.org/cgi/reprint/hlthaff.w5.r18v1.

Kronick, R.G., Bella, M., Gilmer, T.P. *et al.* (2007) *The Faces of Medicaid II: Recognizing the Care Needs of People with Multiple Chronic Conditions*. Center for Health Care Strategies, Hamilton, NJ.

Levit, K., Wier, L., Stranges, E., *et al.* (2009) *HCUP Facts and Figures: Statistics on Hospital-Based Care in the United States, 2007*. Agency for Healthcare Research and Quality, Rockville, MD.

Machlin, S.R. (2009) *Trends in Health Care Expenditures for the Elderly Age 65 and Over: 2006 versus 1996*. Statistical Brief #256. Agency for Healthcare Research and Quality, Rockville, MD.

Machlin, S., Cohen, J.W., & Beauregard, K. (2008) *Health Care Expenses for Adults with Chronic Conditions, 2005*. Statistical Brief #203. Agency for Healthcare Research and Quality, Rockville, MD.

Martin, L.G., Freedman, V.A., Schoeni, R.R., *et al.* (2010) Trends in disability and related chronic conditions among people ages fifty to sixty-four. *Health Affairs*, 29, 725–731.

McGlynn, E.A., Asch, S.M., Adams, J., *et al.* (2003) The quality of health care delivered to adults in the United States. *New England Journal of Medicine*, 348, 2635–2645.

Medicare Payment Advisory Commission. (2010a) *Report to Congress: Aligning Incentives in Medicare*. Medicare Payment Advisory Commission, Washington, DC.

Medicare Payment Advisory Commission. (2010b) *A Data Book: Healthcare Spending and the Medicare Program*. Medicare Payment Advisory Commission, Washington, DC.

National Center for Health Statistics. (2010) *Health, United States, 2009: With Special Feature on Medical Technology*. Centers for Disease Control and Prevention, Hyattsville, MD.

Norris, S.L., High, K., Gill, T.M., *et al.* (2008) Health care for older Americans with multiple chronic conditions: a research agenda. *Journal of the American Geriatrics Society*, 56(1), 149–159.

Ogden, C.L., Carroll, M.D., & Flegal, K.M. (2008) High body mass index for age among US children and adolescents, 2003–2006. *Journal of the American Medical Association*, 299, 2401–2405.

Ostchega, Y., Dillon, C.F., Hughes, J.P., *et al.* (2007) Trends in hypertension prevalence, awareness, treatment and control in older U.S. adults: data from the national health and nutrition examination survey 1988 to 2004. *Journal of the American Geriatrics Society*, 55, 1056–1065.

Paez, K.A., Zhao, L., & Hwang, W. (2009) Rising out-of-pocket spending for chronic conditions: a ten-year trend. *Health Affairs*, 28(1), 15–25.

Partnership to Fight Chronic Disease. (2008) *The Almanac of Chronic Conditions, 2008*. Partnership to Fight Chronic Disease, Washington, DC.

Partnership to Fight Chronic Disease. (2009) *The Impact of Chronic Disease on U.S. Health and Prosperity: A Collection of Statistics and Commentary*. Partnership to Fight Chronic Disease, Washington, DC.

RAND Health. (2002) *The Health Risks of Obesity*. RAND Corporation, Santa Monica, CA.

Rhoades, J.A. (2005) *Overweight and Obese Elderly and Near Elderly in the United States, 2002: Estimates for the Noninstitutionalized Population Age 55 and Older*. Statistical Brief #68. Agency for Healthcare Research and Quality, Rockville, MD.

Russo, A., Wier, L.M., & Elixhauser, A. (2009) *Hospital Utilization Among Near-Elderly Adults, Ages 55 to 64 Years, 2007*. HCUP Statistical Brief #79. Agency for Healthcare Research and Quality, Rockville, MD.

Schoenborn, C.A., & Heyman, K.M. (2009) *Health Characteristics of Adults Aged 55 Years and Over: United States, 2004–2007*. National Health Statistics Reports #16. National Center for Health Statistics, Hyattsville, MD.

Stanton, M.W., & Rutherford, M.K. (2006) *The High Concentration of U.S. Health Care Expenditures*. Research in Action Issue 19. Agency for Healthcare Research and Quality, Rockville, MD.

Thorpe, K.E., & Ogden, L.L. (2010) The foundation that health reform lays for improved payment, care coordination, and prevention. *Health Affairs*, 29, 1183–1187.

Thorpe, K.E., Ogden, L.L., & Galactionova, K. (2010) Chronic conditions account for rise in Medicare spending from 1987 to 2006. *Health Affairs*, 29, 718–724.

U.S. Census Bureau. (2008) *Statistical Abstract of the United States, 2008*. U.S. Government Printing Office, Washington, DC.

U.S. Department of Health and Human Services. (2001) *The Surgeon General's Call to Action: To Prevent and Decrease Overweight and Obesity*. U.S. Department of Health and Human Services, Rockville, MD.

Vogeli, C., Shields, A.E., Lee, T.A., *et al.* (2007) Multiple chronic conditions: prevalence, health consequences, and implications for quality, care management and costs. *Journal of General Internal Medicine*, 22(Supplement 3), 391–395.

Wallace, P.J. (2005) Physician involvement in disease management as part of the CCM. *Health Care Financing Review*, 27(1), 19–31.

Weiss, C.O., Boyd, C.M., & Yu, Q. (2007) Patterns of prevalent major chronic disease among older adults in the United States. *Journal of the American Medical Association*, 298, 1160–1162.

Wilber, S.T., Gerson, L.W., Terrell, K.M., *et al.* (2006) Geriatric emergency medicine and the 2006 Institute of Medicine reports from the Committee on the Future of Emergency Care in the U.S. Health System. *Academic Emergency Medicine*, 13, 1345–1351.

Williams, C. (2004) *Medicaid Disease Management: Issues and Promises*. Kaiser Commission on Medicaid and the Uninsured, Washington, DC.

Wolff, J.L., & Boult, C. (2005) Moving beyond round pegs and square holes: restructuring Medicare to improve care. *Annals of Internal Medicine*, 143, 439–445.

Yang, Z., & Hall, A.G. (2008). The financial burden of overweight and obesity among elderly Americans: the dynamics of weight, longevity, and health care costs. *Health Services Research*, 43, 849–868.

Chapter 2

Overview

Cheryl Schraeder, Paul Shelton, Linda Fahey,
Krista L. Jones, and Carrie Berger

Introduction

As a result of scientific advances and public health initiatives implemented over the past century, American longevity has increased by three decades (Centers for Disease Control [CDC] 2007). Along with this increased longevity, there has been a steady increase in the number of individuals living with one or more chronic illnesses. In the coming decade the number of Americans afflicted by chronic disease is expected to reach 150 million (CDC 2007).

Chronic illness profoundly affects a person's physical, emotional, and mental health status, often making it difficult for them to complete simple tasks or carry on with daily routines, thereby negatively impacting their overall quality of life. These challenges are compounded by an increasingly complex and fragmented health care system in which chronic illness patients receive care from multiple providers who are often unaware of the diagnoses and treatment provided by their colleagues in managing the patients' chronic diseases.

Uncoordinated care results in polypharmacy issues, conflicting advice, contraindication in care regimens, increased medical errors, waste of health services and resources, and ineffective provider billing and reimbursement (Bodenheimer 2008; Pham *et al.* 2007). This chapter will explore the need for comprehensive care coordination, review barriers impacting implementation, and discuss facilitators toward adherence to this strategy.

Comprehensive care coordination defined

Overall, it is obvious that our health care system has failed to embrace and provide comprehensive care coordination. However, a new level of energy was created when the Patient Protection and Affordable Care Act (PPACA) was signed into law in 2010. In this legislation, referred to as federal health care reform, the concept of coordinated care was mentioned 25 times. Unfortunately, a formal definition of coordinated care was not included in the law. An inability to define the process and assert meaning to the benefits

Comprehensive Care Coordination for Chronically Ill Adults, First Edition. Edited by Cheryl Schraeder and Paul Shelton.
© 2011 John Wiley & Sons, Inc. Published 2011 by John Wiley & Sons, Inc.

derived from the coordinated delivery of services to patients, their families and caregivers, combined with the basic structure and focus of the current health care system, will more than likely impact its future adoption.

Our approach to comprehensive care coordination is shaped by the definition of care management employed by Bodenheimer and Berry-Millett (2009a) and Bodenheimer and colleagues (2009b). For our purposes, care coordination is a set of activities that assist patients and their families in self-managing their health conditions and related psychosocial problems more effectively; coordinating their care among multiple health and community providers; bridging gaps in care; and receiving the appropriate levels of care. Care coordination is generally provided by a registered nurse (RN) in collaboration with the patient/family, their primary care provider, and other health and community providers involved in the patient's health care. RN care coordinators maintain a panel of patients over time and primarily see patients face-to-face in the home, in a clinical office setting, or they contact patients by telephone.

The specific activities of care coordination include: (1) assessing the risks and needs of each patient, including knowledge of their health conditions, current level of self-management activities, and their own goals of care; (2) developing a comprehensive care plan that is based upon evidenced-based guidelines and standards of care; (3) ensuring that patients are up-to-date on current recommended health promotion activities; (4) teaching and coaching patients and their families about their health conditions and medications, including self-management activities and how to anticipate and plan for their needs based upon their prior responses to their health conditions and contact with the health care system; (5) empowering and supporting patients to take ownership of their health conditions and management options; (6) coaching and guiding patients and families on how to respond to worsening symptoms in order to avoid emergency department (ED) visits and hospital admissions; (7) proactive patient monitoring to identify changes in their health status or related psychosocial needs; (8) communicating pertinent information to involved providers during care transitions; (9) tracking patients' health status over time with early communication to other providers of any change or psychosocial needs; (10) evaluating the effectiveness of the plan of care, and teaching patients to evaluate self-management activities; and (11) revising care plans to reflect changes in a patient's health status, psychosocial needs, and self-management skills.

Rose is a 78-year-old woman who was diagnosed with type 2 diabetes 10 years ago. She also has a history of incontinence, arthritis, and depression – the latter developing because of the loss of her husband after 55 years of marriage. Five years ago, Rose was diagnosed with hypertension following an episode of acute myocardial infarction (AMI). While hospitalized for the AMI, Rose was placed on a higher dosage and schedule of insulin. As a result, Rose suffered hypoglycemia, further complicating her cardiac condition and prolonging her hospital stay.

Rose sees a primary care physician, urologist, cardiologist, endocrinologist, certified diabetes educator, and psychiatrist. Rose's daughter and grandchildren provide most of her care including taking her to provider appointments. As a result of her co-morbidities and a lack of comprehensive care coordination, she has been the victim of conflicting medical advice and polypharmacy.

Rose's story is one of thousands that exemplify a need for chronic care coordination. In the next section, we address the barriers encountered by care coordinators and patients like Rose when seeking to assure comprehensive service delivery.

Barriers to comprehensive care coordination

Fragmentation

Accessibility and the affordability of patient care are hindered by a complex, fragmented, and overwhelmed system of care. Imagine a time when you had an illness and sought treatment from a primary care provider. Most likely you called to make an appointment with the receptionist or scheduling center. From that point you may have been directed to the Billing Department to assure that you had coverage to pay for the appointment. Upon seeing the primary care provider, you were informed that you required further testing and diagnosis with a specialist. You began the cycle again for the next level of appointments. Imagine you have multiple chronic illnesses, scheduling multiple appointments for diagnosis, treatment, and follow-up care, all the while assuring your providers that your appointments, medications, therapy, and all other forms of treatment are covered by your health insurance.

Approximately 20% of adults have a chronic disability (U.S. Census Bureau 2010). The care of these patients is currently being managed within a fragmented system of multiple specialists and primary care providers at multiple settings, including ambulatory care clinics, private physician offices, the ED diagnostic services (radiology/lab), and hospitals. This fragmentation leads to poor communication across providers and settings, duplication of services, excess utilization of acute care services (particularly the ED), polypharmacy, higher costs, higher rates of non-compliance with treatment, and poorer patient outcomes (Luck *et al.* 2007).

Kroll and colleagues (2006) identified multiple barriers affecting access to primary preventative services for individuals with a chronic disability. They divided these barriers into two primary domains: structural-environmental (conditions in the physical and social environment impacting service delivery), and process (barriers experienced as services were provided to patients).

Examples of structural-environmental barriers include: lack of transportation services to appointments, lack of disabled parking spaces and wheelchair ramps into medical buildings, lack of adaptable equipment such as accessible bathrooms, special weight scales for individuals in wheelchairs, and adjustable exam tables. Many providers are ill-equipped to meet the needs of this disadvantaged population, often citing structural concerns and the need for re-design of medical facilities.

Examples of process barriers include poor communication among providers, failure to receive preventative teaching, and lack of consistent health promotion strategies (Kroll *et al.* 2006). Additionally, patients often experience a lack of flexibility in scheduling appointments, long telephone waits, automated answering systems, failure of providers to return calls in a timely manner, and feeling rushed during provider visits, resulting in an inability to have questions addressed (Coughlin *et al.* 2002).

Bayliss and colleagues (2008; 2003) described challenges faced by elderly patients with multiple chronic illnesses, including access to their primary provider, difficulty scheduling appointments, "telephone tag" with provider offices, lack of e-mail communication, and the frustrations of traveling long distances to see multiple specialists. In addition, patients expressed concerns about physician turnover in large practices and the difficulty with repeating their history over and over to new incoming providers. Limited coordination of care, lack of a cohesive plan to manage their multiple conditions, and an inability on the part of providers to give patients time to have their concerns addressed during appointments, as well as be an active participant in the plan of care, were additional barriers to effective care management.

Adults with multiple chronic illnesses echoed similar barriers. Jerant and colleagues (2005) identified barriers these individuals face to active self-management and in accessing self-management support services. Barriers to active self-management included depression, weight problems, difficulty exercising, fatigue, poor physician communication, low family support, pain, and financial problems. Lack of awareness, physical symptoms, transportation issues, and cost/lack of insurance coverage were barriers to accessing self-management support.

When barriers are faced with the physician office, patients often turn to EDs to fill the gap. Frequent users of the ED tend to have chronic health problems, and while most ED patients identify a place where they usually receive care, few have had contact with their physicians prior to seeking ED care (Milbrett & Halm 2009; Weber *et al.* 2008). Increased use of the ED is associated with a lack of access to primary care services (Rust *et al.* 2008), and a majority of ED visits take place on the weekends or on a weekday after physician office hours (Pitts *et al.* 2010), or by patients who were discharged from the hospital within the last seven days (Burt *et al.* 2008).

If a patient is admitted to the hospital, they are likely to be cared for by a physician they have never met. Over 50% of all hospitals employ hospitalists. Hospitalists are physicians who do not see patients in an office-based setting, and who often provide all inpatient coverage for primary care physicians who have chosen to practice in an outpatient setting. While this model can actually improve timeliness of care in the hospital, continuity of care across settings becomes more challenging (Hamel *et al.* 2009). For example, almost 20% of Medicare patients discharged from hospitals are readmitted within 30 days, and 34% are rehospitalized within 90 days (Jencks *et al.* 2009). However, over 50% of patients who were readmitted within 30 days had not seen their primary physician for a follow-up visit at any time after discharge.

The length of stay for hospitalized patients has decreased dramatically. Over 38% of hospitalized patients are elderly (age 65 and older) and have an average length of stay of only five days. Admissions are driven primarily by Medicare guidelines concerning financial reimbursement. Medicare guidelines allow very little time for physicians and nurses to sort out care issues surrounding and associated with chronic illnesses.

Discharge planning is focused on matching the patient with community services needed after hospital discharge. This can be a challenging task for discharge planners because the non-hospital service providers are under no obligation to accept referrals, and may make choices based solely on the reimbursement available for that service (Popejoy *et al.* 2009). Nursing home placement, home care services, equipment needed at home, or personal services necessary for continued care may not be available. Additionally, patient education tends to be focused on survival skills for that particular diagnosis. In a recent survey of Medicare beneficiaries, 19% indicated that when they were discharged from the hospital they were not provided information about home care services or instructions on follow-up care or problems they might encounter and whom to contact with questions (Centers for Medicare & Medicaid Services [CMS] 2010).

The shortage of primary care physicians, and the delivery structure within their offices, has resulted in work days with patients' appointments scheduled at 15-minute increments, leaving little or no time for coordination of care. Additionally, a lack of involvement with specialists and hospitalists, as well as limited or no involvement in care transitions, impedes the management of their patients with multiple chronic illnesses (Bodenheimer *et al*. 2009c).

In this fragmented delivery structure, obtaining accurate medication lists for patients on hospital admission and ensuring patient discharge with appropriate medications (medication reconciliation) is one of the biggest quality challenges that health systems face. The percentage of patients who have inaccurate or incomplete medication lists at the time of admission can be as high as 69% (Slain *et al*. 2008). Over half of patients (54%) often experience at least one potentially adverse drug event while hospitalized; 70% are attributable to inaccurate admission histories, and 30% to errors in reconciling the medication history with discharge orders when patients are transitioned from a long-term care facility to the acute care setting (Pippins *et al*. 2008). Over 27% of adverse drug events are considered potentially harmful (Pippins *et al*. 2008). The results are particularly concerning in the care of hospitalized elderly adults since the likelihood of adverse drug events steadily increases with the number of co-morbidities (Page *et al*. 2010). A lack of effective care coordination at key transition points can be devastating.

Financing and payment barriers

While it is somewhat difficult to determine a direct causal relationship, our fragmented health system structure is supported by a system of financial incentives that perpetuate a lack of care coordination. In 2007, total health expenditures accounted for 16% of the gross domestic product (National Center for Health Statistics 2010). While there are a number of different health insurance plans and payers, the largest is the federal government. The Medicare program alone accounts for 13% of the annual federal budget (Satiani 2009). With health care spending and federal deficits escalating, the Medicare program has become a political focus for examining the overhauling of health care delivery.

The Medicare program originally was conceptualized as an expansion of Social Security benefits to provide limited coverage of inpatient hospital care for the elderly. It was expanded to include physician and state welfare services and became law in 1965 with Medicare Part A covering hospitals, Medicare Part B covering physician services, and Medicaid providing support to individual states for indigent health care (Blumenthal & Morone 2008). When Medicare was initially enacted into law, the financing structure of health care was largely fee-for-service payments to physicians and hospitals. There was little history on which to base cost estimates, and no controls or standards to define appropriate levels of service. Essentially, the more services a hospital or physician provided, the more they were paid.

In 1984, a new method for hospital reimbursement was enacted for the Medicare program. Hospitals started receiving one payment for an episode of care based on Diagnosis Related Groups (DRGs). Hospitals began assuming financial risk for each hospital stay based on the predicted costs for a particular diagnosis rather than payments for every service performed. DRGs placed emphasis on hospital length of stay and utilization of services, but physician fee-for-service payments did not change. This placed hospitals and physicians on different incentive platforms, since each had different financial incentives and reimbursement mechanisms for the care they provided (Goldsmith 2010). Neither method of payment, however, encouraged care beyond a single episode, thus furthering fragmentation of services.

With the need for even further cuts in Medicare spending, physician payments were redesigned in 1992 with the Resource-Based Relative Value Scale (RBRVS; Johnson & Newton 2002). The RBRVS was a complicated system with a fee structure based on the type of work, practice environment, and malpractice costs of physician services, but it was still a fee-for-service method that did not control quality or necessity of testing (Verrilli *et al.* 1996). In addition, the fee scale tended to support procedures at a much higher rate than physician activities involving patient management and evaluating outcomes. This resulted in declining reimbursement for primary care services, and escalating payments to specialists who performed multiple procedures. With decreasing revenue, primary care physicians increased patient volume, leaving little time for coordination of care necessary for patients with chronic illnesses (Bodenheimer *et al.* 2009c). This payment structure continues today. Additionally, both home health care and skilled nursing facilities (SNFs) now receive payments based on episodes of care with scales designed specifically for those types of services. Pharmacy benefits, as well as managed care options through private insurance companies, have also been added to the Medicare program.

This complicated Medicare payment structure supports a silo delivery system wherein each provider is focused on one episode of care within a defined period of time. For hospitals, the focus is on a single hospitalization. For SNFs, the focus is on skilled needs within a defined timeframe. Home care has a similar focus, with benefits paid based on an acuity adjusted 60-day episode of care (Davitt & Choi 2008). Physicians continue to receive payments for the individual services they provide. Pharmacies function independently with private plans covering Medicare patients. At no point is there any financial incentive for these various providers to work as a team across multiple episodes of care or to achieve continuity of care for an individual patient.

To complicate this picture even further, some Medicare beneficiaries may also qualify for additional benefits through the Medicaid program. Medicaid is a federally supported program designed to help states meet the health care needs of low income citizens, targeting children, adults, and individuals with disabilities. People who reside in residential and long-term care facilities are also eligible for coverage. Medicaid benefits and services vary significantly from state to state. Medicaid beneficiaries must meet annual eligibility requirements, and many states set even more frequent eligibility periods. The recertification process results in patients moving in and out of eligibility based on their current life situations. These interruptions in coverage affecting individuals with chronic illnesses can lead to serious deterioration in disease management and result in multiple hospitalizations (Bindman *et al.* 2008; Hall *et al.* 2008).

Reducing costs and redesigning financing is a major focus of health care reform. The PPACA includes provisions for reimbursement based on quality of care outcomes to health care providers. In addition, the law established criteria to explore and financially support delivery models where coordinated care is provided across all levels and settings of care, especially for individuals suffering from chronic illnesses (Goldsmith 2010). Regardless of whether the payment system is driving care or is simply a by-product of a poorly designed system, there is widespread acknowledgement that current methods for delivery and payment of health care are not acceptable, affordable, or sustainable into the foreseeable future.

Workforce concerns

According to the Institute of Medicine (IOM 2008) the current health care workforce lacks essential education and training in the care of adults – particularly older adults – with chronic illnesses. At the same time, the workforce is not nearly large enough to care for the rapid aging of America, especially with the advancing influx of baby boomers. This scarcity of qualified health care providers is expected to continue to rise along with this aging population. By 2030, it is estimated that we will need an additional 3.5 million health care providers, a 35% increase over current levels, just to maintain the current ratio of providers to the total population (IOM 2008). Providers who are in short supply include nurses, primary care physicians, physician assistants, geriatric social workers, nursing assistants, and home care and home health aids (Bureau of Labor Statistics 2010).

Comprehensive care coordination calls for new models of delivering chronic illness care that will demand new skills and expertise from providers – especially from nurses and primary care physicians – that are not emphasized in today's health care environment (Bohmer 2010; Margolius & Bodenheimer 2010). These skills involve: designing care around the patient (that is, adopting patient-centered care); communicating and collaborating in multidisciplinary care teams; evaluating and continuously improving the quality and safety of patient care; monitoring patients over time, using and sharing information technology; and viewing care from the broadest perspective, which is population-based care.

To address these workforce barriers, various solutions have been proposed. Examples of solutions include: substantial changes in financial incentives for redesigned primary care delivery and reimbursement for primary care physicians and nurse practitioners; substantial increases in funding for medical and nursing education and training with a focus on geriatrics; and legislative proposals that a certain percentage of clinicians practice in primary care with appropriate financial and educational incentives for doing so (Bodenheimer *et al.* 2009b).

Health information technology

As described above, efforts to effectively coordinate and manage chronic illnesses have been hampered by a number of barriers, including a fragmented health care system and the need for more coordination across sites of care; the difficulty which people with chronic illnesses have in paying for their care; the current reimbursement system does not reward key elements of chronic illness care; and the need for enhanced medical and nursing training and education, which places an increasing focus on chronic care.

Our health care system is currently not well equipped to address these concerns. Because of the highly fragmented nature of health care, patient information is stored in many locations, primarily in paper-based forms with limited access. As a result, clinicians often do not have comprehensive patient information at the point of care, when it is most needed. It also impedes having the necessary information to measure performance and facilitate quality improvement of patient populations. Additionally, patients do not have access to necessary information they need to help manage their own health and health care.

Health information technology (HIT) holds great promise for addressing many of these barriers to comprehensive care coordination and is a key component in managing patient populations and complex communications within a team environment (Hillestad *et al.* 2005). HIT facilitates access to and retrieval of clinical data from different entities involved in the care delivery system, which can result in more timely, efficient, effective, equitable, patient-centered care (Marchibroda 2008). For example, HIT can compile individual patient information related to care performed by multiple clinicians, hospitals, and community providers, and provide different views of this information by the interdisciplinary care team, thus enhancing care coordination activities. HIT systems can also trigger individual patient alerts and reminders to support clinicians and patients regarding tests that need to be performed or medications that need to be prescribed or filled. The connection of HIT to personal health records can improve patient engagement, by not only providing additional information to support self-management, but also creating a mechanism for patients to input their own experiences to support the work of the care team. Furthermore, the use of remote devices that connect to personal health records and clinical HIT applications can enable timelier, more accurate capture of specific information that is critical to chronic disease management.

Researchers estimate savings of approximately $81 billion over 15 years (Girosi *et al.* 2005), and as many as 200,000 adverse drug events per year could be prevented (RAND Health 2005) if HIT was widely adopted. Despite the advantages outlined above and potential financial savings, HIT adoption rates are low. Survey estimates indicate that approximately 24% of physician offices, 16% of solo practitioners, and 39% of large physician practices are using electronic health records (EHR; Blumenthal *et al.* 2006). Based on a 2009 study, only 8% of responding hospitals reported basic implementation of an EHR system, while only 2% reported having achieved successful comprehensive integration (Jha 2009). The cost of establishing EHR within a hospital setting can be extensive. Depending on the size of the hospital, EHR systems can cost anywhere between $35,000 to $50,000 per provider (Jha *et al.* 2009; Hildreth 2010). Inadequate capital for purchasing and maintaining the EHR system are often cited as the main reason for transition delays (DePhillips 2007).

Little is known about how to create and successfully implement a comprehensive HIT system that will positively impact comprehensive care coordination for patients with complex chronic illnesses. In a systematic literature review, Dorr and colleagues (2007) identified HIT components important in supporting this concept. Components of an HIT system that were closely correlated with positive outcomes included a connection of an electronic medical record, computerized prompts, population management, including reports and feedback, specialized decision support, electronic scheduling, and personal health records. Barriers included costs, data privacy and security concerns, and failure to consider workflow issues.

Self-management and health literacy

Chronic illnesses are irreversible, latent, and incurable (Lubkin & Larsen 2008). They can profoundly affect a person's physical, emotional, and mental health status and make it difficult to complete simple tasks or carry on with daily routines, thereby negatively impacting their overall quality of life. Although health professionals assume responsibility for the medical management of chronic illness, the patient assumes responsibility for the day-to-day management of his or her own chronic illness. All individuals with chronic illnesses engage in self-management behaviors by deciding what to eat and drink, whether or not to exercise, and if they will take their prescription medications. To help chronically ill patients succeed in improving their health-related behavior, health care providers continually engage in self-management support; patient self-management is a prominent component of comprehensive care coordination (Holman & Lorig 2004).

The purpose of self-management support is to help chronically ill patients become actively involved in their treatment (Bodenheimer *et al*. 2005; Holman & Lorig 2004) and involves two interrelated activities. The first is helping patients to be informed about their chronic illnesses, and the second is trying to work with patients and their caregivers to make informed medical decisions and become more self-motivated. Thus, self-management support involves both information giving and sharing and collaborative decision making to assist patients in their self-directed learning.

Several strategies and techniques have been used in a variety of self-management programs to assist providers and patients in collaborative decision making, including establishing an agenda; information giving (ask, tell, ask); assessing readiness to change (motivational interviewing); and goal setting (Bodenheimer *et al*. 2005). Using a collaborative approach to patient self-management support, an agenda for each visit is negotiated between the patient and clinician, focusing on the patient's needs and/or wants. Elicit, respond, elicit (ask, tell, ask) is a technique for information giving and sharing that seeks to overcome too little information (insufficient) or too much information (overload) given in the teaching/learning encounter that is directed by the patient. Motivational interviewing is a useful technique for assessing readiness to change by focusing on the behavior's importance to the individuals and their confidence in actually making a behavior change (Rollnick *et al*. 2000). Goal setting is used to help patients in agreeing to concrete, short-term goals, accompanied by action plans that are highly specific.

A variety of self-management programs have been developed and implemented for patients with chronic illnesses, especially for older adults with specific illnesses. They have achieved various levels of success, especially for patients with diabetes, hypertension, and arthritis, but there is no agreement on the essential components that make them successful (Chodosh *et al*. 2005). However, self-management support programs have not been evaluated within the context of a multi-component, comprehensive, randomized intervention. Overall, the evidence does suggest that: self-management support does improve health-related behaviors; providing information is a necessary, but not sufficient, intervention to improve health-related behaviors; informed, motivated patients tend to have better health-related behaviors and clinical outcomes; establishing an agenda, goal setting, and motivational interviewing have shown success with older adults (Abramowitz *et al.* 2010; Bodenheimer *et al.* 2005; Flocke *et al.* 2009; Hibbard *et al.* 2004; Paradis *et al.* 2010). Whatever method or technique works best in supporting self-management, patients with multiple chronic illnesses have identified five skills they need to help them manage their diseases: correctly using medications, monitoring important disease symptoms, improving sleep, managing pain, and reducing stress (Noel *et al.* 2007).

Although it is difficult to identify specific components that contribute to the success of self-management support, a person's level of health literacy, or their ability to understand and appropriately act upon health-related information, is directly related to their ability to care for themselves or their loved ones (Villaire & Mayer 2007). Although there is no agreed upon standard definition, health literacy is defined as the ability to read, understand, and act on health information in order to make appropriate health decisions.

It has been estimated that upwards of 45% of the U.S. adult population has literacy skills at or below an eighth-grade reading level. Inadequate health literacy increases steadily with age, from 16% of adults aged 65 to 69 to 58% of those over age 85 (Gazmararian *et al.* 1999). Older adults with low health literacy have trouble reading health information materials, following prevention recommendations, understanding basic medical instructions, and adhering to medication regimes. Health literacy levels are lowest among the elderly, the uneducated, lower socioeconomic levels, minority populations, and those with limited English proficiency (Kutner 2006). Limited health literacy skills are associated with increased risks of mortality, greater difficulty with self-management skills (managing a chronic illness), poor health status, impaired ability to remember and follow treatment recommendations, and reduced medication adherence, as well as a reduced ability to navigate within the health care system and a greater likelihood of hospitalizations due to poor self-management skills (Gazmararian *et al.* 2003; Persell *et al.* 2007; Powell *et al.* 2007; Schillinger *et al.* 2002; Sudore *et al.* 2006).

A patient's inability to understand health care information adds another barrier in establishing a collaborative, clinician–patient relationship and in improving the patient's decision-making skills. For example, compared to adults with higher health literacy, adults with lower health literacy skills tend to ask fewer questions about their illnesses and medical care issues, are more likely to not understand what the clinician said, and are less likely to use medical terminology, refer to their medications by name, or request additional information (Katz *et al.* 2007). Several instruments are available to clinicians to help them assess health literacy and identify patients who have poor literacy skills. The instruments are easy to administer and interpret and do not require undue patient information overload. The Rapid Estimate of Adult Literacy in Medicine, Revised (REALM-R) is a brief screening instrument that can be used to assess a person's ability to read common medical words (Bass *et al.* 2003), and the Medication Knowledge Assessment can be used to determine a person's knowledge about their medications and their ability to read and comprehend information necessary for appropriate medication use, and may serve as the basis of a focused knowledge improvement plan (American Society on Aging and the American Society of Consultant Pharmacists Foundation 2006).

Summary

The barriers to effective care coordination are numerous, but the imperative to succeed is even more compelling. Chronically ill patients suffer for several reasons, including readmissions to hospitals, returns to EDs, and polypharmacy errors. Health care providers are frustrated with a system that does not support the care of these high-need patients, and they have difficulty providing appropriate care with the constraints placed on them by the current reimbursement structure.

Effective coordinated care provides a solution where patients and providers can work together to overcome many of the barriers outlined in this chapter. Through coordination, fragmentation of care can be minimized. Unnecessary costs of care including unnecessary readmissions can be reduced or eliminated. Errors caused by incomplete medication information can be reduced significantly. Primary care physicians and nurses working together with the patient in a realistic delivery model can improve satisfaction for those health care providers and make the roles attractive to help meet future workforce needs. By providing the patients with tools that they need to manage their health and involving them in the process, long-term positive health outcomes are possible. It's time for all of us to learn how to do this.

References

Abramowitz, S.A., Flattery, D., Franses, K., *et al.* (2010) Linking a motivational interviewing curriculum to the chronic care model. *Journal of General Internal Medicine*, 25 (Supplement 4), S620–S626.

American Society on Aging and the American Society of Consultant Pharmacists Foundation. (2006) *Adult Medication: Improving Medication Adherence in Older Adults*. Available at: http://www.adultmeducation.com/downloads/Adult_Meducation.pdf.

Bass, P.F. III, Wilson, J.F., & Griffith, C.H. (2003) A shortened instrument for literacy screening. *Journal of General Internal Medicine*, 18, 1036–1038.

Bayliss, E., Edwards, A., Steiner, J., *et al.* (2008) Processes of care desired by elderly patients with multiple morbidities. *Family Practice*, 25, 287–293.

Bayliss, E., Steiner, J., Fernald, D., *et al.* (2003) Descriptions of barriers to self-care by persons with comorbid chronic diseases. *Annals of Family Medicine*, 1, 15–21.

Bindman, A.B., Chattopadhyay, A., & Auerback, G.M. (2008) Interruptions in Medicaid coverage and risk for hospitalization for ambulatory care-sensitive conditions. *Annals of Internal Medicine*, 149, 854–60.

Blumenthal, D., DesRoches, C., Donelan, K., *et al.* (2006) *Health Information Technology in the United States: The Information Base for Progress*. Robert Wood Johnson Foundation, Princeton, NJ.

Blumenthal, D., & Morone, J. (2008) The lessons of success – revisiting the Medicare story. *New England Journal of Medicine*, 359, 2384–2389.

Bodenheimer, T., MacGregor, K., & Sharifi, C. (2005) *Helping Patients Manage Their Chronic Conditions*. California Healthcare Foundation, Oakland, CA.

Bodenheimer, T. (2008) Coordinating care - a perilous journey through the health care system. *New England Journal of Medicine*, 358, 1064–1071.

Bodenheimer, T., & Berry-Millett, R. (2009a). *Care Management of Patients with Complex Health Care Needs*. Research Synthesis Report 19, Robert Wood Johnson Foundation, Princeton, NJ.

Bodenheimer, T., Chen, E., & Bennett, H.D. (2009b) Confronting the growing burden of chronic disease: can the U.S. workforce do the job? *Health Affairs*, 28 (1), 64–74.

Bodenheimer, T., Grumbach, K., & Berenson, R.A. (2009c) A lifeline for primary Care. *New England Journal of Medicine*, 360, 2693–2696.

Bohmer, R.M.J. (2010) Managing the new primary care: the new skills that will be needed. *Health Affairs*, 29, 1010–1014.

Bureau of Labor Statistics. (2010) *Occupational Outlook Handbook* (2010–11 edition). United States Department of Labor, Washington, DC. Available at: http://www.bls.gov/oco/ocos083.htm.

Burt, C.W., McCaig, L.F., & Simon, A.E. (2008) *Emergency Department Visits by Persons Recently Discharged from U.S. Hospitals.* National Health Statistics Reports, No. 6, National Center for Health Statistics, Hyattsville, MD.

Centers for Disease Control. (2007) *The State of Aging and Health Care in America*. Centers for Disease Control and Prevention, Atlanta, GA.

Centers for Medicare and Medicaid Services. (2010) *Summary of HCAHPS Survey Results/HCAHPS Executive Insight*. Centers for Medicare & Medicaid Services, Baltimore, MD. Available at: http://hcahpsonline.org/executive_insight/Files/Summary%20Scores%20March%182010.pdf.

Chodosh, J., Morton, S.C., Mojica, W., *et al.* (2005) Meta-analysis: chronic disease self-management programs for older adults. *Annals of Internal Medicine*, 143, 427–438.

Coughlin, T.A., Long, S. K., & Kendall, S. (2002) Health care access, use, and satisfaction among disabled Medicaid beneficiaries. *Health Care Financing Review*, 24, 115–136.

Davitt, J.K., & Choi, S. (2008) Tracing the history of Medicare home health care: the impact of policy on benefit use. *Journal of Sociology & Social Welfare*, 35, 247–276.

DePhillips, H. (2007) Initiatives and barriers to adopting health information technology. *Disease Management and Health Outcomes*, 15 (1), 1–6.

Dorr, D., Bonner, L.M., Cohen, A.N., *et al.* (2007) Informatics systems to promote improved care for chronic illness: a literature review. *Journal of the American Medical Informatics Association*, 14, 156–163.

Flocke, S.A., Kelly, R., & Highland, J. (2009) Initiation of health behavior discussions during primary care outpatient visits. *Patient Education and Counseling*, 75, 214–219.

Gazmararian, J.A., Baker, D., Williams, M., *et al.* (1999) Health literacy among Medicare enrollees in a managed care organization. *Journal of the American Medical Association*, 281, 545–551.

Gazmararian, J.A., Williams, M.V., Peel, J., *et al.* (2003) Health literacy and knowledge of chronic disease. *Patient Education and Counseling*, 51, 267–275.

Girosi, E., Meili, R., & Scoville, R. (2005) *Extrapolating Evidence of Health Information Technology: Savings and Costs*. RAND Corporation, Santa Monica, CA.

Goldsmith, J. (2010) Analyzing shifts in economic risks to providers in proposed payment and delivery system reforms. *Health Affairs*, 29, 1299–1304.

Hall, A.G., Harman, J.S., & Zhang, J. (2008) Lapses in Medicaid coverage: impact on cost and utilization among individuals with diabetes enrolled in Medicaid. *Medical Care*, 46, 1219–25.

Hamel, M.B., Drazen, J.M., & Epstein, A.M. (2009) The growth of hospitalists and the changing face of primary care. *New England Journal of Medicine*, 360, 1141–1143.

Hibbard, J.H., Stockard, J., Mahoney, E.R., *et al.* (2004) Development of the patient activation measure (PAM): conceptualizing and measuring activation in patients and consumers. *Health Services Research*, 39 (4, Part 1), 1005–1026.

Hildreth, S. (2010) *Healthcare Electronic Records Technology and Government Funding: Improving Patient Care?* Available at: http://www.b-eye-network.com/view/11201.

Hillestad, R., Bigelow, J., Bower, A., *et al.* (2005) Can electronic medical record systems transform health care? potential health benefits, savings, and costs. *Health Affairs*, 24, 1103–1117.

Holman, H., & Lorig, K. (2004) Patient self-management: a key to effectiveness and efficiency in care of chronic disease. *Public Health Reports*, 119, 239–243.

Institute of Medicine Committee on the Future of Health Care Workforce for Older Americans. (2008) *Retooling for an Aging America: Building the Health Care Workforce.* National Academies Press, Washington, DC.

Jerant, A.F., von Friederichs-Fitzwater, M.M., & Moore, M. (2005) Patients' perceived barriers to active self-management of chronic conditions. *Patient Educating and Counseling*, 57, 300–307.

Jencks, S.F., Williams, M.V., & Coleman, E.A. (2009) Rehospitalizations among patients in the Medicare fee-for-service program. *New England Journal of Medicine*, 360, 1418–1428.

Jha, A., DesRoches, C.M., Campbell, E.G., *et al.* (2009) The use of electronic health records in U.S. hospitals. *New England Journal of Medicine*, 360, 1628–1638.

Johnson, S.E., & Newton, W.P. (2002) Resource-based relative value units: a primer for academic family physicians. *Family Medicine*, 34, 172–176.

Katz, M.G., Jacobson, T.A., Veledar, E., *et al.* (2007) Patient literacy and question-asking behavior during the medical encounter: a mixed-methods analysis. *Journal of General Internal Medicine*, 22, 782–786.

Kroll, T., Jones, G.C., Kehn, M., *et al.* (2006) Barriers and strategies affecting the utilization of primary preventative services for people with physical disabilities: a qualitative inquiry. *Health and Social Care in the Community*, 14, 284–293.

Kutner, M., Greenberg, E., Jin, Y., *et al.* (2006) *Health Literacy of America's Adults: Results From the 2003 National Assessment of Adult Literacy*. U.S. Department of Education, Washington, DC. Available at: http://nces.ed.gov/naal/health_results.asp.

Lubkin, I., & Larsen, P. (2008) *Chronic Illness: Impact and Intervention*. Jones & Bartlett, Sudbury, MA.

Luck, J., Parkerton, P., & Hagigi, F. (2007) What is the business case for improving care for patients with complex conditions? *Journal of General Internal Medicine*, 22 (Supplement 3), 396–402.

Marchibroda, J.M. (2008) The impact of health information technology on collaborative chronic care management. *Journal of Managed Care Pharmacy*, 14 (2 Supplement), S3–S11.

Margolis, D., & Bodenheimer, T. (2010) Transforming primary care: from past practice to the practice of the future. *Health Affairs*, 29, 779–784.

Milbrett, P., & Halm, M. (2009) Characteristics and predictors of frequent utilization of emergency services. *Journal of Emergency Nursing*, 35, 191–198.

National Center for Health Statistics. (2010) *Health, United States, 2009: With Special Feature on Medical Technology*. Centers for Disease Control and Prevention, Hyattsville, MD.

Noel, P.H., Parchman, M.L., Williams, J.W., *et al.* (2007) The challenges of multimorbidity from the patient perspective. *Journal of General Internal Medicine*, 22 (Supplement 3), 419–424.

Page, R.L. II, Linnebur, S.A., Bryant, L.L., *et al.* (2010) Inappropriate prescribing in the hospitalized elderly patient: defining the problem, evaluation tools, and possible solutions. *Clinical Interventions in Aging*, 5, 75–87.

Paradis, V., Cossette, S., Frasure-Smith, N., *et al.* (2010) The efficacy of a motivational nursing intervention based on the stages of change on self-care in heart failure patients. *Journal of Cardiovascular Nursing*, 25, 130–141.

Persell, S.D., Osborn, C.Y., Richard, R., *et al.* (2007) Limited health literacy is a barrier to medication reconciliation in ambulatory care. *Journal of General Internal Medicine*, 22, 1523–1526.

Pham, H., Schrag, D., O'Malley, A., *et al.* (2007) Care patterns in Medicare and their implications for pay for performance. *The New England Journal of Medicine*, 356, 1130–1139.

Pippins, J., Gandhi, T., Hamann, C., *et al.* (2008) Classifying and predicting errors of inpatient medication reconciliation. *Journal of General Internal Medicine*, 23, 1414–1422.

Pitts, S.R., Carrier, E.R., Rich, E.C., *et al.* (2010) Where Americans get acute care: increasingly, it's not at their doctor's office. *Health Affairs*, 29, 1620–1629.

Popejoy, L., Moylan, K., & Galambos, C. (2009) A review of discharge planning research of older adults 1990-2008. *Western Journal of Nursing Research*, 31, 923–947.

Powell, C.K., Hill, E.G., & Clancy, D.E. (2007) The relationship between health literacy and diabetes knowledge and readiness to take health actions. *Diabetes Educator*, 33, 144–151.

RAND Health. (2005) *Health Information Technology: Can HIT Lower Costs and Improve Quality?* RAND Corporation, Santa Monica, CA.

Rollnick, S., Mason, P., & Butler, C. (2000). *Health Behavior Change: A Guide for Practitioners.* Churchill Livingston, Edinburgh, UK.

Rust G., Ye J., Baltrus P., *et al.* (2008) Practical barriers to timely primary care access: impact on adult use of emergency department services. *Archives of Internal Medicine*, 168, 1705–10.

Satiani, B. (2009) A Medicare primer. *Journal of Vascular Surgery*, 50, 453–460.

Schillinger, D., Grumbach, K., Piette, J., *et al.* (2002) Association of health literacy with diabetes outcomes. *Journal of the American Medical Association*, 288, 475–482.

Slain, D., Kincaid, S.E., & Dunsworth, T.S. (2008) Discrepancies between home medications listed at hospital admission and reported medical conditions. *American Journal of Geriatric Pharmacotherapy*, 6, 161–166.

Sudore, R.L., Yaffe, K., Satterfield, S., *et al.* (2006) Limited literacy and mortality in the elderly: the health, aging, and body composition study. *Journal of General Internal Medicine*, 21, 806–812.

United States Census Bureau. (2010) *Population Profile of the United States.* United States Department of Commerce, Suitland, MD. Available at: http://www.census.gov/population/www/pop-profile/disabil.html.

Verrilli, D.K., Dunn, D.L., & Sulvetta, M.B. (1996) The measurement of physician work and alternative uses of the resource based relative value scale. *Journal of Ambulatory Care Management*, 19 (4), 40–48.

Villaire, M., & Mayer, G. (2007) Low health literacy: the impact on chronic illness management. *Professional Case Management*, 12, 213–216.

Weber, E.J., Showstack, J.A., Hunt, K.A., *et al.* (2008) Are the uninsured responsible for the increase in emergency department visits in the United States? *Annals of Emergency Medicine*, 52, 108–115.

Chapter 3

Promising practices in acute/primary care

Randall S. Brown, Arkadipta Ghosh, Cheryl Schraeder, and Paul Shelton

Introduction

Medicare beneficiaries suffering from multiple chronic conditions account for a disproportionate share of Medicare spending, which is often due to inadequate care, poor communications, and weak adherence by patients. Indeed, evidence suggests that beneficiaries with chronic illnesses often receive care that is suboptimal in its frequency, timing, mix, and intensity, which leads to poor clinical outcomes, dissatisfaction with care, and high costs to both the beneficiaries and Medicare (Asch *et al.* 2006; Leatherman & McCarthy 2005; Jencks *et al.* 2003). Even though care coordination programs seem to hold great promise for reducing healthcare costs and improving the quality of life for individuals with chronic illnesses, their effectiveness remains uncertain given the mixed evidence from rigorous evaluations. This chapter aims to synthesize evidence from care coordination interventions for which there is strong, credible evidence that they are effective in reducing hospital use and costs for individuals with chronic illnesses.

A decade of research and demonstrations has developed evidence regarding "care coordination" interventions that are effective in achieving both improved beneficiary outcomes and reduced Medicare expenditures. This chapter synthesizes the evidence on successful care coordination interventions and their essential components, and identifies key issues for future research in this area. A successful intervention for the purposes of this chapter is one that reduces the need for hospitalizations while maintaining or improving other patient outcomes, as hospitalizations account for the bulk of Medicare expenditures. The chapter both draws on and updates the evidence summarized in existing reviews of care coordination programs by Boult *et al.* (2009b), Bodenheimer and Berry-Millett (2009), Brown (2009), and Bott *et al.* (2009). However, unlike some of the earlier reviews, it does not adopt a systematic approach in reviewing the existing literature on care coordination for individuals with chronic illnesses, but it is geared toward synthesizing evidence and lessons drawn from rigorously evaluated programs that have been found to be successful in reducing hospitalizations and expenditures. Also, the emphasis is on care coordination in the "acute care domain" for Medicare FFS beneficiaries with chronic

Comprehensive Care Coordination for Chronically Ill Adults, First Edition. Edited by Cheryl Schraeder and Paul Shelton.
© 2011 John Wiley & Sons, Inc. Published 2011 by John Wiley & Sons, Inc.

diseases; this chapter does not examine employer-based commercial programs or managed care programs. In course of our review, we also address interventions that have generally been shown to be *ineffective*, especially those that were evaluated as part of Medicare demonstrations.

While we mainly focus on care coordination programs for Medicare beneficiaries with chronic illnesses, we also examine care coordination interventions under Medicaid that target beneficiaries with chronic illnesses, including dual-eligibles – that is, beneficiaries covered by both Medicare and Medicaid. Given our objective of synthesizing evidence from successful care coordination interventions for a chronically ill population, these findings will contribute to the ongoing debate and experimentation on two other related and promising models for improving care quality and controlling healthcare cost in patient-centered medical homes (PCMH) and accountable care organizations (ACOs).

Definition of care coordination

We adopt the definition of care coordination presented in Chapter 2, which states that care coordination is a set of activities that assist patients and their families in: self-managing their health conditions and related psychosocial problems more effectively; coordinating their care among multiple health and community providers; bridging gaps in care; and receiving the appropriate level of care. Care coordination is generally provided by a registered nurse (RN) in collaboration with the patient/family, their primary care provider, and other health and community care providers involved in the patient's health care. RN care coordinators maintain a panel of patients over time and primarily see them face-to-face in the home or clinical office settings, or they contact them by telephone.

As discussed in Brown (2009), care coordination for chronically ill Medicare beneficiaries could encompass both health care and social support interventions, depending on a beneficiary's medical and social service needs at a particular point in time. For completeness, we also examine the evidence on disease management programs for this population.

Given the need to slow the rapid and unsustainable increase in health care spending, we classify a program as "successful" only if it significantly reduces Medicare expenditures and sufficiently offsets intervention costs. Because hospitalizations are the major source of expenditures for the chronically ill, we focus on care coordination interventions that reduce participants' needs for hospitalizations (including rehospitalizations).

Overview of the chapter

Our objective in this chapter is to focus primarily on the few studies of care coordination or disease management programs that meet the criteria of providing rigorous evidence of reductions in hospitalization and costs. However, we also review the findings from several other rigorously evaluated interventions – mainly those evaluated as part of Medicare demonstrations – to identify interventions that do not seem to be effective in a Medicare fee-for-service environment. The next section utilizes a logic model to discuss the conceptual framework underlying care coordination interventions, it describes the various components in a typical intervention, and also offers a discussion of three factors that can cause seemingly similar programs to differ in their success. In Section III, we briefly summarize the evidence on what works in care coordination from existing reviews. Section IV summarizes findings from several Medicare care management demonstrations, and Section V contains our detailed review of effective care coordination programs based on findings from rigorous evaluations. In Section VI, we briefly review the evidence on care coordination programs for Medicaid beneficiaries, and also assess the evidence from a recent study of telephonic care management for a commercially insured population that includes individuals with chronic illnesses, with the appropriate caveat that the health conditions and health care needs of a Medicaid or commercially insured population often differ significantly from those of Medicare beneficiaries. Finally, Section VII concludes with a summary of the lessons learned, directions for future research, and the policy relevance of the findings for the currently popular PCMH and ACO models.

Conceptual framework

Care coordination interventions are based on the hypothesis that some combination of the following features will address the barriers to improving patient health, and thereby lead to improved patient health, reduced utilization of expensive acute care services, and reduced costs: (1) improved patient adherence to treatment regimens, (2) increased physician use of evidence-based guidelines for medications and other treatments, (3) improved communication between patients and providers and across providers, (4) better management of transitions between care settings, (5) careful monitoring of patient symptoms and well-being to identify and address health problems and exacerbations earlier than might otherwise occur, and (6) improved access to health-related services. Figure 3.1 shows a logic model for how the different components of a care coordination intervention are expected to improve quality of care and reduce the use of expensive Medicare services, such as hospitalizations, thereby controlling cost.

The approach toward care coordination in an intervention can be captured by looking at a set of key components or features, which we will call "intervention domains." These domains have been identified through an evaluation of the Medicare Coordinated Care Demonstration (MCCD; Peikes *et al.* 2009) and in developing a design for a new care coordination demonstration, the Medicare Chronic Care Practice Research Network (MCCPRN). These domains are based on experiences and the recent literature, in addition to management and through review of project directors of each program identified in Table 2, Chapter 5 (see Schraeder & Shelton 2009). Each of these 14 domains, as identified in Table 3.1, can play a crucial role in affecting the outcomes of an intervention. Also, specific domains are likely to be more important for some patients than others, depending on their healthcare needs, and this may vary over time as their health and social situations change.

As mentioned above, in order to have any hope of generating sufficient medical savings to cover its cost, a care coordination intervention needs to accomplish the difficult task of reducing beneficiaries' needs for hospitalizations. Achieving a sizeable reduction in the number of hospitalizations for a chronically ill population of Medicare beneficiaries is inherently fraught with difficulties, due to the so called "funnel effect," which can

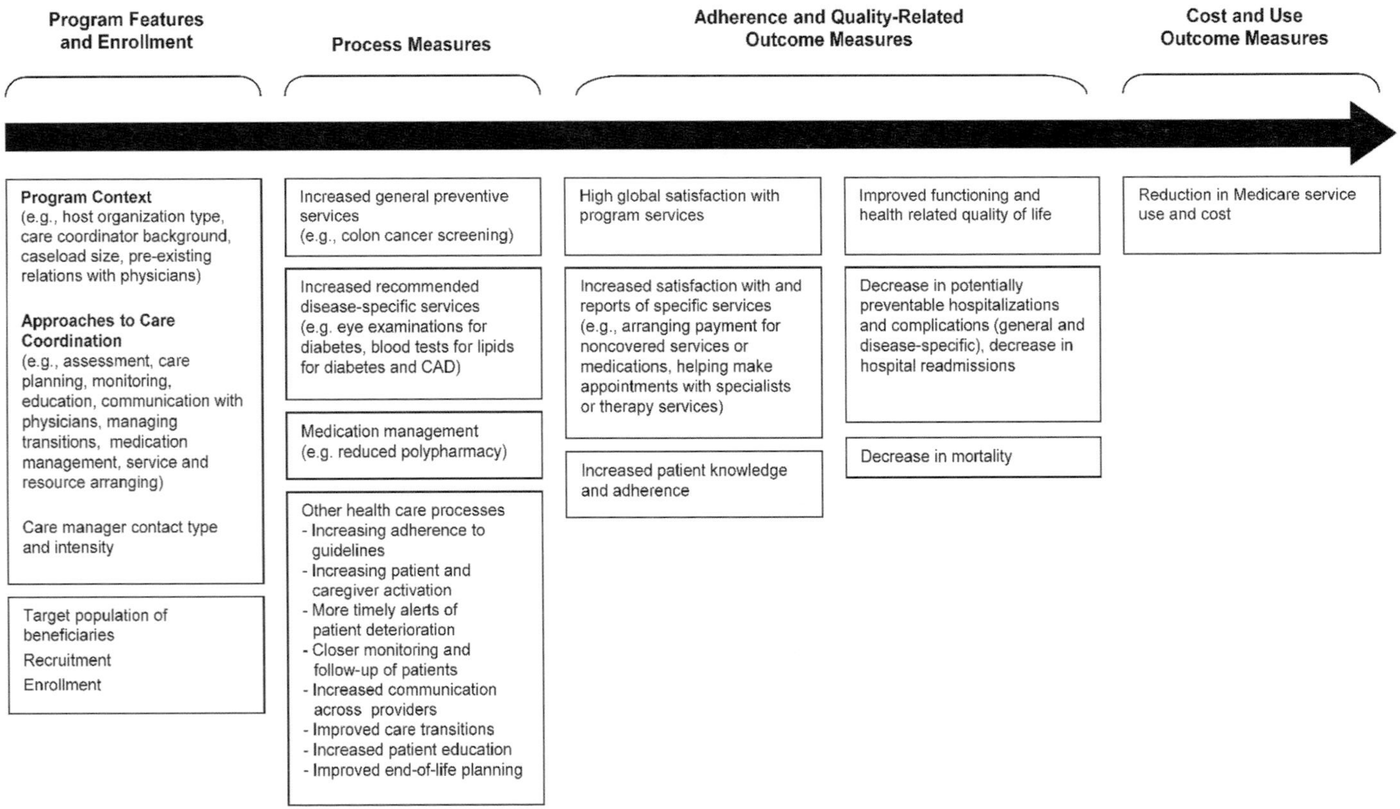

Program Features and Enrollment

Program Context
(e.g., host organization type, care coordinator background, caseload size, pre-existing relations with physicians)

Approaches to Care Coordination
(e.g., assessment, care planning, monitoring, education, communication with physicians, managing transitions, medication management, service and resource arranging)

Care manager contact type and intensity

Target population of beneficiaries

Recruitment

Enrollment

Process Measures

Increased general preventive services
(e.g., colon cancer screening)

Increased recommended disease-specific services
(e.g. eye examinations for diabetes, blood tests for lipids for diabetes and CAD)

Medication management
(e.g. reduced polypharmacy)

Other health care processes
- Increasing adherence to guidelines
- Increasing patient and caregiver activation
- More timely alerts of patient deterioration
- Closer monitoring and follow-up of patients
- Increased communication across providers
- Improved care transitions
- Increased patient education
- Improved end-of-life planning

Adherence and Quality-Related Outcome Measures

High global satisfaction with program services

Increased satisfaction with and reports of specific services
(e.g. arranging payment for noncovered services or medications, helping make appointments with specialists or therapy services)

Increased patient knowledge and adherence

Improved functioning and health related quality of life

Decrease in potentially preventable hospitalizations and complications (general and disease-specific), decrease in hospital readmissions

Decrease in mortality

Cost and Use Outcome Measures

Reduction in Medicare service use and cost

Figure 3.1 Logic Model for Care Coordination Interventions

Table 3.1   Domains of Care Coordination Interventions

Key Program Components
- Comprehensive Care Coordinator training
- Care Coordinators are predominately RNs
- Collaborative relationship with primary care provider
- Use of evidence-based guidelines and protocols
- Use of health information technology (IT) and electronic patient records
- Comprehensive assessment
- Action planning and problem identification
- Longitudinal patient management with frequent face-to-face contacts
- Ongoing monitoring and evaluation
- Patient/caregiver self-management via education and coaching
- Medication management
- Coordinating and arranging health and community services
- Transitional care
- Quality management and outcomes reporting

perhaps be best explained with the following illustration. For a voluntary (opt-in) care coordination intervention targeted at Medicare beneficiaries with one or more serious chronic illnesses such as congestive heart failure (CHF), chronic obstructive pulmonary disease (COPD), or coronary artery disease (CAD), let us assume that patients who enroll in the program have, on average, one hospitalization per member per year. Even if we assume that half of these hospitalizations are theoretically preventable, and the care coordination intervention succeeds in actually preventing 30% of the theoretically preventable hospitalizations, the overall reduction in the number of hospitalizations would only be 15% (which would be expected to produce an associated cost reduction of something around 10%). In other words, even under quite optimistic assumptions about the potential to reduce hospitalizations and the effectiveness of the intervention, it is difficult to achieve a sizeable reduction in the number of hospitalizations for beneficiaries suffering from multiple, serious chronic illnesses.

In spite of such difficulties, some interventions do succeed in reducing hospitalizations and controlling costs, but other similar sounding interventions are not successful on this dimension. Hence, it is important to identify the reasons behind the success of specific interventions. In a recent commentary, Mahoney (2010) identifies three constructs that determine the success of multifactorial fall prevention interventions: content, process, and the choice of target group. These factors are equally applicable to the success of care coordination interventions. Content, according to Mahoney (2010), refers to the components of an intervention that are integral to its success (for example, refer to the domains of care coordination in Table 3.1). Process refers to the way in which the intervention is delivered to induce uptake and behavior change – a particularly difficult task in a fee-for-service environment. The choice of an appropriate target group is equally crucial, if enrollees are at limited risk of hospitalization, it will be difficult to deflect many hospital admissions; conversely, some patients could be so ill that it is too late in the progression of their disease to reduce the need for admissions. It is useful to note here that among the handful of successful care coordination models reviewed in detail in Section VI, including the MCCD results noted above, one common feature was that each of these models succeeded in reducing expenditures only for a *high-risk* subgroup of patients, although the exact definition of high-risk varied from one intervention to another.

Earlier reviews of the literature

Boult *et al.* (2009b) performed a systematic review of models of comprehensive healthcare that have been found to be promising with respect to improving the quality, efficiency, and health-related outcomes of care for elderly patients with chronic diseases. They identified 15 models belonging to the following six model categories that have improved at least one outcome: interdisciplinary primary care (1), models that supplement primary care (8), transitional care (1), models of acute care in patients' homes (2), nurse-physician teams for residents of nursing homes (1), and models of comprehensive care in hospitals (2). We reexamined the evidence presented by Boult *et al.* (2009b) to further limit the set of promising models to those that have evidence of reducing hospitalizations. For instance, evidence from a meta-analysis they reviewed suggests that interdisciplinary primary care teams focused on heart failure can reduce hospitalizations and total costs. However, among models that supplement primary care, the evidence is mixed. Transitional care interventions that facilitate safe transitions from hospital to another healthcare setting or to home have shown clear evidence of reducing hospital readmissions and costs; however, these interventions are short-term in nature. Finally, hospital-at-home programs that provide acute care for certain conditions in patients' homes and nurse-physician teams for nursing home residents have also demonstrated their capacity to reduce inpatient admissions.

Bodenheimer and Berry-Millett (2009) synthesize evidence from a large number of studies on care management for patients with complex healthcare needs, including Medicare care management demonstrations. They offer a useful summary of findings from such studies, including the characteristics of successful care management programs, where success is broadly defined in terms of quality improvement or reductions in hospitalizations and costs. Again narrowing our focus to models for which Bodenheimer and Berry-Millett (2009) find evidence for reductions in hospitalizations, their review shows (like Boult's) that transitional care interventions that target complex patients with multiple diagnoses who are being discharged from hospitals are highly effective in reducing hospital readmissions and total costs. However, the evidence on reductions in hospital use and costs is somewhat mixed for care management interventions in a primary care setting or for care management within integrated delivery systems, and any favorable evidence on cost savings from disease management is based on weak and questionable research methodologies. Bodenheimer and Berry-Millett (2009) also note that Medicare demonstrations of care coordination have usually failed to find evidence for reductions in service utilization and costs. They go on to summarize the characteristics of successful care coordination programs, using a broad definition of success, as previously mentioned: selection of the right patients or the right target group; person-to-person encounters between patients and care managers, including home visits; appropriate training of care managers; a multidisciplinary care management team including physicians; presence of informal family caregivers at home; and the use of coaching techniques as part of care management.

Brown (2009) adopts a more stringent definition of an "effective" care coordination intervention in that to be deemed effective, an intervention should have reduced hospitalizations and costs. His review identifies three types of interventions that have demonstrated effectiveness in reducing hospitalizations for Medicare beneficiaries with multiple chronic diseases: (1) transitional care interventions, in which patients are first engaged within the hospital and then followed intensively over four to six weeks after discharge, to ensure adherence to medication and self-care instructions, recognition of symptoms requiring immediate attention, and in keeping appointments with primary care physicians; (2) self-management education interventions that engage patients for four to seven weeks in community-based programs in order to activate them in the management of their own conditions; and (3) coordinated care interventions that identify patients with chronic conditions at high risk of hospitalizations, conduct initial assessments and care planning, and provide ongoing monitoring of patients' symptoms and self-care, working with the patient, primary care physician, and caregivers to improve the exchange of information. Brown (2009) discusses the implications of the findings from his review for the design of the PCMH model, and for approaches to financing of care coordination models, and ends by identifying issues for ongoing research.

Bott *et al.* (2009) provide a qualitative summary of the findings from seven disease management (DM) demonstrations conducted by the Centers for Medicare & Medicaid Services (CMS) since 1999 involving around 300,000 fee-for-service Medicare beneficiaries. In general, the findings from these demonstrations have not been encouraging in that the results have not consistently shown evidence for improvement in evidence-based care, satisfaction with care, or broad behavior change. Also, very few programs have led to cost savings for Medicare, net of program fees. For instance, the Case Management Demonstration involving beneficiaries with heart failure and diabetes achieved some reduction in hospitalizations and Medicare costs, but cost savings were not sufficient to offset program fees, and in the Care Management for High-Cost Beneficiaries Demonstration, three of the six participating programs achieved financial savings of which only two had sufficient savings to cover program fees and meet the required 5% savings target, net of fees. Bott *et al.* (2009) conclude by noting that several factors will determine the success of future demonstrations involving beneficiaries with chronic diseases, including developing a better understanding of the targeted population and their barriers to getting high-quality care, redesigning future demonstrations based on current evidence, and reassessing ongoing demonstrations to define parameters of success.

Below we update the findings in these existing reviews with findings from recent demonstration evaluations, and then go into more detail about the most successful of the original studies that these reviews have highlighted.

Findings from medicare demonstrations

Over the past decade, CMS has conducted several demonstrations involving thousands of Medicare beneficiaries with chronic illnesses. Barring a few exceptions, the findings from these demonstrations have not been encouraging in that, cost reduction, if any, achieved by any of these demonstrations, was not sufficient to cover intervention costs

(Bott *et al.* 2009). These demonstrations can be grouped into the following two categories based on their mode of beneficiary targeting: (1) population-based disease management programs, and (2) voluntary care management programs. Key features of and findings from several demonstrations falling in either of these categories are summarized below, followed by a brief summary of the lessons learned from the evaluations of these demonstrations.[1]

Population-based disease management

The congressionally mandated *Medicare BIPA Disease Management Demonstration* was intended to provide disease management services and a comprehensive prescription drug benefit to certain chronically ill beneficiaries to test whether disease management in the traditional fee-for-service program led to improved outcomes and lower total costs to Medicare. Medicare FFS beneficiaries with advanced stage CHF, diabetes, or CAD were recruited into three programs operating in Louisiana, Texas, California, and Arizona. The demonstration, which began in 2004, however, did not continue to conclusion, as none of the programs had impacts on the key outcomes of Medicare Part A and Part B expenditures and service use (Chen *et al.* 2008); the programs were therefore terminated before the end of their originally scheduled three-year duration.

Although all three disease management programs in the demonstration used Medicare claims data to identify potentially eligible beneficiaries and recruited beneficiaries through letters, telephone calls, or referrals by physicians and hospitals, they encountered unanticipated difficulties with recruitment, and two programs did not meet their enrollment targets. An independent evaluation found that the programs differed in their timeliness of conducting initial patient assessments and also in their frequency of patient contacts that additionally varied with program maturity. Although, overall, none of the programs had any impacts on hospitalizations, emergency room visits, or Medicare expenditures, one program (XLHealth) reduced hospital admissions and Medicare expenditures among a later cohort of enrollees, specifically those who enrolled after the first six months of program operations. However, even for this later cohort of enrollees in the program, the cost savings were not sufficient to cover program fees (Chen *et al.* 2008). Finally, the programs had limited or no impacts on prescription drug access, patients' satisfaction, functioning, mortality, and potentially preventable hospitalizations.

The *Lifemasters Supported SelfCare Demonstration*, a randomized controlled trial covering the three-year period from January 2005 to December 2007, was a CMS sponsored population-based disease management demonstration program implemented by LifeMasters Supported SelfCare (LifeMasters). The program targeted Medicare fee-for-service beneficiaries who were dually enrolled in Medicaid (dual-eligibles); resided in Florida; and had CHF, CAD, diabetes, or a combination of the three. A sample of Florida beneficiaries meeting the target criteria were randomly assigned to the treatment group, which was eligible to receive the LifeMasters intervention, or the control group, which was not eligible for it; both groups retained their regular Medicare and Medicaid fee-for-service benefits. The LifeMasters intervention included patient assessment and care planning, routine nurse monitoring, patient self-monitoring, patient education, care coordination, and (limited) service arrangement. The intervention was conducted primarily over the telephone by registered nurses, although some nurses also conducted in-person visits to patients classified by the program as frail. LifeMasters classified enrolled treatment group members as either *active* or *inactive*. Active beneficiaries were those who agreed to participate, at some level, in the demonstration and for whom LifeMasters received a monthly management fee. LifeMasters further classified active beneficiaries as *mediated* or *instructional*. Mediated patients participated fully in the disease management program; instructional patients received only a quarterly health magazine and an occasional telephone call from program staff. LifeMasters was at financial risk for this demonstration, meaning that while it would receive a substantial share of any net savings, it was required to reimburse CMS for any net losses (that is, gross savings in Medicare savings minus fees paid). Gross savings were calculated by the Actuarial Research Corporation (ARC) as the difference in average Medicare expenditures per month for the full treatment group (that is, all beneficiaries assigned to the treatment group, regardless of whether they actually engaged with the program) minus average monthly expenditures for the control group, multiplied by the number of treatment group member months.

The formal evaluation of the LifeMasters demonstration, using an intent-to-treat design, found that it did not reduce total Medicare expenditures, hospitalizations or emergency room visits (Esposito *et al.* 2008a; Esposito *et al.* 2008b) for the sample of 36,959 enrollees and 14,797 control group members. However, monitoring reports produced by ARC indicated that the intervention might have had impacts on the subset of beneficiaries with CHF and those who had both diabetes and CAD, and on beneficiaries residing in a subset of the demonstration counties. Therefore, at LifeMasters request, CMS approved a demonstration redesign, to begin in March 2007, for which eligibility criteria were narrowed to include only beneficiaries who resided in select counties and who had CHF only, or at least two of the three targeted conditions (CHF, CAD, and diabetes). Additionally, LifeMasters attempted to enhance its efforts to mediate patients and continued with several program enhancements that were started in the fall of 2006, including wound care, end-of-life planning programs, and complex case management. The evaluation study population for the redesign period of March 2007 through August 2009 included two groups of randomly assigned beneficiaries: those enrolled in the demonstration before March 1, 2007, and eligible for the redesign (Cohort 1) and those enrolled after the start of the redesign (Cohort 2), and thus provided a unique opportunity to study the impact of the intervention on two distinct populations with varying degrees of exposure to the program. An evaluation of the redesign phase of the intervention, however, found that the program had no effects on quality of care, health care utilization, or Medicare expenditures (Stewart *et al.* in press).

The program's failure to generate savings, despite the apparent comprehensiveness of the interventions and the targeting on high-risk beneficiaries who are dually enrolled in Medicaid and have serious chronic illnesses, suggests that it may be difficult for telephonic disease management programs to achieve savings in a Medicare fee-for-service environment. However, even after the redesign, LifeMasters succeeded in contacting only 67.6% to 77.3% of patients in the two cohorts within 13 weeks of enrollment, and no more than 30% of the active treatment group members were mediated (fully engaged) at any point of time during the redesign phase. Furthermore, the program had limited contact with even the mediated patients, and LifeMasters made no use of the Medicaid prescription drug data that it had purchased from the state for its enrollees. Thus the intervention may have been too weak to be effective for this population.

Medicare Health Support (MHS): The Phase I of the MHS Demonstration, was a three-year (2005–2008) pilot designed to test a variety of care management interventions for invited fee-for-service Medicare beneficiaries with CHF or diabetes, tested a range of program models serving diverse populations in urban and rural areas. The programs offered self-care guidance and support to chronically ill beneficiaries to help them manage their health, adhere to their physicians' plan of care, and assure that they obtain medical care that they need to reduce their health risks. The Phase I programs together served approximately 100,000 chronically ill Medicare beneficiaries.

The program was cancelled in August 2008 because experience from Phase I of the MHS program suggested that the program did not meet the statutory requirements of improved clinical quality outcomes, improved beneficiary satisfaction, and financial savings (CMS 2008). An initial evaluation conducted by RTI based on the first six months of program operations for the eight Medicare Health Support Organizations (MHSOs) found few or no significant differences in acute care utilization between the treatment and control groups. The report also notes that negotiated program fees were not covered by reductions in Medicare expenditures over the first six months, and without a reduction in these fees programs may not be budget neutral in the long run (McCall *et al.* 2007). While the early report noted an unexpected and growing divergence between the treatment and control groups from the time of random assignment to the time of program start-up in monthly Medicare expenditures that could affect the ability of the MHSOs to meet their savings targets, none of the analyses suggested that the programs reduced hospitalizations or costs.

The *Care Management for High Cost Beneficiaries (CMHCB)* demonstration, originally approved for three years, was launched by CMS in 2005 with sites in different areas of the country. It tests provider-based intensive care management services as a way to improve quality of care and reduce costs for fee-for-service beneficiaries with one or more chronic illnesses (with the primary focus on CHF, diabetes, and chronic kidney disease [CKD] and high Medicare costs). Six organizations were selected to provide disease management services to a large number (1,800 to 15,000) of beneficiaries. CMS pre-selected beneficiaries for the demonstration according to eligibility criteria, but participation in the demonstration is voluntary. Program services were intended to increase adherence to physician prescribed care, reduce unnecessary hospital stays and emergency room visits, and help participants avoid expensive and debilitating complications. Each of the six organizations chose their own care management interventions that ranged from a distributed network of personal visiting physicians (PVPs) who see patients urgently and routinely in their homes and nursing facilities, or intensive disease management directed by nephrologists in supplementary clinics to use a technology platform in patients' homes to coach them about their health, collect vital signs, and transmit risk-stratified results to multispecialty medical groups. While detailed results from the evaluation of the CMHCB demonstration is awaited, CMS granted three-year extensions to three of the six original programs in the demonstration, based on the initial success of these programs in meeting or exceeding the savings required by the demonstration agreement (CMS 2009a). These three organizations, serving beneficiaries in New York, Massachusetts, Oregon, and Washington, would be subject to monthly operational monitoring and quarterly financial evaluations of performance with the demonstration being extended one year at a time based on their financial status or yearly projected savings. Savings were not measured using a randomized design, but rather were based on projections.

Voluntary care management for high-risk patients

The *Medicare Case Management Demonstrations* studied the appropriateness of providing case management services to beneficiaries with catastrophic illnesses and high medical costs. It tested case management as a way of controlling costs in the fee-for-service sector. These demonstrations were implemented in three Midwestern sites (Indiana, Iowa/eastern Nebraska, and suburban Detroit) in October 1993 and continued through November 1995. The three programs chose different target populations, (for example, those with CHF only, CHF or COPD, or any of eight conditions), and the style and focus of case management differed greatly across the three programs, specifically in their levels of in-person contact, use of nurses and social workers, degree to which case management was structured or allowed to evolve, and their emphasis on education and service coordination. However, the programs also shared a number of key activities, such as client assessment and periodic reassessment, service coordination and monitoring, condition-specific self-care education, and emotional support to clients and their informal caregivers.

An evaluation of the *Case Management Demonstrations* found that although the programs succeeded in identifying and enrolling Medicare beneficiaries at risk of high Medicare spending, participation rates were much lower than expected for all three programs, with beneficiaries older than 85 years and those who died within six months of the participation decision being less likely to participate (Schore *et al.* 1999). Also, in spite of high levels of satisfaction among eventually participating beneficiaries, none of the programs improved patient self-care or reduced hospital admission rates and Medicare spending. In fact, there was a significant increase of 10% points in the proportion of patients admitted to the hospital in one site, which was a hospital; the number of hospital admissions increased by 34%. While the evaluation was unable to conclude whether the observed increase in hospitalizations in this site was a true program effect, it did note that since the program was hosted by a hospital, it might have been more receptive to admitting program clients for observation or treatment. The paper noted four possible reasons for the lack of intended impacts on health behavior or Medicare service use and expenditures: no involvement of clients' physicians in the interventions, lack of a clear focus in the interventions and goals, lack of staff with sufficient case management experience and clinical knowledge, and inadequate financial incentives to reduce Medicare spending.

The *Community Nursing Organization (CNO) Demonstration* tested a capitated, nurse-managed system of care that provided a specified package of community-based services, in conjunction with case management, under a capitated payment methodology. In 1993, CMS selected four organizations in Illinois, Arizona, Minnesota, and New York to provide community nursing and ambulatory care services to Medicare beneficiaries. Services covered as part of the CNO service package included home health services, medical supplies, appliances, and devices, durable medical equipment, ambulance services, outpatient physical therapy, services provided by a clinical psychologist or a clinical social worker, and case management services–defined as services which assist enrollees in gaining access to and coordinating/approving utilization of needed medical, social, educational, and other services. Each of the CNO sites was free to define and configure the process of case management in the way it judged to be most beneficial to the members and efficient for the organization. Methods of assessment, resources devoted to planning and monitoring, as well as the number of members whose care was actively managed, therefore, differed from site to site.

Applicants to the CNOs were randomized to treatment (CNO) or control (traditional Medicare) groups, and based on this randomized research design, the preliminary evaluation report covering the period from January 1994 through 1999, found that Medicare spending per person per month was higher for members of the treatment group than for members of the control group in each of the programs, with these differences being statistically significant at three of the four sites. Furthermore, average monthly Medicare spending in the treatment group kept increasing relative to the population over the course of the demonstration (Frakt *et al*. 2003). However, based on data collected from two sites on beneficiary satisfaction, the final report also found that an overwhelming majority of enrollees at both sites were satisfied with the care received and felt that their nurse consultant was available when needed.

The *Informatics for Diabetes Education and Telemedicine (IDEATel) Demonstration* tested the effects of providing home-based telemedicine services to 1,093 eligible Medicare beneficiaries in two cohorts who had diabetes mellitus and lived in medically underserved areas in New York City and upstate New York. The demonstration began in February 2000, and was originally scheduled to end in February 2004. However, Congress extended the demonstration and the evaluation for a second four-year period and the demonstration ended in February 2008. In both phases eligible Medicare beneficiaries from New York City and upstate New York who volunteered to participate in the demonstration were randomly assigned to either the treatment or a control group. During the demonstration, control group members in both sites received usual diabetes care from their primary care physicians. Treatment group participants also continued to see their primary care physicians *and* additionally received a home telemedicine unit (HTU), which they could use to (1) measure and monitor blood pressure and blood sugar and transmit their measurements to a nurse case manager, (2) communicate with a nurse case manager via audio/videoconferences, known as televisits, and (3) access web-based chat rooms and educational materials available only to participants.

The evaluation of IDEATel (Moreno *et al*. 2008; Moreno *et al*. 2009) found that the intervention as delivered was neither as intensive nor as technologically sophisticated as originally designed, since the Consortium delivering the intervention encountered unexpected challenges and deliberately departed from its plans in some areas. Most importantly, a relatively low proportion of treatment group members made consistent use of the HTUs, and very few used a wide range of its functions. While IDEATel improved clinical outcomes in one site, it had no statistically discernable impact on Medicare Part A and Part B expenditures or the use of expensive services, such as hospital admissions in either phase of the demonstration, in either site. Furthermore, the high intervention costs of the demonstration – more than $8,000 per participant per year – exceeded the control group's combined Part A and Part B expenditures in upstate New York, and were far higher than the costs of comparable home telemedicine programs. Given the absence of effects on costs or services, even a less expensive version of this demonstration would not have produced sufficient Medicare savings to offset demonstration costs (Moreno *et al*. 2008).

The *Medicare Coordinated Care Demonstration (MCCD)*: In early 2001, CMS selected 15 demonstration programs for the MCCD out of 58 applicants in a competitive awards process under which each program was allowed to define, within broad boundaries, its own intervention and target population. Each program began enrolling patients between April and September of 2002, and was authorized to operate for four years. Eleven of the 15 programs later requested, and were granted, two-year extensions, and continued to operate into 2008. The program hosts included disease management companies, community hospitals, academic medical centers, integrated delivery systems, hospice, and an upscale retirement community, which were located in geographically diverse areas. Although the care coordination interventions of the 15 programs varied widely, all programs assigned patients to a nurse care coordinator–usually a registered nurse–and in all programs the care coordinator assessed patients and developed patient care plans.

The evaluation of the 15 original MCCD programs showed that none generated net savings to Medicare (Peikes *et al*. 2008) and 14 programs showed no statistically significant differences in hospitalizations. However, one program (Mercy Medical Center) significantly reduced hospitalizations and had a sizable yet statistically insignificant reduction in Part A and B expenditures, and another program (Health Quality Partners [HQP]) showed promise, with both hospitalizations and expenditures about 11% lower in the treatment group, though these decreases were not statistically significant (Peikes *et al*. 2009). CMS subsequently granted these two programs extensions to operate for two more years. A Report to Congress on these two promising MCCD programs (Mercy and HQP) found that they significantly reduced hospitalizations among a *high-risk subgroup* (enrollees with COPD, CHF, or CAD and at least one hospitalization in the year before randomization, or with any of 12 chronic conditions and at least two hospitalizations in the prior two years). HQP also achieved significant cost reductions for this subgroup (Schore *et al*. 2010). Further, ongoing analysis of data from 11 of the original 15 programs over 2002–2008 shows that four of these programs significantly lowered hospitalizations by 8% to 33% among a high-risk subgroup of beneficiaries (Peikes *et al*. 2010). The implications of these recent findings from the ongoing analysis of data from the MCCD are discussed in greater detail in Section V below.

Lessons learned from the evaluations of medicare demonstrations

The findings from the Medicare demonstrations, whether the population based disease management programs or voluntary care management, are, in general, disappointing in that none of these meet our criteria for a successful intervention that reduces the number of hospitalizations and Medicare expenditures. Also, some of these demonstrations, such as the Disease Management and the Case Management Demonstrations encountered difficulties in beneficiary recruitment and participation, while for some others such as the IDEATel demonstration, intervention costs were too high to lead to any savings in Medicare expenditures. Although full evaluation results for the CMHCB demonstration are awaited, none of the other demonstrations met their budget neutrality requirements.

Valuable lessons, however, have emerged from the evaluation of the MCCD, in particular from recent findings that four programs reduced hospitalizations and costs among a high-risk subgroup of beneficiaries. Also, as briefly discussed above in Section III, these four successful programs share certain intervention characteristics that are lacking in some of the other MCCD programs. Overall, the findings from the ongoing analysis of data from the MCCD suggest that care coordination can generate savings to Medicare if the *right interventions are targeted to the right people*. In other words, following Mahoney's (2010) framework, identifying an appropriate target group, carefully developing the content of an intervention tailored to the needs of the target population, and delivering the intervention in a patient-centered way by triaging and activating patients are the key determinants of success in a care coordination program. Also, as noted by Bott *et al.* (2009) in their review of disease management demonstrations in Medicare, reassessing ongoing demonstrations to define parameters of success in future demonstrations, and striking a balance between program costs and expected savings or between program costs and value in terms of improvements in quality and outcomes would be crucial to future success in Medicare demonstrations.

Successful programs/models

Very few care coordination or care management programs that used a randomized design to compare an intervention group with an equivalent control group have reported significant impacts on hospitalizations or costs of health services. Effective care coordination program models that have reported impacts in hospitalizations or cost fall into one of three categories: (1) transitional care interventions (Naylor *et al.* 2004; Coleman *et al.* 2006), (2) self-management interventions (Lorig *et al.* 1999; Lorig *et al.* 2001; Wheeler *et al.* 2003) and (3) care coordination interventions (Care Management Plus, the Geriatric Resources for Assessment and Care of Elders, Guided Care, and four sites that participated in the CMS Medicare Coordinated Care Demonstration [MCCD]). In the next section we briefly describe these programs and their outcomes.

Transitional care

Some of the strongest evidence of care transition interventions that reduce hospitalizations and costs are two well-tested models designed to reduce readmissions to hospitals. The transitional care intervention developed by Naylor *et al.* (2004) targeted patients who were hospitalized for CHF and used highly trained advanced practice nurses (APNs) to administer the intervention. The intervention was highly structured and effective. The APNs met with patients in the hospital and in their homes shortly after discharge to provide intense coaching and education on medications, self-care, and symptom identification. The intervention lasted a total of 12 weeks, and patients were followed for one year. The intervention was evaluated with a randomized design and intent-to-treat approach. During the year following the hospital discharge, the number of rehospitalizations per patient year was 34% lower in the treatment group than the control group. In addition, rehospitalization rates in the treatment group were 44.9% compared to 55.4% in the control group, a difference of 10.5%. At one year, treatment group patients also had mean total costs 39% lower than control group patients ($7,636 versus $12,481). The total intervention cost was $115,856 ($982 per patient).

The other successful transitional care model, developed by Coleman *et al.* (2006), also used advanced practice nurses as the care coordinators (referred to as "transition coaches"), but targeted hospitalized patients with a range of chronic conditions. Under Coleman's model, the one-month intervention provided patients with (1) tools to promote cross-site communication, (2) encouragement to take a more active role in their care, and (3) continuity of care and guidance from their transition coach. The intervention was evaluated with a random design. Intervention patients had lower rehospitalization rates than control subjects at 30 days (8.3% versus 11.9%) and 90 days (16.7% versus 22.5%), as well as lower rehospitalization rates for the same condition that precipitated the initial hospitalization at 90 days (5.3% versus 9.8%) and 180 days (8.6% versus 13.9%). In addition, mean hospital costs were $488 lower for intervention patients than controls at 180 days ($2,058 versus $2,546). The annual cost of the intervention was $74,310 ($196 per patient), resulting in a net cost savings of approximately $147,797 over the six-month follow-up.

Self-management

Another model that has been shown to generate reductions in hospitalizations is one that focuses on educating patients in how to self-manage their conditions. Kate Lorig and John Wheeler both developed self-management models and produced studies with favorable results. The programs focus on four factors: (1) identifying patients' goals; (2) improving their self-management skills; (3) building their sense of self-efficacy; and(4) assessing their mastery of these skills.

Lorig *et al.* (1999; Lorig *et al.* 2001) offered a community-based self-management program to patients who were 40 years of age or older and had a physician-confirmed diagnosis of heart disease, lung disease, stroke or arthritis. In seven weekly group sessions, course leaders provided program participants with instruction on exercise, cognitive symptom management techniques, nutrition, fatigue and sleep management, use of medications, dealing with emotions, communication, problem-solving, and other topics.

The program was evaluated with a six-month randomized, controlled trial with an intent-to-treat approach. Compared to control subjects, treatment subjects demonstrated improvements at six months in weekly minutes of exercise, cognitive symptom management, communication with physicians, and other healthy practices. Treatment subjects also had one-third fewer hospital stays (0.17 versus 0.25) and spent, on average, half as many nights in the hospital as control subjects (0.8 versus 1.6). Treatment subjects also generated $820 less in average six-month health care costs than control subjects. The cost of the intervention was only $70 per participant, which produced health expenditure savings of approximately $750 per participant over the six-month follow up.

Wheeler's (2003) model is similar to Lorig's work. Drawing from six hospital sites, Wheeler administered the program to women who were 60 years or older and had a diagnosis of cardiac disease. The four-week program featured weekly group meetings in which health educators taught program participants to manage cardiac problems such as diet, exercise and taking medicine. The program was assessed with a randomized design, and an intent-to-treat approach. The results show that over a 21-month period following the intervention's conclusion, the treatment group experienced 39% fewer in-patient days and 43% lower in-patient costs than women in the control group. The program cost about $374 per patient, resulting in a ratio of medical expenditure savings to program costs of approximately 5 to 1.

Care coordination

Care Management Plus (CMP) is a primary care based interdisciplinary team model from Intermountain Healthcare and Oregon Health and Science University. CMP includes care managers, either registered nurses (RNs) or social workers, located on-site, working in health care teams and using information technology (IT) to help care for patients with complex chronic illness. CMP prioritizes health care needs through structured protocols and tools to assist patients and caregivers to self-manage their chronic diseases. Specialized IT tools allow clinicians to access individualized care plans and receive reminders about best practices, and they facilitate communication among the health care team and with other providers such as subspecialists. RN care managers typically have a caseload of approximately 350 to 500 patients and provide individualized assessment and care planning, using disease management guidelines; teaching/coaching self-management skills; assisting in care transitions and coordinating services with different providers; and proactive monitoring and providing ongoing guidance and support (Dorr *et al.* 2006; Dorr *et al.* 2007a). CMP has demonstrated several benefits to chronically ill patients. It reduced annual mortality rates by more than 20% and hospital admission rates by 24% to 40% for patients with diabetes and depression (Dorr *et al.* 2008), and improved quality of care through higher adherence to clinical testing guidelines and increased physician productivity (Dorr *et al.* 2007b).

In the Geriatric Resources for Assessment and Care of Elders (GRACE) program, on-site support teams, comprised of an advanced practice nurse and social worker, provide comprehensive, home-based primary care for low-income seniors receiving care through community health centers. The support team meets with off-site geriatrics interdisciplinary teams to review each patient at least quarterly (Counsell *et al.* 2006). Each support team has a caseload of approximately 100 to 125 patients and are seen face-to-face by the support team at least every two months. The focus of the intervention is on an initial in-home assessment and individualized care plan; the use of specific clinical protocols; an electronic medical record, and a web-based care management tracking tool; the integration of affiliated pharmacy, mental health, home health and community-based and inpatient geriatric services; and the coordination and continuity of care among all health care providers and sites of care. GRACE has demonstrated improvements in quality of care, reductions in hospital admissions, and cost savings for a pre-defined subgroup of patients (Counsell *et al.* 2007; 2009) at high risk of hospitalization when they entered the program based on a PRA score greater than or equal to 0.4 (Boult *et al.* 1993). Overall, GRACE reduced emergency department visits by 17% for all intervention patients and 35% for high risk patients, reduced hospital admissions by 44% for high risk patients, and reduced expenditures (not including program costs) by 23% for high risk patients one-year post intervention.

In Guided Care, two to five primary care physicians partner with an on-site RN to provide comprehensive primary care to 55 to 60 of their elderly, chronically ill patients at high risk for using costly health services in the upcoming year. The RN conducts a comprehensive in-home assessment and then monitors and contacts patients every month, engages them and their caregivers in self-management activities, provides transitional care when needed, and coordinates important health-related services across different provider settings (Boyd *et al.* 2007; Boult *et al.* 2009a). The RN also helps patients to create a personal care guide and action plan and provides emotional support on an on-going basis. Preliminary data indicate that Guided Care improves quality of care (Boult *et al.* 2008; Boyd *et al.* 2010), reduces family caregiver strain (Wolff *et al.* 2010), improves physician satisfaction with chronic care (Marsteller *et al.* 2010), and reduces the use and cost of expensive health services (Leff *et al.* 2009; Boult *et al.* in press).

As noted above, although the 15 original MCCD national sites did not show net savings to Medicare (Peikes *et al.* 2009), ongoing analysis identified four programs that significantly reduced hospitalizations by 11% and Medicare expenditures (including program costs) by $178 per patient per month among their high risk patients (Peikes *et al.* 2010). High risk patients were defined as having chronic obstructive pulmonary disease (COPD), congestive heart failure (CHF) or coronary artery disease (CAD), and having at least one hospitalization in the prior year or any of 12 chronic illnesses and two or more hospitalizations in the previous two years. The four programs were implemented in four different geographical settings: (1) a hospital that is part of an integrated delivery system in rural northern Iowa (Mercy Medical Center, Mason City), (2) an urban academic medical center (Washington University, St. Louis), (3) a hospice and home health care provider (Hospice of the Valley, greater Phoenix area), and (4) a quality improvement service provider in suburban and rural Pennsylvania (Health Quality Partners). While the programs were different, they had core similarities. All four programs used RNs trained in comprehensive care coordination and focused on improved self-care, chronic symptom recognition and management, improved medication management, and improved transitional care and physician communication.

Two common features highlight the successful care management/care coordination models. The first was that transitional care and self-management education were integral components of the model. The second is that they all succeeded in reducing expenditures for a *high-risk* subgroup of patients, although the exact definition of high-risk varied from one intervention to another. The lessons learned from these successful models form the basis of essential care coordination components discussed in Chapter 5. We return to the identification of *high-risk* patients in the concluding section of this chapter.

Selected studies on medicaid and commercial populations

In this section, we critically evaluate findings from two studies that evaluate care coordination programs in Medicaid and a commercially insured population respectively. Although the demographic and health profiles of Medicaid beneficiaries differ from that of Medicare beneficiaries in important ways, including the higher prevalence of younger beneficiaries, homelessness, substance abuse, and mental and behavioral health problems among the former, a sizeable number of patients with chronic illnesses are enrolled in Medicaid, either with or without Medicare coverage. Hence, we are interested in interventions funded by Medicaid that served a similar population of beneficiaries with chronic illnesses. Similarly, even though a commercially insured population is likely to be younger and healthier on average, we review a recent evaluation of a telephone-based care management strategy for a commercially insured population that included beneficiaries with chronic illnesses.

Indiana chronic disease management program (ICDMP)

The ICDMP, assembled by Indiana Medicaid and implemented in 2003, had several components and was primarily designed to improve the quality and cost effectiveness of care for Medicaid beneficiaries with CHF, diabetes, asthma, and other conditions (Rosenman *et al*. 2006). The ICDMP was implemented in three stages: it was launched on July 1, 2003, in central Indiana for eligible participants with diabetes or CHF, and northern and southern parts of Indiana as well as a statewide asthma disease management program were added to ICDMP during 2004. ICDMP for adults with diabetes or CHF had several components: identification of eligible participants through their ongoing participation in the state's primary care case management programs (PCCMs) for Medicaid beneficiaries and through queries of Medicaid claims to identify people with specific conditions; risk stratification based on predicted costs whereby the highest-risk (20%) of eligible participants were assigned to nurse care managers and the remaining (80%) to telephonic care management; use of information systems for decision support; and the creation of quality improvement collaboratives for primary care practices. It is interesting to note that more than 40% of the participants in the ICDMP who had diabetes or CHF were dually enrolled in both Medicare and Medicaid.

Holmes *et al*. (2008) evaluate the net fiscal impact of the ICDMP, based on a randomized research design, in which eligible Medicaid beneficiaries who had CHF, or diabetes, or both received chronic disease management services or standard care, based on the random assignment status of their Indianapolis-based primary medical provider's practice. The study uses multivariate methods controlling for baseline differences in age, sex, risk status, prescription drug use, Medicare coverage, and levels of claims paid during the pre-ICDMP period to find that ICDMP significantly reduced claims paid by Medicaid for all beneficiaries with CHF, especially the low-risk beneficiaries with CHF, but it did not have any cost-saving effect for beneficiaries with diabetes. However, the study's findings and conclusions are questionable due to several methodological issues.

The first problem with the study is that in spite of random assignment, the treatment and control groups were not balanced in their baseline characteristics – in particular, they differed widely in average Medicaid expenditures during the year prior to enrollment. While this difference can be controlled for statistically, the advantage of randomization is not realized in this study—the sizeable difference in pre-enrollment expenditures raises concerns that the two groups differed along unobserved or unmeasured characteristics, which could bias the impact estimates obtained by the authors. Moreover, the authors do not examine treatment-control differences in pre-intervention *trends* in Medicaid claims that could highlight potential differences in the claims pattern over time between the two groups, although they report having 21 months of pre-ICDMP data for each patient in the analysis sample. This problem arises due to the small sample size of individuals with CHF, only 186 beneficiaries, resulting in imprecise estimates that are heavily influenced by outliers. The problem is exacerbated by the finding that the effects are limited to the subset of 117 sample members who are in the low-risk subgroup of beneficiaries with CHF.[2] Finally, the authors do not examine any other outcomes, such as service utilization outcomes, which would provide a reasonable robustness test and guide as to the potential source (for example, reduction in hospitalizations) of the estimated cost savings. The surprising findings of no cost savings for high-risk beneficiaries and favorable program impacts on only the low-risk beneficiaries with CHF are at odds with virtually all of the other studies discussed above, in which impacts are observed only for the high-risk subgroup of sample members.

Telephone-based care management for a commercially insured population

A recent population-based randomized study by Wennberg *et al.* (2010) evaluated a telephone-based care management strategy for a commercially insured population that included patients with selected chronic conditions, such as heart failure, COPD, CAD, diabetes, and asthma. In this study, 174,210 subjects were randomly assigned to either a usual support group (control) or an enhanced support group (treatment). The study team used predictive models to predict health service utilization and the likelihood of surgical intervention for a beneficiary with a preference-sensitive condition. The key difference between the two groups was in the extent of outreach – a greater proportion of patients received outreach through health coaches or interactive voice-response calls in the enhanced support group through the lowering of cutoff points for predicted health care costs or utilization. The intervention content delivered to the two groups – that reached 10.4% of the patients in the enhanced support group and 3.7% of the patients in the usual support group – was otherwise similar, and consisted of telephonic contacts by health coaches providing behavioral change and motivational counseling, and promoting shared decision making. The study finds that telephonic care management led to a statistically significant 4% reduction in total healthcare expenditures that was mainly driven by a significant 10% reduction in hospital admissions in the treatment group. Additionally, there were significant reductions in hospital admissions for at least two beneficiary subgroups, those with selected chronic conditions and those with high-risk conditions other than the selected chronic or preference-sensitive conditions. With low program costs of $2 per person per month, the results suggest that the net savings from the program was about $6 per person per month.

    In spite of these impressive findings and an apparently strong research design, there are several problematic aspects of this study that make these results suspect. First, given that the treatment in reality is the differential outreach to the two groups, we believe that the analysis should have ideally been limited to those who met the new (lowered) threshold for the intervention but did not meet the original higher threshold, in both the treatment and comparison groups. Such a strategy would have ensured that (1) the analysis included only beneficiaries for whom the program could conceivably have had any effect, by excluding the 82% of sample members for whom it was irrelevant; (2) the study had the correct counterfactual – those eligible for the intervention who did not receive it; (3) the analysis was still an intent-to-treat approach in that all beneficiaries in both the treatment and control groups who met the target eligibility criteria were included in the analysis regardless of whether they actually received the intervention or not; and (4) despite the much smaller sample size, the analysis would have had more statistical power, given that the impacts have to be concentrated in the individuals selected.[3] However, the authors conduct their analysis on all beneficiaries in both groups regardless of whether they were eligible for the intervention (that is, met the lower cutoff for predicted costs or utilization). This in turn leads to the second issue of whether these effects are reasonable or not. Given the nature of eligibility for the intervention, the effects detected for the full sample of beneficiaries can arise only from the greater proportion of beneficiaries in the treatment group who received the telephonic care management services, in other words, for the additional 18% or so of beneficiaries who became eligible to be contacted in the treatment group due to the lowering of the threshold or cutoff,[4] or more specifically for the additional 6.7% of beneficiaries who were actually contacted in the enhanced support group (10.4% versus 3.7% in the usual support group). Since the effects observed for the full sample can only arise from this small percentage of patients in the treatment group who actually received services, the actual effects for this subgroup of treatment group patients must be extremely large.[5] Such effects are not only highly unlikely for such a weak intervention, but are totally at odds with findings from previous randomized controlled trials that report little or no improvements in outcomes from telephone-based care management. The weak methodology raises major concerns regarding the validity of the findings.

Conclusions

CMS-funded demonstrations and empirical work over the last few years has yielded a wealth of new information on the effectiveness of various forms of care coordination/care management for patients with chronic illnesses. The importance of these findings for getting U.S. health care costs under control cannot be overstated. Some of the lessons learned are drawn from studies that have shown certain interventions to be ineffective, while others are drawn from singularly successful interventions. This non-systematic review of the evidence from recent studies published in the literature or in federally funded reports leads us to a number of conclusions:

1. Reducing the need for hospitalizations (and therefore, costs) among individuals with chronic illnesses is extremely difficult to do in a fee-for-service setting, and probably in any setting.
2. Telephonic-only disease management programs are unlikely to generate such savings.
3. Transitional care interventions show the most promise for reducing hospitalizations and costs enough to generate net savings.
4. Self-management models can be successful, but may not work for Medicare beneficiaries with cognitive problems.

5. While several care coordination programs have had positive results and the findings about what factors are most important for their success are quite consistent across the studies, the evidence base is still weak. Most of the successful programs have only been implemented in a single setting, in a single replication, and sample sizes are typically modest.
6. The effects of successful care coordination programs are nearly always confined to the high risk subset of the original target population. Unless the individuals are at a substantially higher risk of hospitalization than the Medicare population at large, care coordination programs are unlikely to succeed in reducing hospitalizations and costs.
7. In general, for a program to be successful, care coordinators must (1) have a substantial amount of in-person contact with patients, (2) build a collaborative relationship with patients' primary care provider through in person contacts, (3) be highly trained problem solvers who implement the care management process utilizing evidence based guidelines and protocols, (4) focus on self-management, medication management, and transitions of care, (5) utilize information systems to document practice, (6) receive and utilize quality and outcome reports to improve patient/panel management, (7) receive comprehensive training in care coordination, (8) have access to other professionals, such as social workers, gerontologists, pharmacists, and dieticians, either as members of a team or on a consultative basis, and (9) facilitate and coordinate communication between multiple health and community providers. (See Chapter 5 for more detailed discussion.)
8. One size does not fit all, the care plan and monitoring of each patient must be tailored to the patient's needs at the given time, in the given setting, and for the patient's given conditions, severity of symptoms, and personal desires.
9. The random assignment demonstrations sponsored by CMS have greatly enhanced our knowledge of what works, and what doesn't, in the area of care coordination for beneficiaries with chronic illnesses. PCMHs, ACOs, and other attempts to bend the medical cost curve are unlikely to be successful if they do not build on these critical lessons regarding how to reduce the need for expensive hospitalizations among those with chronic illnesses, who account for the lion's share of national health care expenditures.

While this knowledge has been gleaned from many studies, much still remains unknown about successful care coordination. Most importantly, we do not know how replicable the findings from the GRACE, Guided Care, Care Management Plus, or MCCD demonstrations are. How dependent were these studies on their leaders? Which of the many aspects of the interventions and how they were performed are critical, and which are unimportant? How important is fidelity to the original intervention, and do we know enough of the details about those that were successful to implement them in the same way? How generalizable are the findings to other settings, do the interventions only work in academic medical centers? Or only in urban areas? How important is the exact definition of "high risk" to the success of the study?

Our collective ignorance about what works extends to other important issues, including the optimal length of time to retain patients in the intervention (ongoing, like many of the models; short term, like the self-management and transitional care interventions; or somewhere in-between). The issue of replicability and generalizability of favorable interventions is extremely important for policymakers in deciding how to move forward. As noted earlier, Mahoney (2010) has described differences in process, content, and targeting that can lead to some interventions failing while other similar ones have succeeded. A recent article in the New Yorker (Lehrer 2010) noted the seemingly mystifying and disconcerting fact that even many randomized controlled trials that have been replicated are being found later to "lose" their potency. This failure of later studies to replicate the success of earlier ones could be due to a number of factors commonly observed, including failure to faithfully implement key components of the original intervention in the same manner and with the same types of staff, differences in the target population, changing alternatives ("counterfactuals") to which the control group is exposed, publication bias, testing of many hypotheses with the same data set without properly controlling for the multi-test bias that results, Hawthorne effects, and selective reporting of results. Thus, we are left in the uncomfortable position of needing to build on past evidence, but being fearful that the "truths" from those earlier studies no longer hold.

The resolution to this conundrum is not to abandon past studies, but to assess critically each piece of new "evidence" to determine its credibility and likely generalizability, and then build new interventions from these firm foundations to refine our knowledge of what works. We also need to learn the lessons from "failed" interventions, and assess whether the inability to reduce hospitalizations was experienced was due to failures of design, process, targeting, or other factors. This assessment should be done in part by contrasting features of the failed intervention with those of successful models. However, such comparisons must look beyond surface descriptions of the interventions and focus on the details of how the intervention was conducted.

Two final points are worth noting. First, the CMS Congressionally mandated Innovations Center has as a primary goal of speeding up the learning process. While understandable, this emphasis on speedy results must be heavily tempered by the critical importance of getting the decisions right, which will often mean taking more time than we wish to develop and sift the evidence. The problem is difficult to solve, so we must measure our risk of serious mistakes when implementing new policies based on evidence developed quickly. We must also continue to monitor and evaluate the new interventions adopted to make sure they continue to be as effective as new alternatives. The second point to note is that new demonstrations are being designed and planned by CMS to test the replicability of transitional care and care coordination interventions that do, in fact, build on some of the studies cited above. This encouraging development is a welcome change to the past practice of simply discarding interventions that do not work and moving on to the newest popular idea, which often has little grounding in hard evidence.

Notes

1. One care management demonstration, the Physician Group Practice Demonstration, was not included in this review. The demonstration, which ran from April 2005 through March 2010, provided performance payments to ten participating physician group practices based on their attaining performance targets on quality measures and achieving

savings in Medicare expenditures. We exclude this from our review since it did not focus on beneficiaries with chronic illnesses and had a relatively weak quasi-experimental research design in which PGP participants' outcomes (expenditure growth, quality measures, and so on) are contrasted to beneficiary outcomes in the comparison groups, which were composed of beneficiaries in the same geographic areas as the PGP participants, but for who the PGP did not provide the plurality of services (Kautter *et al.* 2007; CMS 2009b).

2. It is also not clear why the estimated overall effect for beneficiaries with CHF (−$283) is greater in magnitude than both the estimated effects for the high (−$150) and low-risk beneficiaries (−$247) with CHF, since the overall effect should be a weighted average of the effects for the high- and low-risk beneficiaries.

3. For problems with non-participation, the variance of the estimate of the true impact on those who could have been affected (the participants) increases with the square of the inverse of the participation rate when the full sample is used, but increases only in proportion to the inverse of the participation rate when the sample is restricted to the relevant cases. Thus, even though the restricted sample size is much smaller, the precision of the estimates of impacts on participants is greater, because irrelevant cases have been excluded.

4. As reported by the authors, 7.8% of beneficiaries in the usual support group were targeted for outreach, versus 25.8% of beneficiaries in the enhanced support group.

5. For example, among the subset of beneficiaries who had chronic illnesses, the treatment-control difference in number of hospitalizations was −31 per 1,000 patients, which implies an effect four times larger for a subset of people who could have been affected by the demonstration (the treatment-control difference in the proportion contacted for the intervention). Dividing that estimated impact of −124 admissions per 1,000 by the mean for the control group with chronic conditions (226) yields an estimated impact of 55%, a magnitude that seems highly unlikely for a telephonic only intervention, based on methodologically strong evaluations of similar interventions.

References

Asch, S.M., Kerr, E.A., Keesey, J., *et al.* (2006) Who is at greatest risk for receiving poor-quality health care? *New England Journal of Medicine*, 354, 1147–1156.

Bodenheimer, T., & Berry-Millett, R. (2009) *Care Management of Patients with Complex Health Care Needs.* Synthesis Project, Report No. 19, Robert Wood Johnson Foundation, Princeton, NJ.

Bott, D., Kapp, M., Johnson, L., *et al.* (2009) Disease management for chronically ill beneficiaries in traditional Medicare. *Health Affairs*, 28(1) 86–98.

Boult, C., Reider, L., Frey, K., *et al.* (2008) Early effects of guided care on the quality of health care for multimorbid older persons: a cluster-randomized controlled trial. *Journal of Gerotology: MEDICAL SCIENCES*, 63A, 321–327.

Boult, C., Giddens, J.F., Frey, K., *et al.* (2009a) *Guided Care: A New Nurse-Physician Partnership in Chronic Care.* Springer Publishing Company, New York, NY.

Boult, C., Green, A.F., Boult, J.T., *et al.* (2009b) Successful models of comprehensive care for older adults with chronic conditions: evidence for the Institute of Medicine's "Retooling for an Aging America" report. *Journal of the American Geriatrics Society*, 57, 2328–2337.

Boult, C., Reider, L., Leff, B., *et al.* (in press) The effect of guided care teams on the use of health services: results from a cluster-randomized controlled trial. *Archives of Internal Medicine*.

Boyd, C.M., Boult, C., Shadmi, E., *et al.* (2007) Guided care for multimorbid older adults. *The Gerontologist*, 47, 697–704.

Boyd, C.M., Shadmi, E., Conwell, L.J., *et al.* (2008) A pilot test of the effect of guided care on the quality of primary care experiences for multi-morbid older adults. *Journal of General Internal Medicine*, 23, 536–542.

Boyd, C.M., Reider, L., Frey, K., *et al.* (2010) The effects of guided care on the perceived quality of health care for multi-morbid older persons: 18-month outcomes from a cluster-randomized controlled trial. *The Journal of General Internal Medicine*, 25, 235–242.

Brown, Randall. (2009) *The Promise of Care Coordination: Models That Decrease Hospitalizations and Improve Outcomes for Medicare Beneficiaries with Chronic Illness*. Report Commissioned by the National Coalition on Care Coordination. Mathematica Policy Research, Princeton, NJ.

Centers for Medicare and Medicaid Services. (2008) *Completion of Phase I of Medicare Health Support Program*. Fact Sheet. Centers for Medicare and Medicaid Services, Baltimore, MD. Available at: https://www.cms.gov/CCIP/downloads/EOP_Fact_Sheet_FINAL_012808.pdf.

Centers for Medicare and Medicaid Services. (2009a) *Care Management for High-Cost Beneficiaries*. Summary. Centers for Medicare and Medicaid Services, Baltimore, MD. Available at: http://www.cms.gov/DemoProjectsEvalRpts/downloads/CMHCB_summary.pdf.

Centers for Medicare and Medicaid Services. (2009b) *Physician Group Practice Demonstration Evaluation Report*. Report to Congress. Centers for Medicare and Medicaid Services, Baltimore, MD. Available at: http://www.cms.hhs.gov/Reports/Downloads/RTC_Sebelius_09_2009.pdf.

Chen, A., Brown, R., Esposito, D., *et al.* (2008) *Report to Congress on the Evaluation of Medicare Disease Management Programs*. Mathematica Policy Research, Princeton, NJ.

Coleman, E.A., Parry, C., Chalmers, S., *et al.* (2006) The care transitions intervention: results of a randomized controlled trial." *Archives of Internal Medicine*, 166, pp. 1822–1828.

Counsell, S.R., Callahan, C.M., Buttar, A.B., *et al.* (2006) Geriatric resources for assessment and care of elders (GRACE): a new model of primary care for low-income seniors. *Journal of the American Geriatrics Society*, 54, 1136–1141.

Counsell, S.R., Callahan, C.M., Clark, D.O. *et al.* (2007) Geriatric care management for low-income seniors: a randomized controlled trial. *Journal of the American Medical Association*, 298, 2623–2633.

Counsell, S.R., Callahan, C.M. Tu, W., *et al.* (2009) Cost analysis of the geriatric resources for assessment and care of elders care management Iintervention. *Journal of the American Geriatrics Society*, 57, 1420–1426.

Dorr, D.A., Wilcox, A., Burns, L., *et al.* (2006) Implementing a multidisease chronic care model in primary care using people and technology." *Disease Management*, 9(1), 1–15.

Dorr, D.A., Wilcox, A. Jones, S., *et al.* (2007a) Care management dosage. *Journal of General Internal Medicine*, 22, 2007a, pp.736–741.

Dorr, D.A., Wilcox, A., McConnell, K.J., *et al.* (2007b) Productivity enhancement for primary care providers using multicondition care management. *American Journal of Managed Care*, 13(1), 22–28.

Dorr, D.A., Jones, S.S., & Wilcox, A. (2007c) A framework for information system usage in collaborative care. *Journal of Biomedical Informatics*, 40, 282–287.

Dorr, D.A., Wilcox, A.B., Brunker, C.P., *et al.* (2008) The effect of technology-supported, multidisease care management on the mortality and hospitalization of seniors." *Journal of the American Geriatrics Society*, 56, 2195–2202.

Esposito, D., Schore, J., Brown, R., *et al.* (2008a) *Evaluation of Medicare Disease Management Programs: LifeMasters Interim Report of Findings*. Mathematica Policy Research, Princeton, NJ.

Esposito, D., Brown, R., Chen, R., *et al.* (2008b) Impacts of a disease management program for dually eligible beneficiaries. *Health Care Financing Review*, 30(1), 27–45.

Frakt, A.B., Pizer, S.D., & Schmitz, R.J. (2003) *Phase II Evaluation of CNO Demonstration: Final Report to Congress*. Abt Associates, Cambridge, MA.

Holmes, A.M., Ackermann, R.D., Zillich, A.J., *et al.* (2008) The net fiscal impact of a chronic disease management program: Indiana Medicaid. *Health Affairs*, 27, 855–864.

Jencks, S.F., Huff, E.D., & Cuerdon, T. (2003) Change in the quality of care delivered to Medicare beneficiaries, 1998–1999 to 2000–2001. *Journal of the American Medical Association*, 289, 305–312.

Kautter, J., Pope, G.C., Trisolini, M., *et al.* (2007) Medicare physician group practice demonstration design: quality and efficiency pay-for-performance. *Health Care Financing Review*, 29(1), 15–29.

Leatherman, S., & McCarthy, D. (2005) *Quality of Health Care for Medicare Beneficiaries: A Chartbook*. Commonwealth Fund, New York, NY. Available at: http://www.cmwf.org/publications/publications_show.htm?doc_id=275195.

Leff, B., Reider, L., Frick, K.D., *et al.* (2009) Guided care and the cost of complex healthcare: a preliminary report. *American Journal of Managed Care*, 15, 555–559.

Lehrer, J. (2010) The truth wears off: is there something wrong with the scientific method? *The New Yorker*, December 13, 52–57.

Lorig, K., Sobel, D., Stewart, A., *et al.* (1999) Evidence suggesting that a chronic disease self-management program can improve health status while reducing hospitalization. *Medical Care*, 37(1), 5–14.

Lorig, K.R., Ritter, P., Stewart, A.L., *et al.* (2001) Chronic disease self-management program: 2-year health status and health care utilization outcomes. *Medical Care*, 39, 1217–1223.

Mahoney, J.E. (2010) Why multifactorial fall-prevention interventions may not work? *Archives of Internal Medicine*, 170, 1117–1119.

McCall, N., Cromwell, J., & Bernard, S. (2007) *Evaluation of Phase I of Medicare Health Support (Formerly Voluntary Chronic Care Improvement) Pilot Program Under Traditional Fee-for-Service Medicare*. Report to Congress. RTI International, Washington, DC.

Marsteller, J., Hsu, Y.J., Reider, L., *et al.* (2010) Physician satisfaction with chronic care processes: a cluster-randomized trial of guided care. *Annals of Family Medicine*, 8, 2010, 308–315.

Moreno, L., Shapiro, R., Dale, S., *et al.* (2008) *Final Report to Congress on the Informatics for Diabetes Education and Telemedicine (IDEATel) Demonstration, Phases I and II*. Mathematica Policy Research, Princeton, NJ.

Moreno, L., Dale, S., Chen, A., *et al.* (2009) Costs to Medicare of the IDEATel home telemedicine demonstration: findings from an independent evaluation. *Diabetes Care,* 32, 1202–1204.

Naylor, M.D., Brooten, D.A., Campbell, R.L., *et al.* (2004) Transitional care of older adults hospitalized with heart failure: a randomized, controlled trial. *Journal of the American Geriatrics Society*, 52, 675–684.

Peikes, Deborah., Brown, R., Chen, A., *et al.* (2008) *Third Report to Congress on the Evaluation of the Medicare Coordinated Care Demonstration*. Mathematica Policy Research, Princeton, NJ.

Peikes, D., Chen, A., Schore, J., *et al.* (2009) Effects of care coordination on hospitalization, quality of care, and health care expenditures among Medicare beneficiaries: 15 randomized trials. *Journal of the American Medical Association*, 301, 603–618.

Peikes, D., Peterson, G., Schore, G., *et al.* (2010) *Effects of Care Coordination on Hospitaliza-tions, Mortality, and Health Care Expenditures Among High-Risk Medicare Beneficiaries: 11 Randomized Trials.* Unpublished Report, Mathematica Policy Research, Princeton, NJ.

Rosenman, M.B., Holmes, A.M., Ackermann, R.T., *et al.* (2006) The Indiana chronic disease management program." *The Milbank Quarterly*, 84(1), 135–163.

Schore, J., Brown, R., & Cheh, V. (1999) Case management for high-cost Medicare beneficiaries. *Health Care Financing Review*, 20(4), 87–101.

Schore, J., Peikes, D., Peterson, G., *et al.* (2010) *Fourth and Final Report to Congress on the Evaluation of the Medicare Coordinated Care Demonstration.* Draft Report. Mathematica Policy Research, Princeton, NJ.

Schraeder, C., & Shelton, P. (2009) *Design for a Care Coordination Demonstration.* Medicare Chronic Care Practice Research Network. Available at: http://www.mccprn.com/Documents/.

Stewart, K.A., Esposito, D., Holt, J.A., *et al.* (in press) *Evaluation of the LifeMasters Disease Management Demonstration Program for Dual Eligible Beneficiaries.* Final Report. Mathematica Policy Research, Princeton, NJ.

Wennberg, D.E., Marr, A., Lang, L., *et al.* (2010) A randomized trial of a telephone care-management strategy. *The New England Journal of Medicine*, 363, 1245–1255.

Wheeler, J.R., Janz, N.K., & Dodge, J.A. (2003) Can a disease self-management program reduce health care costs? the case of older women with heart disease. *Medical Care*, 41, 706–715.

Wolff, J.L., Giovannetti, E.R., Boyd, C.M., *et al.* (2010) Effects of guided care on family caregivers. *The Gerontologist*, 50, 459–470.

Chapter 4

Promising practices in integrated care

Patricia J. Volland and Mary E. Wright

Introduction

As health care reform continues to take shape, care coordination has arrived center stage as a means to help avert a potential health care crisis brought on by a rapidly aging population whose health and long-term care needs are not best served under the current system. Chronic conditions are known to increase with age: currently more than eighty percent of adults over age 65 suffer from at least one chronic medical condition, and 50% have at least two chronic medical conditions (Centers for Disease Control and Prevention 2002). Three quarters of Medicaid spending by states is dedicated to providing health and long-term care services to persons with chronic conditions, with costs driven by hospital care, physician services, prescription drugs, and home health services (Mollica & Gillespie 2003). As the population ages in the years ahead, with the fastest growing cohort being the oldest old, the alarm has been sounded that we must act quickly both in terms of developing innovative models of care that depart from an outmoded system focused on acute care, and preparing a trained workforce equipped to deal with the oncoming "silver tsunami."

To date, the care coordination has often been focused on the medical needs of older adults, with less attention paid to the social support and long-term care needs that are commonly associated with old age. Long-term care needs arise from limitations of activity in older adults and are intimately tied to some combination of chronic disease, injuries such as falls, and acute illness. In spite of this close association between illness and functional limitations, the long-term care and social support needs of older adults are widely reported in the public media as a caregiver issue. Caregivers are the backbone of the long-term care system, and for the year 2007, caregiving services were estimated at approximately $375 billion (American Association of Retired Persons 2008). Even though there is an enormous societal cost when caregivers must quit their jobs or succumb to illness themselves, due to increased levels of stress, the long-term care needs of older adults are all too often not included as part of the medical care and health paradigm.

Why is this? Certainly any health or social service provider understands that frail, chronically ill older adults often need *both* long-term social supports *and* medical care, in order to maintain optimal health and support the desire to remain within home and community, and that neither older adults nor their caregivers are necessarily equipped to deal with the situation at hand. However, over the years the system has developed so that different public funding streams provide payment for long-term care (most often associated with Medicaid) and medical care (primarily associated with Medicare), with the exception of some waiver programs that integrate the two. Long-term care needs may also be addressed by a patchwork of home and community-based services available to older adults through state and area agencies on aging (AAA), funded primarily through the Older Americans Act, and aging and disability resource centers which seek to coordinate state long-term care services through a single point of entry. The home and community-based services provided on the state and local level play key roles in extending the services that enable older adults to remain in the home, but are rarely coordinated with medical care, and can be confusing to both older adults and their caregivers in terms of availability and access.

The silos that have grown up around the financing and delivery of acute care versus long-term care have led to a poorly coordinated system for which there is no real justification. In fact, the fee-for-service nature of Medicare, the arbitrary assignment of most long-term care services to Medicaid, and a cobbled together system of home and community-based services on the state and local level, has led to fragmentation and gaps in service, lack of communication among providers, poor outcomes for beneficiaries, and ultimately increased program costs. In addition, long-term care under Medicaid demonstrates a strong bias toward institutional care, in opposition to both consumer interest and the potential cost advantages of remaining within a home and community-based setting.

Effective care coordination can bridge the gap between these two financing and service delivery systems by integrating health and long-term care services. Many years of research and demonstration programs developed under the authority of the Centers for Medicare & Medicaid Services (CMS) have provided information and feedback on models of care that integrate health and long-term care to varying degrees. In its most robust incarnation, care coordination for older adults includes comprehensive assessment, an interdisciplinary team of medical and social service professionals, and a holistic approach to patient care that involves clinical, psychosocial, and environmental follow up. Care coordination programs vary in their particulars and degree of integration between health and long-term care, but the purpose is fundamentally the same: to establish the most quality-oriented, cost-effective method of meeting the complex health and social service needs of older adults, using interdisciplinary teams that are organizationally equipped to manage an unwieldy system of multiple providers and services.

Evidence from care coordination programs must be further developed in order to establish whether the integration of health and long-term care enables beneficiaries to better maintain physical functioning and independence, avoid unnecessary hospital admissions and readmissions, and avoid premature institutionalization. Waiver and other programs for dual-eligibles, which extend services to older adults who are eligible for both Medicare and Medicaid, have helped lay the groundwork for models that integrate health and long-term care services. Managed health care plans, state- and county-operated programs, and Veterans Administration programs also provide examples of entities that seek to coordinate medical care, behavioral health, and long-term social support services. In this chapter we shall present an analysis of ten programs using care coordination models that take different approaches to integrating health care and long-term care services and have demonstrated positive outcomes with respect to quality improvement and cost effectiveness. To date, care coordination programs have come in many different shapes and sizes, and the challenge before us is to understand which of these programs have been the most effective in achieving their aims, and which show the greatest potential for future support and expansion.

Evidence for integrated care coordination programs

The analysis of care coordination programs presented in this chapter builds on the work of the National Coalition on Care Coordination (N3C), established by the Social Work Leadership Institute of the New York Academy of Medicine and the American Society on Aging in 2008. A national coalition of consumer, aging, social service, health care, family caregiver, and professional organizations, N3C works to promote better coordinated health and social services for older adults with multiple chronic conditions as an essential part of health care reform. From its inception N3C has recognized the importance of establishing the effectiveness of care coordination through evidence-based analysis. Among its key initiatives, N3C commissioned several papers to synthesize evidence on effective care coordination models and on options for providing and paying for such programs: (1) "The Promise of Care Coordination: Models that Decrease Hospitalizations and Improve Outcomes for Medicare Beneficiaries with Chronic Conditions," authored by Randall Brown (2009); and (2) "Structuring, Financing, and Paying for Effective Care Coordination," authored by Robert Berenson and Julianne Howell (2009).

Brown's (2009) analysis of medically focused care coordination programs found substantial evidence for the effectiveness of approaches that included transitional care interventions, self-management care interventions and selected programs from the Medicare Coordinated Care Demonstration that began implementation in 2002. Measures of the effectiveness of these programs came from randomized control trials that offered evidence for interventions that reduced the rate of participants' hospitalizations (including rehospitalizations) as a measure of improved health outcomes, as well as an indicator of reduced expenditures.

An analysis of programs that integrate health and long-term care by definition needs to take a more expansive look at outcomes in order to evaluate whether or not a given program has achieved success. While integration of social support and long-term care may have a positive effect on rates of hospitalization, of equal importance is analyzing how these programs help avoid or delay institutional care, which reflects both the desire of individuals with functional limitations to reside within the home and community and has a positive impact on cost. In the analysis of ten programs put forth in this chapter, we will take a broader look at the types of evidence that describe care coordination outcomes, using as a guide the Agency for Healthcare Research and Quality (AHRQ) guidelines on evidence ratings that include "strong," "moderate," and "suggestive" (AHRQ 2009). The major focus in this chapter is on strong and moderate evidence, based on either randomized control trials or evaluations that utilize a quasi-experimental design to make comparisons to similar populations in the same state or geographical locale. Where appropriate, qualitative outcomes are also included to illustrate successful aspects of integrated programs.

Programs for inclusion were identified through a search of several research databases, the New York Academy of Medicine's Grey Literature Report archive, and discussions with national policy experts. The basic criteria for including a program in the analysis were that the care coordination model integrates medical with long-term care support, albeit to varying degrees, and demonstrates positive outcomes related to both quality and cost effectiveness. An additional criterion for programs is that they meet the N3C definition of care coordination: *a person-centered, assessment-based, interdisciplinary approach to integration of health care and social support services in which the care coordination function is integral to managing and monitoring an individual's needs and preferences based on a comprehensive care plan.* These programs have also been selected for their prominence in having gained national attention for their innovative role in using care coordination to integrate care, and are sufficiently established to have provided a sound footing for evaluation.

Ten programs for analysis

Four categories were created to elucidate different models, based on the degree of integration and the primary focus of the program:

- *Fully integrated models* are health plans that coordinate medical care and long-term social support services in a comprehensive manner. These models integrate all Medicare and Medicaid services, most often under a capitation system that provides a single funding stream and thus a flexibility of choice on how to provide the appropriate services. The major hindrance to the expansion of fully integrated programs, which to a great extent focus on the high-risk dual eligible population, is that they are time consuming and complex to plan and implement. As a result, they have achieved a modest enrollment over time, although they have been essential to the development of promising care coordination practices and are effective in achieving positive outcomes.
- *Community-based socially oriented models* are programs primarily focused on the provision of long-term social support services, with varying levels of integration with medical care. Socially oriented programs are designed to provide management and coordination of home and community-based long-term care services but in general do not directly address medical care. This limited approach to integration is typically focused only on obtaining information from physicians about health status, diagnosis, medications, and treatments. In community-based programs that utilize single point of entry systems to coordinate care, there may be access to multiple funding streams: state funded services, Medicaid state plan and waiver services, social services block-grant funds, and Older Americans Act funds.
- *Patient-Centered Medical Homes* offer a medical model that utilizes a primary care physician practice as the source of health care with, in some instances, explicit linkages to community based social support services. When first developed, patient-centered medical homes had little or no integration with long-term care and social supports. Recently there has been a movement toward integration with community-based supports, although the medical nature of the model still dominates. Like socially oriented

models, though in opposite direction, they offer a fertile ground for development of a more robust integration.

• *Other Models* consist of two integrated models of care that are somewhat anomalous, primarily because of funding sources or eligibility criteria – the Veterans Administration Geriatric Evaluation and Management program and Hospice. Both programs have provided evidence for the efficacy of care coordination in achieving positive outcomes, and have targeted specific populations in need that are outside the more familiar realm of high-risk beneficiaries who are either dual-eligibles or who meet the criteria of being eligible for nursing home placement.

The ten programs chosen for inclusion are summarized in Table 4.1 and are briefly described below.

Fully integrated managed care models

The Arizona Long Term Care System, Minnesota Senior Health Options, the Wisconsin Partnership Program, and the Program for All-Inclusive Care for the Elderly (PACE) are all well-established programs that primarily serve the dual eligible population on a statewide basis, or in the case of PACE, nationally.

Arizona Long Term Care System (ALTCS)

In 1989, Arizona created the Arizona Long Term Care System (ALTCS), a mandatory managed care program under which contractors provide a range of acute and long-term care services for individuals who are Medicaid eligible and at risk of institutionalization (McCall 1997). Coverage for medical care includes doctor's office visits, hospitalization, prescriptions, lab work, and behavioral health services. ALTCS is targeted to individuals who fall into any one of the following categories: age 65 or over, blind, or disabled. The individual must be in need of ongoing long-term care. Approximately 48% of ALTCS participants live in their own homes or an assisted living facility and receive needed in-home services. ALTCS uses a formula for determining case load, and the Arizona Health Care Cost Containment System (AHCCCS) sets a specific rate for case management services separate from the capitated rate that covers health care services. ALTCS requires case managers to be in contact with clients living in the community at least once every 90 days, which differs from most plans that do not stipulate such a high frequency of contact.

ALTCS pays contractors prospectively on a capitated, per member, per month basis. Using utilization trend data and medical cost inflation factors, the blended rate is established by taking into consideration acute care, home and community-based care, institutional care, behavioral health care, and administrative costs. Two different capitation rates are established, based upon whether or not members have Medicare benefits (CMS 2007). Some of the eight contracted programs also have special established payment arrangements for disease-specific conditions (CMS 2007).

Minnesota Senior Health Options (MSHO)

The Minnesota Senior Health Options (MSHO) program began as a Medicaid 1115 demonstration in 1997 and was designed to test the cost and quality-related outcome

Table 4.1 Programs Analyzed

Program/Plan	Start Date	Current Authority	Fully Inte-grated Managed Care Models	Community Based Socially Oriented Models	Community Based Patient Centered Medical Home	Other
Arizona Long Term Care System (ALTCS)	1989	Medicaid 1115 Waiver	X			
Minnesota Senior Health Options (MSHO)	1997	Medicare SNP	X			
Wisconsin Partnership Program (WPP)	1995	Medicaid/Medicare Integrated Care Model	X			
Program for All-Inclusive Care for the Elderly (PACE)	1997	Medicare Plan option/ Managed Care Model	X			
Ohio PASSPORT Program (PASSPORT)	1984	Medicaid 1915 (c) Waiver		X		
Wisconsin Family Care Program	1998	Medicaid 1915 (c) & (b) Waiver		X		
Community Care of North Carolina (CCNC)	1998	Medicaid Managed Care			X	
Vermont Blueprint Integrated Pilot (BIP)	2008	Mixed			X	
Geriatric Evaluation and Management (GEM)	1976	Veterans Administration				X
Hospice	1979	Medicare benefit				X

effectiveness of an integrated Medicare/Medicaid service benefit for dually eligible seniors in four counties in Minnesota. Participating health plans were converted to Medicaid 1915 waivers in 2003 and became Medicare Advantage (MA) Special Needs Plans in 2006. The program continues to operate under Medicare Section 402 demonstration authority to allow for payment differences from other MA plans (CMS 2007; Malone 2004). Over 35,000 members are enrolled in MSHO (CMS 2007); of those, approximately 38% reside in nursing homes. Another 32% meet the criteria for nursing home placement but are being served in the community through home and community based services. MSHO contracts with non-profit health organizations to provide a full range of Medicaid acute, behavioral health, home and community-based services and also the full range of Medicare Part A, B, and D benefits (CMS 2007). The model's centerpiece is its use of care coordination as the tool to improve quality and ensure efficiency. Each member is assigned a care coordinator, who works closely with both the primary care physician and the beneficiary to coordinate all medical and social service needs.

Wisconsin Partnership Program (WPP)

The Wisconsin Partnership Program (WPP), also a managed care plan for dually eligible individuals, began in 1995 with funding from the Robert Wood Johnson Foundation. WPP was converted into an integrated Medicare/Medicaid waiver program in 1999. It was designed to serve nursing-home eligible people over the age of 65 and adults (age 18+) with physical disabilities. Interdisciplinary teams coordinate all primary, acute, mental health, and long-term care services, with a nurse practitioner serving as the primary coordinator.

Capitation contracts are awarded to health organizations by the state to provide or arrange for the provision of all Medicaid-covered primary and acute care services, community based long-term care services, and nursing facility services. The Medicaid payment is 95% of the weighted average of payments made to fee-for-service participants, resulting in the State realizing an automatic 5% savings. In addition, there is an annual case mix adjustment to the rates. Medicare payments are based on hierarchical condition category (HCC) methodology, in addition to a "frailty adjuster" to account for the frailty of the population being served (CMS 2007).

Program for all-inclusive care for the elderly

OnLok Senior Health Services in San Francisco was the first program in the country to test a combined Medicare and Medicaid capitated approach to meeting the health and social support needs of nursing-home eligible, community-dwelling elders. The Program for All-Inclusive Care for the Elderly (PACE) was modeled after OnLok and was authorized under the Balanced Budget Act of 1997 (White *et al.* 2000).

PACE provides and coordinates the entirety of medical and social services for its members using an interdisciplinary team approach composed of a primary care physician, nurses, social workers, rehabilitation therapists, dieticians, and direct care workers. The team develops the care plan and delivers all services (acute care, medical, social, and when necessary, nursing facility care) in a seamless, ongoing and integrated manner. PACE centralizes its services around an adult day center.

PACE is a capitated benefit for older adults (age 55 or older) who, based on an assessment, are deemed to require a nursing-home level of care. PACE members can be eligible for Medicare or Medicaid or both. Medicare recipients who are not eligible for Medicaid pay monthly premiums equal to the Medicaid capitation amount. PACE organizations receive capitated Medicare payments from the Centers for Medicare and Medicaid Services and Medicaid payments from the state. At this time, the Medicare rate includes the "frailty adjuster" which accounts for the relative frailty of the member population. The Medicaid rate is reimbursed below a traditional fee-for-service equivalent. PACE providers assume full financial risk for participants' care without limits on amount, duration, or scope of services.

Community-based socially oriented models

This analysis also looked to evidence from programs that are traditionally categorized as socially oriented, long-term care programs, but that also formally include coordination with at least some integration of medical health services provided to the recipients. Two programs met the criteria for inclusion, the Ohio PASSPORT program and the Wisconsin Family Care Program.

Ohio passport program

The Ohio PASSPORT Program (Pre-Admission Screening System Providing Options and Resources Today) is a Medicaid 1915(c) waiver established in 1984. It is the oldest Ohio waiver program and one of the largest waiver programs in the country. PASSPORT's goal is to provide long-term services and supports to nursing-home eligible individuals to help them remain safely in their own homes. PASSPORT has two arms: first, a point-of-entry system that offers pre-admission telephone screening to determine Medicaid eligibility, assess care needs, and provide information about available service options, and second, a home care system, which includes case management and monitoring services. Once a person is determined eligible, a case manager is assigned to that person and works with the individual to craft an individualized care plan. The case manager primarily coordinates long-term support services but also arranges for some medical aspects of the person's care (medical equipment purchasing and transportation for medical appointments). In order to facilitate integration of the medical and social support dimensions, the person's physician must be made aware of and agree to the care plan created. Certainly, there is room for growth in the level of coordination with the health care needs of the older adult, since the current level of integration is minimal. The ground work for effective care coordination is in place, however, and lends itself to an enhanced connection with health care needs.

In support of the goal of making the program cost effective, Ohio requires that the PASSPORT program for each participant must not exceed 60% of the cost of comparable nursing home care. The Ohio Department on Aging with oversight by the Ohio Department of Job and Family Services established contracts with 13 agencies to administer the PASSPORT program. The administrative agency is not permitted to be the home care service provider and must contract out for services. In addition to the services provided in the PASSPORT care plan (primarily personal care), participants receive traditional medical Medicaid services.

Wisconsin Family Care Program (WFC)

The Family Care Program in Wisconsin (WFC, a combined 1915c and 1915b waiver) began in 1998, authorized to serve people with disabilities (developmental and physical) and frail elders. Its goals are to provide consumers with choices in services/residences, improved access to services, improved quality related to outcomes, and cost effectiveness. WFC has two organizational components: aging disabilities resource centers (ADRCs) and managed care organizations. The ADRCs serve as a point of entry into the long-term care system and provide an array of telephone-based and in-home services.

Managed care organizations (MCOs) offer the Family Care Benefit for both institutional and community dwelling individuals. The benefit does not include coverage for medical services (unlike ALTCS and MSHO) but does blend funding streams to offer consumers an individualized and flexible long-term care benefit. MCOs receive a capitated per person payment to manage and purchase services for their members. The Family Care benefit requires MCOs to use an interdisciplinary team approach to assessment and coordination.

Although medical services are not covered by the Family Care Benefit, these services are coordinated by the Family Care interdisciplinary team. Nurses on the interdisciplinary team coordinate the care directly with the medical providers and also may accompany the member to appointments. Any recommendations made by medical practitioners are brought back to the team, and the team then assists the member in following the recommendations.

Patient-centered medical homes

An evolving model of coordinated care is the patient centered medical home. The primary care physician practice serves as the central point for the delivery of services to its patients, and care is delivered in a holistic, person-centered way. Although many of these models are primarily medically focused, two have explicitly integrated medical care and long-term social support services: Community Care of North Carolina and the Vermont Integrated Care Pilot Program.

Community Care of North Carolina

Community Care of North Carolina (CCNC) began in 1998 with its foundations in the Medicaid program. The program is structured as an enhanced fee-for-service model with a designated dollar amount per member/per month to support care management activities. To expand the model to recipients of Medicaid and dually eligible individuals with chronic conditions and long-term care needs, CCNC has established a chronic care program that targets Medicaid eligible beneficiaries who are elderly, blind or disabled. This program also targets a defined subset of high risk/high utilization individuals for comprehensive case management. The model is structured so that primary care physicians are supported by a network of other community providers, including hospitals, health centers, and community social service departments (Steiner *et al.* 2008). CCNC currently includes 14 non-profit networks with over 3,000 physicians managing approximately 900,000 Medicaid recipients (80% of North Carolina's Medicaid population). Case management is a core function of the networks, and case managers, employed by the networks, follow a standardized protocol to identify at-risk patients, assess the patients' needs, and determine the level of intensity case management required.

Using case management and information technology systems as vehicles, the Chronic Care Program includes services such as disease management, prevention strategies for avoidable emergency department (ED) visits, hospital admissions, and readmissions (Wilhide & Henderson 2006). While CCNC does not explicitly address long-term care, it maintains a community focus and includes mental health referrals, social case management, family/caregiver involvement, and collaboration with community providers.

Vermont Blueprint Integrated Pilot

The Vermont Blueprint Integrated Pilot (BIP) shares similarities with the CCNC model, as it utilizes the patient-centered medical home as the source of primary care, with local interdisciplinary "Community Care Teams" composed of nurse coordinators, public health prevention specialists, Office of Vermont Health Access care coordinators, social workers, dietitians, and community health workers. This ambitious program does not restrict itself to older adults, although its focus on chronic conditions such as arthritis, heart disease, and diabetes ensures that older adults, who have a disproportionate amount of chronic illness compared to their younger counterparts, stand to benefit from these pilots. A linchpin of this system reform is the establishment of patient-centered integrated care models and the integration of health care, public health, and supporting social services to support population health. As with CCNC, the community-based nature of the program provides for social support and mental health services, but lacks an explicit focus on long-term care.

Financial integration is to be achieved through the mandatory participation of the three major commercial insurers and Medicaid, with a sliding care management fee linked to ten NCQA Patient-centered Medical Home criteria and plans for participation on the national level by Medicare. Finally, the program has a strong focus on the incorporation of health information technology as a means to improve the quality of care and facilitate a thorough evaluation of outcomes.

Other models of care coordination

Two additional programs are included in this analysis: the Veterans Administration Geriatric Evaluation and Management Program and Hospice (as a Medicare benefit). They are grouped for convenience as neither fits neatly in the preceding categories.

Geriatric Evaluation and (Case) Management (GEM)

Geriatric Evaluation and (Case) Management (GEM) is a widely evaluated model of case management and health care service delivery. The Veteran's Administration (VA) began implementing the model with positive results in 1976. Although the VA has taken the lead and is most commonly associated with it, GEM has spread rapidly in the United States and abroad. GEM can be implemented in an inpatient unit, outpatient clinic, or primary care setting. It is based upon a multidimensional bio-psycho-social assessment conducted by an interdisciplinary team (most commonly comprised of a social worker, nurse practitioner and geriatrician). Using the Comprehensive Geriatric Assessment, the team creates a care plan that then coordinates medical/health, rehabilitation, education, and social service interventions with the aim of improving the quality of life for targeted individuals in a cost efficient manner.

Hospice

The Medicare Hospice Benefit is intended to provide compassionate and cost-effective care for Medicare beneficiaries with incurable advanced illnesses. Medicare's very large expenditures on dying beneficiaries, combined with federal funding pressures, have given new prominence to end-of-life care. Hospice provides a combination of services designed to address not only the physical needs of patients, but also the psychosocial needs of patients and their caregivers. The team of providers engaged in hospice care includes doctors, nurses, home health aides, social workers, clergy/spiritual counselors, therapists, and volunteers.

Hospice has been a Medicare benefit for almost three decades, starting in 1979 when the Health Care Financing Administration (now CMS) invited and supported 26 hospice care demonstrations. Hospice became a Medicare benefit (temporarily) in 1984, and permanently in 1986. In 1985, Medicaid programs were given the option to cover Hospice as a benefit. Many private insurance plans also include a hospice benefit. Under Medicare, Hospice is a capitated benefit with daily prospective (and regionally adjusted) rates established for routine home care, continuous home care (24-hour care), inpatient respite care, and general inpatient care. Medicaid uses the same categorization. Physician services are reimbursed separately.

Analysis of outcomes and program effectiveness

For all of the programs under analysis, the respective evaluations report changes in utilization patterns that demonstrate effective approaches to integrating health and long-term care services: decreases in hospitalizations, readmissions, and/or ED use, and decreases in nursing home utilization and costs. The methodology used for measuring these outcomes differed by program: some used a control group, others compared outcomes to another state's utilization statistics and expenditures for a similar population, and yet others compared the community-based program costs to projected nursing home costs. Table 4.2 summarizes the outcomes found for each program, followed by brief descriptions of the most significant studies and findings for each program. Of the programs selected for inclusion, evaluation outcomes for Vermont's Blueprint Integrated Pilots are not yet available, although a comprehensive evaluation is in progress and an outline of this evaluation will be provided. We have chosen to include this program based on the innovative aspects of its program

Table 4.2 Program Outcomes

Program	Hospitals: Fewer/decrease in hospitalizations	Hospitals: Lower rates of admissions	Hospitals: Fewer days/1000	Hospitals: Shorter length of stay	Hospitals: Lower inpatient costs	Hospitals: Fewer/decrease in ED visits	Nursing Homes: Lower rate of NH admissions	Nursing Homes: Less expensive than NH care	Nursing Homes: Lower NH costs	Home Care: Slower increase in costs	Costs: Lower overall costs
ALTCS (3)			X								X
MSHO (4)	X	X		X		X					X
WPP (5)		X		X		X	X				
PACE (6)		X				X	X				
PASSPORT (7)								X			
WFC (8)					X				X		X
CCNC (9)	X	X				X				X	X
GEM			X (10)			X (11)			X (14)	X (15)	X (12)
Hospice	X (13)										X (16)

Notes:
(3) When compared to traditional Medicare beneficiaries in New Mexico (McCall 1997)
(4) When compared to 2 control groups (Kane 2004)
(5) When compared to a similar population (CMS 2007)
(6) When compared to control groups (MacAdam 2008)
(7) When compared to costs related to nursing home care (Ciferri 2007)
(8) When compared to control group (APS Healthcare 2005)
(9) When compared to a control group in asthma, diabetes care, or compared to ACCESS without control mechanisms (CCNC Website)
(10) When compared to patients in usual care (Engelhardt 2006)
(11) When compared to a control group, GEM patients were less likely to use ED (Englehardt 2006; Boult et al. 1994, 2001)
(12) When compared to patients in usual care (Englehardt 2006)
(13) When compared to models not using a social worker (Reece 2004)
(14) When compared to models not using a social worker (Reece 2004)
(15) When compared to models not using a social worker (Reece 2004)
(16) Medicare costs were less for those receiving Hospice for beneficiaries with 1 of 16 diagnoses (Ascribe 2004)

design, the robust use of information technology to measure outcomes, and its potential as a model of the future to address the care needs of older adults through a PCMH model.

Compared to traditional Medicaid in New Mexico, ALTCS beneficiaries were found to use significantly less institutional care and more, but not significantly, ambulatory care. When compared to New Mexico, ALTCS beneficiaries had more home visits (case management and evaluation); however, the number of hospital days per thousand, per year was 22% lower (McCall 1997). Over a five year period (1989–1993) a comparison of traditional Medicaid in New Mexico to Arizona Long Term Care System (ALTCS) found ALTCS total costs, including medical, long-term support services, and administrative costs, to be 16% less. If only medical costs were considered, an 18% savings was achieved, totaling almost $290 million. The savings increased over time (McCall 1997). Community-dwelling Minnesota Senior Health Options Plan (MSHO) patients had significantly fewer preventable hospitalizations and ED visits when compared to patients in two control groups (Kane 2004). MSHO enrollees living in a nursing home had significantly fewer ED room visits, hospital admissions, shorter lengths of stay when hospitalized, and fewer preventable hospitalizations than control group enrollees (Kane 2004).

For people who had physical disabilities, The Wisconsin Partnership Program demonstrated a statistically significant decrease in hospital admissions when compared to a similar population. Lower rates of preventable emergency services were also achieved (CMS 2007). For specific diseases/conditions, the rate of hospital admissions for diabetes, congestive heart failure (CHF), bacterial pneumonia, and chronic obstructive pulmonary disease diminished compared to the year prior to enrollment. The length of stay during an admission for these conditions decreased 18.6% for diabetes and 71.6% for CHF (Landkamer 2005).

PACE achieved lower rates of hospital use, nursing home admissions, ED visits, and mortality rates and better quality of life than the control groups (MacAdam 2008). Ambulatory service rates were higher than the control group (MacAdam 2008). In a study by Abt Associates, PACE was found to show lower total overall costs - with lower Medicare and higher Medicaid costs than compared to the control group (White *et al.* 2000).

With regard to qualitative measures, Ohio's PASSPORT program successfully targeted the population in need of their services, based on specific eligibility criteria, such as financial need and functional limitations. Further, it was found that case management function was a linchpin of the program's success, and that the assessment process adequately covers consumer needs and contributes to an appropriate service plan. Overall, an independent evaluation of the program found that PASSPORT "is a cost-neutral, effectively targeted, quality-oriented, thoroughly monitored, consumer-responsive care program" (Ciferri 2007).

On the cost savings front, the home and community-based care options proved less expensive than nursing home care. In 2006, the average Medicaid cost per person for nursing home care was $55,751 (including health care expenditures, medication and long-term supportive services); the average cost for a PASSPORT client was $23,703 (including traditional Medicaid health care expenditures, medication and PASSPORT long-term supportive services). Even when considering all public sources of funding (SSI, food stamps, housing, HEAP), the costs of caring for a PASSPORT recipient were less than for a similar beneficiary living in a nursing home (Ciferri 2007).

The stated goals of the Wisconsin Family Care Program (WFC) are to provide "Choice, Access, Quality and Cost-Effectiveness." Qualitatively, members demonstrated a high level of satisfaction (92% of the survey respondents) with the care management and overall quality of services provided. WFC was also successful in supporting the desire of members to gain access to their residential choice (almost always home and community), with 82.4% of Family Care Members residing in their preferred living arrangement (Wisconsin Department of Health and Family Services [WDHFS] 2009).

In an independent assessment, researchers found that the overall Medicaid costs were lower for Family Care beneficiaries in the four non-Milwaukee county managed care organizations and within each of the target groups. Costs were also lower than in a comparison group when looking at frail elders in Milwaukee County. Researchers determined that the savings were related to two factors: controlling service costs and indirectly, favorably affecting beneficiaries' health and abilities to function (thus needing fewer services). For all but one of the counties studied, the average monthly long-term care costs were significantly less than those in comparison groups. The only group where this was not the case was in the developmentally disabled population in Milwaukee County. Although home health costs (home health care, personal care, and supportive home care) increased over the study period, the increase was significantly slower in the Family Care beneficiaries group than in the control group, except in Milwaukee County. Inpatient hospital costs significantly decreased over the study period for the Family Care beneficiaries in all counties, even though the costs for this group averaged more than the control group at baseline (WDHFS 2007).

The Community Care of North Carolina (CCNC) currently has an evaluation underway of its Chronic Care Program, which is specifically targeted to older adults. This evaluation will incorporate outcomes that are related to global costs/utilization, outreach and enrollment, and case management, as well as outcomes related to specific chronic diseases. In the meantime an evaluation of CCNC's Asthma Disease Management Initiative has demonstrated cost effectiveness related to ED use and hospital admission rates, compared with children in a control group (CCNC 2003). Researchers estimated a $3.5 million dollar savings resulting from the asthma program and $2.1 million savings with the diabetes management program. In estimating the impact of the whole CCNC program, Mercer (2009) found when comparing what the access model would have cost in SFY04, without any concerted efforts to control costs, the program saved approximately $60 million in SFY03, $124 million in SFY04, and $231 million in SFY05 and SFY06.

The Vermont Blueprint Integrated Pilot, first implemented in 2008, has an evidence-based evaluation in progress, which will be based on variety of data sources, including electronic medical records for individual patient care, medical claims from insurers and Medicaid, and public health surveys, among other sources. Uses of the data will cover a broad range of outcomes focused on clinical results, resource utilization, health care expenditures, and overall quality improvement. From the program's inception, health information technologies have been incorporated into the planning both as a tool for quality improvement and as a means to measure outcomes. Thus far, the Vermont pilot programs have been well received by patients, physicians and staff, while the formal evaluation is being conducted. Vermont legislation mandates statewide expansion by July of 2011, and the estimated cost savings is $115 million per year in five years from implementation (Connecticut Health Policy Project 2010).

In one of the longest-running programs, VA Geriatric Evaluation and Management, GEM patients were less likely to use the ED as compared to those in a control group (Engelhardt *et al.* 2006; Boult *et al.* 1994, 2001). In a 24-month period, results showed that GEM patients incurred significantly lower costs (primarily attributable to fewer hospital days of care) than patients receiving routine care (Engelhardt *et al.* 2006).

Turning to Hospice, one study found that when a social worker was involved in hospice care, there were a lower number of hospitalizations per patient; lower home health aide costs, lower nursing costs, lower labor costs, and lower average pain management cost per patient (Reese & Raymer 2004). In another evaluation performed on the Advanced Illness Coordinated Care Program (AICC), a study commissioned by the National Hospice and Palliative Care Organization, found that patients with one of sixteen diagnoses receiving hospice services cost Medicare less than those with the same diagnosis not receiving hospice (Ascribe 2004).

Common elements of successful programs

Despite the varied degree of integration and system of origin, the care coordination approaches described in this paper have several common elements: targeted intervention, in-person assessment/meetings, comprehensive initial assessment, a team approach to care coordination, family involvement, and focus on community-based services (Table 4.3).

Targeted intervention

Most of the programs target a specific population or segment within it. Hospice is specifically designed for patients in the final stage of a terminal illness. GEM is offered to a

Table 4.3 Common Components of Models Analyzed

Component	Definition
Targeted Intervention	Targeting at-risk older adults according to specific focus of model (e.g., dual-eligible, veteran, disease focus, etc.).
Face-to-Face Contact	In-person meetings with client and caregiver, may be conducted in home to better assess environmental considerations.
Comprehensive Initial Assessment	Initial assessment follows specific guidelines and includes some combination of medical, social support, long-term care, and psychosocial needs.
Team Approach	Interdisciplinary approach provides backbone of care coordination by integrating care across treatments and settings.
Family Involvement	Recognition of caregiver support in person-centered approach to care.
Focus on Community-Based Services	Utilization of community-based services to avoid or delay institutional based care and support consumer desire to remain in home and community based setting.

select group of medically complex, frail veterans, although some programs around the country have broadened their scope in order to promote health and prevent disease. While Community Care of North Carolina serves almost the entire Medicaid population of North Carolina, the case management intervention is based on an assessment that assigns a status/level of intensity (Heavy, Medium, Light, Very Light, and Deferred). Vermont's BIP also serves a broad swath of the population, although the program is targeted toward individuals with chronic care needs and utilizes Wagner's Chronic Care Model as a building block. The Wisconsin Family Care Benefit requires that the participant have at least one chronic condition that is expected to last more than 90 days. The other models involve specific eligibility criteria, in particular requiring that an individual need a nursing home level of care in order to qualify for community-based services and care coordination that can prevent institutionalization.

Face-to-face contact and comprehensive assessment

All of these models utilize an assessment, either performed by a designated care coordinator or on the team level. The initial assessment is conducted in person. Most care coordination models also involve telephone contact, including periodic follow-up calls to monitor the care plan and ensure satisfaction, among other tasks. As noted above, the initial assessment is often conducted in the person's place of residence (own home or a residential care facility). Providing in-home assessment allows the care coordinator to directly observe the person's environment, identifying and possibly alleviating barriers the individual may have in receiving services. The PACE assessment is conducted at the adult day center (the epicenter of the model), Community Care of North Carolina assessments are done at the medical home, and GEM's assessments are conducted in outpatient clinics.

Team approach and family involvement

Every program uses an interdisciplinary team approach to coordinating care and/or creating a care plan with the person. A team approach to assessment and care planning recognizes the specialized knowledge and assessment skills provided by different disciplines and encourages multidisciplinary solutions. The Arizona Long Term Care System and the Minnesota Senior Health Options employ a small team (case manager and primary care physician), with the case manager serving as a liaison to the physician. Other programs also use one member of the team as the primary coordinator of services – in GEM, primarily a social worker, in Hospice, a nurse. This central source of coordination decreases the likelihood of miscommunication, gaps in service, and other forms of fragmentation. By contrast, PACE and the Wisconsin Partnership Plan use the entire interdisciplinary team to fulfill the care coordination function.

Direct involvement of the primary care physician, although it was not a universal practice, has positive impacts on rate and length of hospitalizations, cost, and nursing home admissions based upon outcome data from Community Care of North Carolina, PACE, the Wisconsin Partnership Program, GEM, and Hospice. In each instance, the primary care physician does not serve as the care coordinator; instead, this role was most often filled by a nurse or social worker. At least two models involve the family (where appropriate) as a member of the team in the decision making, assessment and coordination of care (Minnesota Senior Health Options and PACE). Some programs also provide supportive services for family caregivers, including support groups and training (PACE, Hospice, and GEM).

Focus on home and community-based services to avoid institutionalization

Focus on home and community-based services that help delay or avoid institutionalization is a key design element in all of the programs. The Arizona Long Term Care System provides incentives for providers to prevent premature institutionalization. Similarly, both the Wisconsin Partnership Program and the Wisconsin Family Care Program stress the importance of early education, early assessment, and early and correct service provision to prevent hospitalization, delay institutionalization, and avoid unnecessary services. PASSPORT is designed specifically for frail homebound seniors with the goal of keeping the senior living independently in the community, rather than place the individual in a nursing home. GEM targets individuals with higher rates of service use such as ED visits, in order to decrease these over time. Hospice strives to keep the person as stable as possible in the home and often uses as a desirable outcome measure, death at home rather than in the hospital.

Care coordinator characteristics

As summarized in Table 4.3, the integrated care coordination programs use registered nurses and/or social workers as care coordinators, working as part of an interdisciplinary

Table 4.4   Care Coordination Team

Program	Care Coordinator
Arizona Long Term Care System	RNs, SWs, or individuals with 2 years of case management experience with older adults and disabled
Minnesota Senior Health Options	Primarily RNs
Wisconsin Partnership Program	APN as head of team with RN and SW or independent living coordinator
PACE	Interdisciplinary team
PASSPORT	RN or SWs
Wisconsin Family Care Program	RN with 1 year experience working with the population served or approved by the Department of Health
Community Care North Carolina	RNs, SWs, or other clinicians
Vermont Blueprint Integrate Pilot	Varies by pilot (care integration coordinator, RN lead manager)
GEM	Interdisciplinary team comprised of APN, geriatrician, and social worker
Hospice	RN is primary coordinator; team approach espoused

Notes: APN = advanced practice nurse; RN = registered nurse; SW = social worker team. In a few cases, the whole team is responsible for performing care coordination. Most programs require bachelor's level (or higher) education as a minimum requirement for care coordinators. The care coordinators are employed by a variety of different entities, ranging from the Veteran's Administration for GEM to community agencies that are part of the networks in Community Care of North Carolina to the Office of Vermont Health Access in the Vermont Blueprint Integrated Pilot.

Other programs of interest

In order to establish an evidence base for care coordination models that integrate the health and long-term care needs of older adults, we have made deliberate choices to include programs that offer representative examples of integrated care and have undergone evaluations that describe key indicators with respect to hospital utilization, use of institutional care and cost outcomes. These are certainly not the only measures that can be used to evaluate the success of a given program, although they do provide significant information about positive results and are closely allied with policy concerns about preventable hospital admissions, rebalancing of long-term care to home and community-based alternatives, and the potentially huge increase in the cost of care brought on by an aging population.

In selecting ten programs that meet the criteria previously outlined, it is important to note that there are a number of other programs that seek to integrate health and long-term care, and are doing so with positive results; in some cases these programs are using different evaluation techniques that are particularly relevant to the health and long-term care issues of older adults. As one example, Missouri has made significant strides towards integrating medical care with community-based social support for older adults through its Aging in Place Program (AIP) which has improved on a state-funded HCBS program called Missouri Care Options, a program designed to provide an alternative to institutionalization. The AIP model uses a nurse care coordinator who performs a comprehensive assessment and creates a care plan for the participant that coordinates the interventions of physician, nurse, and other health providers with the Missouri Care Options services of personal care and homemaking. The most current evaluation of AIP utilizes a quasi experimental design to compare outcomes between older adults who reside in nursing homes with those who received services in the AIP program. The clinical outcomes measured were activities of daily living, cognitive function, depression, incontinence and pressure ulcers. By integrating home care with medical services, the AIP program generated positive results for this set of clinical outcomes, which are of particular relevance to the health of frail and vulnerable older adults (Marek *et al*. 2005).

Another model of integrated care that has generated interest among health and aging professionals is the Senior Health and Clinic (SHC) model, which is used to establish primary care clinics with a geriatric focus on serving older adults with multiple chronic conditions and social support needs. The first Senior Health and Wellness Clinic, a geriatric outpatient clinic in Eugene, Oregon, has been in continuous operation since 2000. Many elements of the SHC model are based in the principles and design of the Chronic Care Model (CCM), which stipulates a true interdisciplinary care approach. The interdisciplinary team is typically composed of a geriatrician, nurse practitioner, social worker, nurse, and dietitian. Ad hoc members may include a chaplain, physical therapist, and home health nurse. Senior Health and Wellness Center patients had lower average Medicare charges, as a result of same or reduced utilization of outpatient, hospital, and ED use (John A. Hartford Foundation 2007). The SHC model has also led to improvements in health-related quality of life (HQRL) outcomes (Stock *et al.* 2008). A hindrance to the expansion of the model, although it is designed for export to any state or region, has been its reliance on Medicare payments – it has no waiver authority or state-supported alternative reimbursement structure – which means that a split billing method has to be employed in order to support the delivery of coordinated, integrated care (Silow-Carroll *et al.* 2006).

Conclusions and policy implication

The historic passage of H.R.3590 – the Patient Protection and Affordable Care Act – is good news for those who believe that care coordination is an essential part of improving the flawed delivery of health and long-term care services to older adults. This act contains provisions that specifically target the development and implementation of models of care that have care coordination principles built in to their design. The continuing dissemination of these models is supported by a number of measures. The establishment of the Centers for Medicare and Medicaid Innovation Center (CMI) has a directive to test innovative payment and service delivery models that improve or maintain quality while controlling costs. Preference will be given to models that promote care coordination by transitioning health care providers away from fee-for-service based reimbursement; models that utilize geriatric assessment and comprehensive care plans to coordinate the care (including through interdisciplinary teams) for individuals with multiple chronic conditions; and models that establish community-based health teams to support small-practice medical homes by assisting the primary care practitioner in chronic care management. The bill also provides for the establishment of a CMS Coordinated Health Care Office that will specifically target dual-eligibles. Some of the goals of this office will be to more effectively integrate benefits under the Medicare and Medicaid programs, improve the quality of health care and long-term services, and support state efforts to align medical and long-term care services for dual-eligibles.

A focus on care coordination has over 30 years of history to build on, with care coordination strategies as a centerpiece of programs serving Medicaid beneficiaries, beneficiaries dually eligible for Medicare and Medicaid, selected veterans in programs administered by the Veterans Administration, and other targeted populations of older adults. As described in this chapter, these types of programs have been essential to the development of models that bridge the medical care and long-term social support service domains and are supported by the evidence for their efficacy. At the same time, many of the problems that have prevented system reform are still entrenched and will require constant vigilance and effort to overcome. One problem is the ongoing medical bias of care coordination, as is often the case with the patient-centered medical home, or the relative weakness of socially oriented models in achieving a meaningful integration of medical care. As mentioned in the introduction, the silos of care that separate medical, long-term care and social supports continue to present roadblocks to change. Dissemination of programs to reach meaningful numbers of the older adult population is also an ongoing problem, and will require fundamental changes to reimbursement mechanisms in order to support models of care that do not fit in to the traditional fee for service system that rewards acute, episodic care. The programs that are the most effective in achieving a full integration of care also tend to be the most time consuming and complex to implement – so more streamlined, flexible ways of achieving full integration will need to be explored.

The findings of this study regarding the components of care coordination that lead to positive outcomes are an important lesson of our analysis: the fundamental role of targeting; the importance of face-to-face contact between the care coordinator and the recipient of care as well as between the care coordinator and the primary care physician; and the central role of assessment and a comprehensive care plan in guiding care. This analysis also highlights the importance of community-based services in the broad array of cost-related outcomes achieved by these diverse programs. Overall, the programs evaluated here showed reductions to hospitalization, ED visits, nursing home admissions, and the total cost of care. These more wide-ranging outcomes were possible because ongoing linkages to social service and other community-based resources help to improve or stabilize the medical conditions of many patients. Care coordination models that address the social support dimensions and link them to medical care are generally designed so that broad-based interdisciplinary teams have the capability to address both the treatment of chronic disease and associated functional limitations that define long-term care needs.

Evidence in support of care coordination and integrated care will have to continue to be developed in order to persuade policy makers and health and social service professionals that integrated models of coordinated care in fact achieve the desired combination of improvements to quality and either cost neutrality or cost savings. It will be important for newer models of care to incorporate a well-thought out evaluation plan from the beginning of their development, and for evaluation experts to agree upon the most relevant and important outcomes. If integrated models of care are able to consistently produce positive results across different settings and populations, this will greatly facilitate the broad dissemination of models of care that effectively target the needs of older adults.

References

American Association of Retired Persons Public Policy Institute. (2008) *Valuing the Invaluable, The Economic Value of Family Caregiving, 2008 Update.* Available at: http://assets.aarp.org/rgcenter/il/i13_caregiving.pdf.

Agency for Healthcare Research and Quality. (2009) *Innovations Exchange.* Agency for Healthcare Research and Quality, Rockville, MD. Available at: http://www.innovations.ahrq.gov/evidencerating.aspx.

APS Healthcare Inc. (2005) *Family Care Options for Long-Term Care: Family Care Independent Assessment: An Evaluation of Access, Quality and Cost Effectiveness for CY 2003–2004.* Available at: http://dhs.wisconsin.gov/ltcare/ResearchReports/IA.pdf.

Ascribe Newswire. (2004) *Hospice Costs Medicare Less and Patients Often Live Longer, Research Shows.* Ascribe Newswire: Medicine, 9/22/2004, p 2–4. Available at: http://search.ebscohost.com/login.aspx?direct=true&db=heh&AN=14533297&site=ehost-live.

Berenson, R., & Howell, J. (2009) *Structuring, Financing and Paying for Effective Chronic Care Coordination*. A Report Commissioned by the National Coalition on Care Coordination (N3C). Available at: http://www.urban.org/UploadedPDF/1001316_chronic_care.pdf.

Boult, C., Boult, L., Murphy, C., *et al.* (1994) A controlled trial of outpatient geriatric evaluation and management. *Journal of the American Geriatrics Society*, 42, 465–470.

Boult, C., Boult, L., Morishita, L., *et al.* (2001) Randomized clinical trial of outpatient geriatric evaluation and management. *Journal of the American Geriatrics Society*, 49, 351–359.

Brown, R. (2009) *The Promise of Care Coordination: Models That Decrease Hospitalizations and Improve Outcomes for Medicare Beneficiaries with Chronic Illness*. Available at: http://www.socialworkleadership.org/nsw/Brown_Full_Report.pdf.

Centers for Medicare and Medicaid Services. (2007) *Long-Term Care Capitation Modes: A Description of Available Program Authorities and Several Program Examples*. Available at: http://www.cms.hhs.gov/IntegratedCareInt/Downloads/LTC_Capitation.pdf.

Centers for Disease Control and Prevention. (2003) Public health and aging: trends in aging—United States and worldwide. *Morbidity and Mortality Weekly Report*, 52, 101–106.

Ciferri, W., Kunkel, S., McGrew, K., *et al.* (2007) *Program Evaluation of PASSPORT: Ohio's Home and Community Based Medicaid Waiver.* Available at: http://sc.lib.muohio.edu/handle/2374.MIA/62.

Connecticut Health Policy Project (2010) *Development of a Vermont Pilot Community Health System to Achieve the Triple Aims*. Available at: http://www.cthealthpolicy.org/webinars/20100223_jhester_webinar.pdf.

CCNC: Community Care of North Carolina. Community Care of North Carolina, Raleigh, NC. Available at: http://www.communitycarenc.com.

Community Care of North Carolina. (2003) *Progress Report: Asthma Initiative*. Community Care of North Carolina, Raleigh, NC. Available at: http://www.communitycarenc.com.

Engelhardt, J.B., McClive Reed, K.P., Toseland, R.W., *et al.* (2006) Effects of a program for coordinated care of advanced illness on patients, surrogates, and healthcare costs: a randomized trial. *The American Journal of Managed Care*, 12, 93–100.

The John A. Hartford Foundation. (2007) *Geriatric Interdisciplinary Teams in Practice: Senior Health and Wellness Clinic Model.* Available at: http://www.jhartfound.org/ar2007html/pdf/Hart07_SENIOR_HEALTH_AND_WELLNESS_CLINIC_MODEL.pdf

Kane, R., Homyak, P., Bershadsky, B., *et al.* (2004) Patterns of utilization for the Minnesota Senior Health Options Program. *Journal of the Geriatrics Society* 52, 2039–2044.

Landkamer, S., & Landsness, R. (2005) *Integrated Health and Long-Term Care Services: The Wisconsin Partnership Program*. Available at: http://ici.umn.edu/products/impact/181/.

MacAdam, M. (2008) *Frameworks of Integrated Care for the Elderly: A Systematic Review*. CPRN Research Report. Available at: http://www.cprn.org/documents/49813_EN.pdf.

Malone, J., Morishita, L., Paone, D., *et al.* (2004) *Minnesota Senior Health Options (MSHO) Care Coordination Study*. Minnesota Department of Human Services, Minneapolis, MN. Available at: http://www.dhs.state.mn.us/main/groups/healthcare/documents/pub/dhs_id_028242.pdf.

Marek, K.D., Popejoy, L., Petroski, G., *et al.* (2005) Clinical outcomes of aging in place. *Nursing Research*, 54, 202–211.

McCall, N. (1997) Lessons from Arizona's Medicaid managed care program. *Health Affairs*, 16 (4), 194–199.

Mercer. (2009) *CCNC/ACCESS Cost-Savings – State Fiscal Year 2007 Analysis*. Mercer Government Human Services Consulting, Atlanta, GA. Available at: http://www.communitycarenc.com.

Mollica, R., & Gillespie, J. (2003) *Care Coordination for People with Chronic Conditions*. National Academy for State Health Policy, Portland, ME.

Reese, D. & Raymer, M. (2004) Relationships between social work involvement and hospice outcomes: results of the National Hospice Social Work Survey. *Social Work*, 49, 415–422.

Silow-Carroll, S., Alteras, T., & Stepnick, L. (2006) *Patient-Centered Care for Underserved Populations: Definition and Best Practices*. Economic and Social Research Institute, Washington, DC.

Steiner, B.D., Denham, A.C., Ashkin, E., *et al.* (2008) Community Care of North Carolina: improving care through community health networks. *Annals of Family Medicine*, 361–367.

Stock, R., Mahoney, E. R., Reece, D., *et al.* (2008) Developing a senior healthcare practice using the chronic care model: effect on physical function and health-related quality of life. *Journal of the American Geriatrics Society*, 56, 1342–1348.

White, A., Abel, Y., & Kidder, D. (2000) *Evaluation of the Program of All-Inclusive Care for the Elderly Demonstration: Comparison of the PACE Capitation Rates to Projected Costs in the First Year of Enrollment*. Abt Associates, Cambridge, MA (HCFA Contract No. 500-01-0027).

Wilhide, S. & Henderson, T. (2006) *Community Care of North Carolina: A Provider-Led Strategy for Delivering Cost-Effective Primary Care to Medicaid Beneficiaries (Executive Summary)*. American Academy of Family Physicians. Available at: http://www.aafp.org/online/etc/medialib/aafp_org/ documents/policy/state/medicaid/ncexecsumm.Par.0001.File.tmp/ncexecsummary.pdf.

Wisconsin Department of Health and Family Services. (2007) *Wisconsin Partnership Program Census Graphs*. Available at: http://dhfs.wisconsin.gov/WIpartnership/census.htm.

Wisconsin Department of Health and Family Services, Division of Long Term Care. (2009) *Long-Term Care in Motion: 2008 Annual Report of Wisconsin's Managed Long-Term Care Programs*. Available at: http://dhs.wisconsin.gov/ltcare/ResearchReports/PDF/2008annualreport.pdf.

Chapter 5

Intervention components

Cheryl Schraeder, Cherie P. Brunker, Ida Hess,
Beth A. Hale, Carrie Berger, and Valerie Waldschmidt

Introduction

Care coordination seeks to bridge the gap between the needs of people with complex chronic health management issues and the health system's fragmented mix of multiple sectors and providers. Comprehensive care coordination is a patient/family system approach that puts the patient and family at the center of the care coordination team. The focus of the patient/family centered care coordination team is to decrease fragmentation of care with the ultimate goal of decreasing the need for and the cost of health care. This is accomplished by assisting patients and families in self-managing their chronic disease(s) and related psychosocial problems (Bodenheimer & Berry-Millett 2009).

The goals of care coordination include improving patients' functional health status and outcomes, improving self-management abilities and healthy lifestyle practices, enhancing the coordination and continuity of care, eliminating the duplication of services, and reducing the need for expensive medical services. Employing registered nurses (RNs) as the care coordinators on the care coordination team helps to accomplish these goals. The team includes the patient/family unit, the patient's primary care provider, the nurse care coordinator, and ancillary or support persons involved in the day-to-day care management of the patient. Together, the team works to identify and address the patient's full range of needs, monitor and improve the person's health status and self-management abilities, and decreases the need for and the fragmentation of health care.

The Chronic Care Model

The Chronic Care Model (CCM) has been used as a guide for effective chronic care management (Bodenheimer *et al.* 2002a; Bodenheimer *et al.* 2002b; Wagner *et al.* 1999). The premise of the CCM is that individuals with chronic illnesses typically face long-term disease management challenges such as fluctuating illness patterns and multiple treatment regimens. While the etiology of each chronic illness is different, the clinical and self-management strategies for each have many similarities (Wagner 2002; Corbin & Strauss 1991).

Comprehensive Care Coordination for Chronically Ill Adults, First Edition. Edited by Cheryl Schraeder and Paul Shelton.
© 2011 John Wiley & Sons, Inc. Published 2011 by John Wiley & Sons, Inc.

There are six components of the CCM: (1) the health care organization; (2) community resources and policies; (3) self-management support; (4) decision support; (5) delivery system design; and (6) clinical information systems. The first two components emphasize an organization's commitment to new ways of chronic care delivery and community integration. The other components provide the foundation for effective chronic illness management.

The model emphasizes that optimal chronic care management should be organized, coordinated, and delivered by care management teams. It embraces a population-based approach to care with the care team accepting accountability for affecting change in patient outcomes (Wagner 2000; Wagner *et al.* 1999). CCM team members include patients and families, primary care providers, RN care coordinators, and additional clinicians as needed. This approach requires team members to have the ability to collaborate, share patient care responsibilities, emphasize preventive care, and participate in focused efforts to improve care. Patients assume active roles in identifying their needs and goals of care, and they actively participate in planning care. The primary care providers use evidence-based guidelines to guide their medical care. Similarly, RN care coordinators follow clinical nursing guidelines and protocols to guide coordination of patient care and provide proactive case and disease management (Wagner 2000).

Care coordination teams

Care coordination teams that have effective, meaningful communication among team members, strong leadership, and respect for the contributions and diversity of other team members allow for the development of comprehensive assessments, complex, evidence-based care plans, and quality research designs (Boult *et al.* 1999; Keogh *et al.* 2002; Shortell *et al.* 2004). Research documents the effectiveness of care coordination teams in heart failure, diabetes, care of frail elders, chronic pain, and integrated mental health services (Ahmed 2002; Dorr *et al.* 2007; Peleg *et al.* 2008; Dickenson *et al.* 2010; Reiss-Brennan *et al.* 2010). Team research illustrates that other health professionals and office staff can manage certain aspects of chronic illness care as well as physicians. Hence, care coordination teams can help with workload distribution issues for patients with certain health care needs (Vickery *et al.* 2006; Callahan *et al.* 2006). Care coordination teams have also been shown to reduce the cost of care, emergency department (ED) visits, and disease-related complications (Boult *et al.* 2009; Dorr *et al.* 2005; Counsell *et al.* 2009).

The effective care coordination team has, at its center, the patient/family. This focus supports the Institute of Medicine's (IOM) vision for the future, which stressed the need for patients to become active partners in their own care (IOM 2008). Each team member is accountable for his or her contributions to care and shares responsibility for intervention and follow-up. Team members collaborate to identify patient problem areas, identify barriers to care, create plans of care, make appropriate decisions, solve problems, and set goals. Effective team relationships develop over time and require ongoing communication and interaction.

The success of the coordinated care team is dependent upon each team member's mutual respect and understanding of each member's roles. Over time, team members develop trust in each other's skills and acknowledge each other's areas of expertise and contributions to the management of the patient's care coordination. Additional factors that strongly influence the ability of the team to work together include long-term working relationships of team members; familiarity with each other and understanding gained through experience of practice patterns; role security of team members and confidence in individual skill-sets; and administrative leadership and support of the team concept.

Team member roles

Each member of the care coordination team plays a unique and vital role. The primary care physician (PCP) provides skilled geriatric care and serves as the primary entry point for access to medical services. Integral to the team's ongoing, open dialogue, the patient/family is encouraged to express their opinions, concerns and goals of care to the team. The RN care coordinators support the team by facilitating effective and appropriate contributions from each team member, including their own contributions.

Serving as the keystone to the care coordination team, the care coordinators accomplish many activities. They assess the risks and needs of each patient/family and develop a comprehensive care plan based on guidelines and standards of care and the individualized feedback from the PCP. They ensure patients are knowledgeable and up-to-date on current, recommended health-promotion activities. Care coordinators teach and/or coach the patient/family regarding disease processes, medications, self-management activities, and how to anticipate and plan for future needs. They work to empower and support patients to take ownership of their health conditions and management options. The individual roles of each team member are displayed in Table 5.1.

Team development

Interdisciplinary team development requires dedicated, coordinated work. How a team operates relates to its institutional location and structure. These can range from primary care, clinic-based comprehensive interdisciplinary teams to two-person teams, or to virtual teams made up of a network of health care providers located at a variety of institutions (Dorr *et al.* 2006; The John A. Hartford Foundation, 2007a; Weiss *et al.* 2010).

No matter the structure or the location, an essential team strategy must uphold respectful, concise inter-professional and intra-professional communication. Effective communication must occur to ensure consistency between the goals of the patient/family, the care coordinator, the physician, and other team members. Consistent, respectful communication supports the development and implementation of effective care plans. Active participation by all team members in program and protocol development, patient care coordination, and ongoing program evaluation helps build cohesiveness and respect for each team member's expertise (Dorr *et al.* 2006; Dorr *et al.* 2007; Xyrichis & Ream 2007).

Table 5.1 Care Coordination Components and Roles of Team Members

Care Coordination Components	Primary Care Provider	Patient	Care Coordinator
Assessment	• Diagnose and evaluate patient and perform specified procedures. • Interpret test results with the patient/family. • Assist patients in synthesizing information regarding health status and recommendations for care.	• Provide accurate information to the care coordinator, primary care provider, and other health/community providers. • Alert the team to changes in their life situation or health status. • Prioritize health problems with team.	• Complete assessments and care plans in the home or office, depending on patient need. • Integrate objective and subjective data from medical records, face-to-face visits, primary care provider reports, office staff comments, family and patient reports, and health and community provider reports to build the initial assessment and care plan.
Guidelines/ Protocols	• Utilize evidence-based guidelines/protocols to guide practice.	• Follow guidelines/protocol recommendations from team.	• Utilize evidence-based guidelines/protocols to guide practice.
Care planning	• Develop medical plan of care interven-tions with input from the health care team.	• Identify goals and assist team in personalizing and prioritizing plan recommendations.	• Develop plan of care with patient, family, and team.
Implementation	• Reinforce recommendations from guidelines/protocols. • Reinforce recommendations for care coordinator/service provider.	• Responsible for follow-through on agreed upon action in order to manage plan of care.	• Support patient/family in implementing plan of care by assisting with identification of barriers to implementation and problem solving.
Teaching/ Coaching	• Provide basis for prescribed treatments and recommendations/introductory teaching.	• Responsible for personal health and make appropriate lifestyle changes. • Complete self-management activities and adhere to recommended care protocols.	• Teach/coach patient/family about disease processes, medications and evidence-based self-management strategies. • Reinforce positive steps when implementing self-management strategies.

Referral	• Refer as appropriate to health providers.	• Utilize correct level of service with assistance from team.	• Refer to appropriate disease specific organizations, self-help groups, and other community services.
Coordinating	• Coordinate care (primary through tertiary) in a variety of settings.	• Alert team to use of health/community services, any recommendations, or issues encountered.	• Coordinate health and community services.
Monitoring and Evaluation	• Evaluate health status and follow through on plan of care.	• Alert team to difficulties following the plan of care and change in health status or new needs/problems.	• Proactively monitor patients on a regular basis. • Evaluate and document patient progress. • Reassess patients at each contact, (comprehensively every 12 months), following hospital and emergency department admits, and revise the plan of care. • Adjust plan of care based on change in status, information from team members and patient preferences.
Communication	• Communicate effectively with team members using multiple formats.	• Communicate effectively with team members.	• Maintain a patient panel over time. • Serve as a conduit for continual communication among care team members using multiple formats.
Advocacy	• Advocate for the value of the care coordinator's contribution to the team. • Advocate for patient services.	• Express viewpoint concerning needs, problems, and services.	• Advocate for the patient/family needs and services.

Care management teams can improve the quality of care for patients with complex, chronic health needs. Their success, however, is determined not only by their ability to function effectively on an interpersonal level, but also on the ability to target appropriate clients for the care management process.

Targeting the appropriate population

Central to the success of any model of care coordination is the ability to identify patients who need, and potentially might benefit from, more comprehensive care. Although the general consensus is that targeting higher-risk patients is important, no commonly agreed upon criteria exists for identifying these potential patients. As a result, some care management models target patients with specific diseases, some rely on physician and other provider referral, and others rely on a combination of clinical, demographic, psychosocial, and utilization data to select high-risk patients.

Instruments used to identify high-risk patients include the Pra (probability of repeated admission) and PraPlus. These screening instruments identify older individuals at risk of future health service use over a two- to four-year time period (Pacala *et al*. 1995; Pacala *et al*. 1997; Boult *et al*. 1998; Boult *et al*. 2001). They have been used with a variety of populations over 15 years by researchers and health care organizations to prospectively identify individuals at risk for substantial health care utilization and higher costs. Another example is the Vulnerable Elders Survey (VES-13), which assesses an individual's functional disability (Saliba *et al*. 2000; Saliba *et al*. 2001). The VES-13 is a simple, function-based screening tool for identifying community-dwelling older adults at risk for health deterioration. The instrument can be administered in person or over the phone by non-clinicians in a variety of settings. The VES-13 has been shown to be an accurate predictor of functional decline and mortality in older, ambulatory care patients over a five year period (Min *et al*. 2009). Higher VES-13 scores of elderly individuals have been associated with increased utilization of ED visits and inpatient and outpatient hospital services (McGee *et al*. 2008). Research suggests that the VES-13 can be useful in identifying community-dwelling older adults who need assessment and coordinated care interventions, as well as a pre-screening tool for identifying elderly cancer patients for comprehensive geriatric assessment (Kellen *et al*. 2010), but additional prospective studies are needed to assess its overall clinical utility.

Another example of a screening instrument that has been widely used is the Charlson Comorbidity Index (CCI; Charlson *et al*. 1987), originally designed as a severity of illness measure. The CCI was originally constructed to predict longitudinal mortality risks for hospitalized patients based upon weighted scores assigned to 22 co-morbid conditions. The original index was calculated via medical record review, but was subsequently adapted so that International Classification of Diseases, Ninth Revision (ICD-9) codes could be used to calculate the score (Deyo *et al*. 1992). Additionally, a self-report CCI score has been developed (Chaudhry *et al*. 2005). Recently, an adapted version of the CCI was used with community-dwelling, primary care patients to predict total annual health care expenditures (Charlson *et al*. 2008). Using this approach, the researchers identified advanced age (Medicare and/or Medicare eligible), multiple co-morbidities (based on a

CCI score of 3 or higher), and previous hospitalizations as significant predictors of higher resource utilization and higher annual costs.

Researchers have also used a sequential approach to identify patients at risk for high health care use. A two-step sequence that selectively administers laboratory tests based on findings from a short self-report questionnaire has been successful in identifying elderly candidates for care coordination (Reuben *et al.* 2003). The difficulty with this type of approach is that it is predicated on the ability to obtain readily available and up-to-date laboratory values from the surveyed patient population.

An example of a computerized, predictive modeling system is hierarchical condition categories (HCC; Pope 2004), which produces diagnosis-based clinical measures based on disease burden and places individuals into risk categories. An example of HCC is the Adjusted Clinical Groups Predictive Model (ACG-PM), which is part of the John Hopkins ACG Case Mix System (Weiner *et al.* 2003). The ACG-PM software uses administrative data to compute the probability that individuals will rank in the highest 5% of the population for medical expenses during the following 12 months. The ACG-PM has been used in several studies to identify potential patients for coordinated care interventions (Sylvia *et al.* 2008; Leff *et al.* 2009). Two other examples of diagnosis-based computerized systems are the Adjusted Clinical Groups (ACGs) and Diagnostic Cost Groups (DCGs; Rosen *et al.* 2005).

Patient surveys, provider referrals, and predictive modeling can be effective, but may be both expensive to initiate and based on inaccurate subjective and clinical data. Regardless of the risk-based targeting method or strategy used, care coordination programs are more likely to have success if they target patients who are at very high risk of hospitalization(s) in the coming year and have multiple chronic illnesses, including congestive heart failure (CHF), coronary artery disease (CAD; acute myocardial infarction and ischemic heart disease) and chronic obstructive pulmonary disease (COPD) (Miller & Wiessert 2000; Peikes *et al.* 2009; Sylvia *et al.* 2006). Additional characteristics that should be considered include fair or poor self-rated health (Idler & Benyamini 1997), impaired functional ability (one or more ADL or IADL limitations; Sylvia *et al.* 2006), cognitive difficulties (dementia and depression), and other mental health needs.

Brown (2009) examined successful care coordination interventions and concluded that programs have a higher likelihood of success if they identify patients at substantial risk of being hospitalized in the coming 12 months, but not necessarily in the highest cost categories. Peikes and colleagues (2010) identified two target groups of elderly adults who appear to be likely candidates for care coordination programs. The first group is comprised of individuals who have been hospitalized one or more times in the past year and have been diagnosed with CHF, CAD and/or COPD. These target patients are potentially attractive for care coordination programs because they represent 18% of the current Medicare fee-for-service population, and they account for approximately 37% of expenditures in the 12 months after identification and 32% over the three years after identification. The second group consists of patients who have been hospitalized at least twice in the previous 24 months and have any of the following chronic illnesses: Alzehimer's disease/dementia, arthritis, atrial fibrillation, cancer, chronic kidney disease, CHF, COPD, depression, acute myocardial infarction/ischemic heart disease, diabetes, osteoporosis, and stroke/transient ischemic attack. The researchers suggest that these eligibility criteria have clinical validity and individuals can be readily identified using a variety of methods, including provider claims, patient self-report, and physician referrals.

Care coordination process

This section describes the essential care coordination processes synthesized from research reviews of methods, documents, and tools with programs that have demonstrated reduced hospital admissions and Medicare expenditures. The interventions were identified by Boult and colleagues (2009), Brown (2009), and Bodenheimer and Berry-Millett (2009). Successful interventions included components of transitional care (Naylor *et al.* 2004; Coleman *et al.* 2006), as well as comprehensive care management programs, including Care Management Plus (Dorr *et al.* 2007; Dorr *et al.* 2008), Geriatric Resources for Assessment and Care of Elders (GRACE; Counsell *et al.* 2007; Counsell *et al.* 2009), Guided Care (Boyd *et al.* 2007, Boult *et al.* 2008; Sylvia *et al.* 2008; Boyd *et al.* 2009; Leff *et al.* 2009), and four sites that were part of the Centers for Medicare & Medicaid Services Medicare Coordinated Care Demonstration (Brown 2009; Peikes *et al.* 2009; Peikes *et al.* 2010). (See Table 5.2 for a synopsis of the processes for each of the seven programs). The care coordination process includes targeting the appropriate patient population (described above), a comprehensive assessment, care planning, guideline development, teaching/coaching patient and family self-management skills, transitional care, provider coordination, proactive monitoring and evaluation, along with ongoing guidance and support. Patients are encouraged to assume an active role in the management of their chronic health conditions. It has been shown that collaborative partnerships can increase the efficiency and effectiveness of health care services, enhance accessibility of care, maintain or improve quality of care, decrease costs, and improve patient and provider satisfaction (Bodenheimer *et al.* 2002a, 2002b).

Comprehensive assessment

Comprehensive assessment is essential to understanding the health care needs of medically complex patients. A comprehensive assessment is completed by the care coordinator for each patient and applicable caregiver. The assessment begins in an initial face-to-face meeting (in-home, primary care provider's office, or medical clinic). If possible, the assessment is completed in the patient's home. The assessment may be completed during multiple visits with the patient and caregiver, if necessary. In care management, the assessment is both interdisciplinary and multidimensional, and addresses functional abilities in physical, social, and psychological domains. Comprehensive geriatric assessments are usually done at initial enrollment into a care coordination program, after hospitalizations for acute illness, when a change in living status is being considered (for example, nursing home placement), after any abrupt change in physical, social, or psychological functioning, when a second opinion is needed on a suggested intervention or treatment protocol, and at predetermined intervals for the person with complex health needs (Tabloski 2006; Schraeder *et al.* 2008).

Table 5.2 Care Coordination Components Evidence

Care Coordination Program	Guided Care (1)	Grace (2)	Care Management Plus (3)	MCCD: Hospice of the Valley (4)	MCCD: Health Quality Partners (4)	MCCD: Mercy Medical Center (4)	MCCD: Washington U (4)
Care Coordination 1. TARGET POPULATION	Over age 65 with high risk of using health services, as estimated by claims-based hierarchal condition category predictive model (HCC Score 1.2 or higher)	Over age 65, established patient of a site primary care clinician, income less than 200% federal poverty	Over age 65 with chronic care needs or younger with high risk of disability, referred by participating physician and enrolled in Medicare Part B one year prior to enrollment	Advanced CHF, COPD, cancer, neurological conditions and at least one hospital admission in the year prior to enrollment	Chronic heart and lung conditions, diabetes, and uncontrolled hyperlipidemia or hypertension; this criteria is for all patients served in MCCD. The criteria for our high-risk group include FFS Medicare beneficiaries; over age 65; a diagnosis of CAD, or an inpatient hospitalization in the prior year and a diagnosis of COPD, HF, or diabetes.	CHF, chornic lung disease, liver disease, stroke, other vascular diseases, or renal failure and hospital admission or emergency room visit in the year prior to enrollment	At least one chronic medical condition and at high risk of incurring substantial medical costs within the next year (prior to 2006 based on proprietary screening algorithm)

(Continued)

Table 5.2 (Continued)

96

Care Coordination Program	Guided Care (1)	Grace (2)	Care Management Plus (3)	MCCD: Hospice of the Valley (4)	MCCD: Health Quality Partners (4)	MCCD: Mercy Medical Center (4)	MCCD: Washington U (4)
2. EXCLUSION CRITERIA	Low HCC score	Residence in nursing home, living with participant in trial, receiving dialysis, severe hearing loss, English language barrier, no access to telephone, severe cognitive impairment without an available caregiver to consent	Live in nursing home	Under age 65, have end-stage renal disease, or receive Medicare hospice benefits	Learning difficulties due to psychosis or dementia, under age 65, organ transplant candidates, cancer, or long-term nursing home residents, ALS, ESRD, Hospice	Long-term nursing home residents, receiving Medicare hospice benefit, or end-stage renal disease	Receiving hospice services, organ transplant candidates
3. CARE COORDINATOR (CC) PRIMARILY LOCATED							
– Office in community (not in clinic, hospital, or home health agency)					x		x
– Primary Care Provider Office/Geriatric Service	x	x	x			x	
– Hospital							
– Home Health				x			

4. CC RELATIONSHIP WITH PRIMARY CARE PROVIDER (PCP)						
— Collaborative; informal and formal communication with primary care provider, team care planning	x	x			x	
— Consultative/parallel; consult with patients experiencing change			x	x		x
5. PERCENT OF CC CASELOAD THAT IS SHARED WITH PCP						
— Active Collaboration	x 100%	x 80%	x 40%	x 63%	x 80%	x 20%
— Update Communication as needed	x 100%	x 20%	x 25% x 50%	x 63%	x 50% x 30%	x 10% x 10%
— No/Limited Contact			x 25%	x 37%	x 20%	x 80%
6. AVERAGE FREQUENCY OF CC CONTACTS WITH A PATIENT PCP						
— Weekly	x Some patients weekly, if emerging issues are present x 100%	x 15%, 100% of new referrals during the first few months x 70%	x If patient presents with active issues	x Some patients weekly, if emerging issues	x Some patients with emerging issues	
— Monthly			x (for physicians contacted)		x 100%	
— Quarterly		x 15%		x Or less		
— Annually	x Or more as needed; average 3 visits per patient (range, 0–14) in first year.					

(Continued)

Table 5.2 (Continued)

Care Coordination Program	Guided Care (1)	Grace (2)	Care Management Plus (3)	MCCD: Hospice of the Valley (4)	MCCD: Health Quality Partners (4)	MCCD: Mercy Medical Center (4)	MCCD: Washington U (4)
— No schedule					x Average 2.5 per patient over their care coordination participation; for patient cases requiring collaborative contacts, averge was 3.9 over 53.8 months		x No regular schedule
7. SOCIAL WORK SERVICE FOR PERCENT OF PATIENTS	x 0–50% of total patients; varies with availability in the community	x 100% of total patients	x 5% of total patients (from home health or hospital)	x 30% of total patients	x 0% of total patients; uses community-based social services	x 25% of total patients	x 75% of total patients
8. PATIENT CONTACT LOCATIONS							
— Home	x	x	x	x	x	x	x
— Hospital	x	x	x	x	x	x	x
— Office (PCP, CC)	x	x	x		x	x	x
— Telephone	x	x	x	x	x	x	x

98

	Col 1	Col 2	Col 3	Col 4	Col 5	Col 6	Col 7
9. AVERAGE PATIENT CONTACTS	Once per month	1.5 per month (Average 18 contacts per year in first year; range, 1–65; 40% face-to-face, 60% telephone)	Once per month	Once per 30–45 days	1.6 per member month or 19.4 per member year.	Once per month	Once per month
10. FREQUENCY OF FACE-TO-FACE MEETINGS	Once every 3 months	Approximately once every 2 months	Once per month	Once per 30–45 days	.85 per member month or 10.3 per member year	Once per month	Twice per year
11. CASELOAD	50–60 patients per CC	100–125 patients per CC per SW	150 patients per CC	45 patients per CC	High-risk: 75–85 patients per CC; mix of high-, moderate-, and low-risk caseload: 110 patients per CC	80 patients per CC	85–95 patients per CC
12. CARE COORDINATION INTERVENTION							
12a. Assessment							
– Standardized	x	x	x	x	x	x	x
– Comprehensive	x	x	x 70%	x	x	x	x
– Brief/targeted	x As needed	x As needed	x As needed	x As needed	x As needed	x As needed	x As needed
12b. Initial Assessment Location							
– Home	x	x	x 90%	x 100%	x	x	x 2.5%
– Office			x 10%		x		x 2.5%
– Telephone							x 95%
12c. Reassessment							
– 6-Month			x 30%	x 100%			x
– Annual	x	x	x 20%		x	x	x
– As Needed	x	x	x 50%	x	x	x	x

(Continued)

99

Table 5.2 *(Continued)*

Care Coordination Program	Guided Care (1)	Grace (2)	Care Management Plus (3)	MCCD: Hospice of the Valley (4)	MCCD: Health Quality Partners (4)	MCCD: Mercy Medical Center (4)	MCCD: Washington U (4)
13. EVIDENCE-BASED CLINICAL GUIDELINES/PROTOCOLS							
— Chronic conditions with self-management strategies (e.g., CHF, Diabetes, COPD)	x		x	x	x	x	x
— Geriatric problems w/self-management strategies (e.g., falls, incontinence)	x	x	x	x	x	x	x
14. CARE PLANNING							
— Establish Mutual Goals	x	x	x	x	x	x	x
— Establish Action Plan	x	x	x	x	x	x	x
15. PATIENT MONITORING/EVALUATION							
— Weekly	x	x	x 15%	x As needed	x As needed	x As needed	x 50%
— Monthly			x 65%	x 90%	x	x	x 50%
— Bi-Monthly			x 5%				
— Quarterly			x 10%				
16. PATIENT EDUCATION/ COACHING/ SELF-MANAGEMENT							
16a. CC Trained/Use							
— Behavioral Change Theory		x			x	x	x
— Readiness to Change		x		x	x	x	x
— Motivational Interviewing	x	x			x	x	x

Item						
16b. CC Evaluates						
– Adherence to agreed to strategies	×	×	×	×	×	×
– Facilitators	×	×	×	×	×	×
– Barriers	×	×	×	×	×	×
16c. Self-Management With:						
– Individual/Family Practice	×	×	×	×	×	×
– Group of Patients (Conducted by CC)		× (Depending on care manager)	×	×	×	
– Community Group	x Referred to local Chronic Disease Self-Management Program	x Referred to local disease management programs and community groups as needed	x Referred to community groups	x Referred to community groups	x Referred to community groups	
17. MEDICATION MANAGEMENT						
17a. Updating Med List						
– Review w/patient each contact	×	×	×	×	×	×
– From Electronic clinic/hospital record	×	×	×	×	×	×
– From discharge summaries	×	×	×	×	×	×
17b. Identify Med Problems by Using/Having:						
– Evidence-based guidelines	x If available	×	×	×	×	×
– Pharmacy review	×	×	×	×	×	×
– Physician review	×	×	×	×	×	×
– Medication software	×	×	×	×	×	×

(Continued)

Table 5.2 (*Continued*)

Care Coordination Program	Guided Care (1)	Grace (2)	Care Management Plus (3)	MCCD: Hospice of the Valley (4)	MCCD: Health Quality Partners (4)	MCCD: Mercy Medical Center (4)	MCCD: Washington U (4)
17c. Approach to managing medications							
– Develop self-management strategies w/patient/family (for understanding, purpose, obtaining, taking, monitoring side effects, reporting to providers)	x	x	x	x	x	x	x
17d. Evaluate implementation strategies at each contact	x		x	x	x	x	x
17e. Resolving Med Affordability							
– Discuss less costly alternative	x	x	x	x	x		x
– Refer to pharmacy assistance program	x	x	x	x	x	x	x
17f. Reconciliation Post-Discharge							
– Compares discharge list w/program/patient list	x	x	x	x	x	x	x
– Consult with PCP	x	x	x	x	x	x	x
– Coach patient on discussing w/providers and taking med list to visits	x	x	x	x	x	x	x
17g. Resolving Med Problems Across Physicians							
– Telephones/e-mails PCPs and other relevant physicians	x	x	x	x	x	x	x
17h. Routinely Provides Updated Med List To:							
– Primary care Providers	x	x	x	x	x	x	x
– Other Health/Community Providers	x	x	x	x	x	x	x

18. TRANSITIONAL CARE

Item							
18a. Notification of ER/Hospital Admit		x	x	x	x	x System in place- it had some faults	x
— Report from Hospital (paper)	x Some	x	x (Recommended if possible)	x	x	x Office manager report	x
— Electronic alert to CM info system	x Some	x		x	x	x	x
— Patient/family notification	x	x	x (recommended to patients)	x	x	x	x
18b. Percent Hospitalizations Known About	x 90%	x 90%	x 60%	x 25%	x 75% estimated	x 80%	x 95%
18c. Visits Patient in Hospital	x	x As needed	x 5%	x	x As needed	x As needed	x
18d. Provides information to Hospital Staff	x	x	x 60% (available in EMR)	x	x	x	x
18e. Assists with Discharge Planning	x Available when questions arise	x	x 30%–100%, depending on hospital connection	x	x As needed with complex issues		x
18f. Requests Discharge Instructions from:							
— Hospital	x	x	x (available in EMR)	x	x	x EMR available	x
— Patient/family	x	x	x	x	x	x Usual	x
18g. Contacts Patient Shortly After Discharge				x depending on severity of hospitalization			
— Telephone	x	x	x	x	x	x	x
— Home Visit	x	x		x	x	x	x

(Continued)

Table 5.2 (*Continued*)

Care Coordination Program	Guided Care (1)	Grace (2)	Care Management Plus (3)	MCCD: Hospice of the Valley (4)	MCCD: Health Quality Partners (4)	MCCD: Mercy Medical Center (4)	MCCD: Washington U (4)
18h. Transition Protocol	x	x		x Contact patient within 48 hours; visit dependent upon hospitalization reason	x		x
18i. Monitors Use of Protocol	x	x		x	x		x
18j. Reviews Hospital/ED Admits							
– CC Team Meeting		x			x	x	x on individual basis
– Review with PCP	x	x	x If questions	x if questions			
19. COORINDATES COMMUNICATION							
19a. Primary Care Provider – CC Communication							
– Attends visits with patient (percent of caseload)	x 50%	x as needed (<10%)	x 20%	x 75%	x 19.1%	x 80%	x 4%
– Update on problems and change plan (e.g., meds, symptoms; percent of caseload)	x 100%	x 100%	x 80%	x 80%	x 62.5%	x 100%	x 5%

	1	2	3	4	5	6	7
19b. Mode of contact (percent of time with each mode)							
— E-mail/Faxed Report	x 50%	x 50% (EMR)	x 80%	x	x 11.3%	x 5%-CC not in practice and in practice	x 1%
— Telephone	x 25%	x 25%	x 10%	x	x 81.3%	x 70% – CC not in practice 20% – CC in practice	x 98%
— Meeting	x 25%	x 25%	x 10%	x	x 7.4%	x 25% – CC not in practice 75% – CC in practice	x 1%
20. COMMUNITY PROVIDER-CC COMMUNICATION							
20a. Update on problem(s), status (percent of caseload)	x 100%	x 100%	x 5%	x	x 37.5%	x 50%	x 1%
20b. Update on change in plan (percent of caseload)	x 100%	x 100%	x 10%	x		x 80%	x 5%
20c. Mode of contact (percent of time with each mode)							
— E-mail/Faxed Report	x 50%	x 20%	x 85%	x	x 2.2%	x 20%	x 1%
— Telephone	x 40%	x 70%	x 10%	x	x 93.8%	x 80%	x 98%
— Meeting	x 10%	x 10%	x 5%	x	x 4%		x 1%
21. CC TRAINING							
— Standardized	x	x	x	x	x	x	x
— Comprehensive	x	x	x	x	x	x	x

(Continued)

105

Table 5.2 (Continued)

Care Coordination Program	Guided Care (1)	Grace (2)	Care Management Plus (3)	MCCD: Hospice of the Valley (4)	MCCD: Health Quality Partners (4)	MCCD: Mercy Medical Center (4)	MCCD: Washington U (4)
22. CM INFORMATION SYSTEM	x	x	x (Integrated Care Coordination Information System: quality metrics, caseload monitoring, tickler system, assessments, clinical summary, decision support)	x	x (Access database and statistical proces reporting software to monitor cohort, patient caseloads and nurses performance)	x	x
23. PROGRAM TRACKS/REPORTS TO CC							
– Utilization	x	x	x	x	x	x	x
– Clinical indicator	x	x	x		x		x
– CM Performance	x	x	x	x	x	x	x

[1]Boult, C., Reider, L., Frey, K., *et al.* (2008). Early effects of "guided care" on the quality of health care for multimorbid older persons: A cluster-randomized controlled trial. *Journal of Gerontology: Medical Sciences*, 63A: 321–327.
[2]Counsell, S.R., Callahan, C.M., Clark, D.O., *et al.* (2007). Geriatric care management for low-income seniors: A randomized controlled trial. *Journal of the American Medical Association*, 298: 2623–2633.
[3]Dorr, D.A., Wilcox, A.B., Brunker, C.P., *et al.* (2008). The effect of technology-supported, multidisease care management on the mortality and hospitalization of seniors. *Journal of the American Geriatrics Society*, 56: 2195–2202.
[4]Brown, R. (2009). The pomise of care coordination: Models that decrease hospitalizations and improve outcomes for Medicare beneficiaries with chronic illness. A report commissioned by the National Coalition on Care Coordination. Available at: http://www.socialworkleadership.org/nsw/Brown_Executive_Summary.pdf.

Comprehensive assessments are beneficial to both patients and clinicians. For patients and families, they allow goals, needs, and concerns to be made explicit. Assessments highlight risk factors that may need to be addressed so proactive strategies can be developed to anticipate change and reduce caregiver stress. For the clinician, comprehensive assessments can improve diagnostic accuracy by monitoring the patient's status, identifying problems early and collaborating with interdisciplinary team members to develop appropriate interventions (Tabloski 2006; Cress 2007; Schraeder *et al*. 2008).

Care coordinators assess their clients through the systematic collection of both subjective and objective data. This data includes analysis and application of information provided from discipline-specific assessments (for example, nutritionists). The data can include physiological, psychological, sociological, cultural, developmental, and spiritual information (Weber 2008) as well as demographics, financial, environmental, functional, caregiver services, and utilization data.

There are two methods commonly used by care coordinators to assess behavioral attitudes toward lifestyle change: readiness to change and motivational interviewing. Readiness to change is identified through a transtheoretical assessment of the five stages a patient moves through as they seek change in their lives (Prochaska & Velicer 1997). Precontemplation is the stage in which patients are not ready to make any changes and may deny that they need to change. Contemplation is the stage in which the patient becomes aware the behavior exists and is weighing its consequences. Preparation to change occurs when the patient may have changed their behavior for a short time but reverted, and is not sure they want to change. When the patient is actively working toward a change, they are in the Action stage. Maintenance is the stage in which the change has occurred and the patient is focused on not relapsing. Relapsing is the stage in which the patient returns to previous behaviors.

Motivational interviewing is an effective strategy used by some care coordinators to both improve communication and stimulate behavior change (Anstiss 2009). The use of motivational change techniques help patients consider the possibility of change, analyze the risks and benefits of change, and prepare them to move forward if they decide to change (Rollnick 2008). In applying the motivational interviewing technique, the patient is asked to identify the most significant concern related to their health and examine their readiness to make changes to improve their health status. The care coordinator focuses on the patient's vision, values, and goals.

The information collected documents the patients' perspectives on the most difficult aspect of managing their illnesses; the reason they came to see the team; their biggest fears; what they already know or have been told about their conditions; and their goals for care. This information helps the care coordinator determine both the focus of care and the priority of patient issues. The care coordinator can provide education and address misinformation that may be increasing the patient's anxiety. Experienced care coordinators find that effective use of motivational interviewing allows them to not only empower patients with self-management strategies, but also build a relationship of trust and communication (Larsen 2009).

Assessing patients and families

Comprehensive caregiver/family assessments are very challenging and require practitioners to develop effective relationships with both patients and caregivers. These relationships allow the team to monitor changes in health status, work within existing funding constraints, and help the family coordinate care from a mix of providers through periods of acuity, maintenance, rehabilitation, and transition.

When working with caregivers, family-focused care management strategies include attention to their cultural background, health literacy, and social support. Research on caregiver assessment supports the need to focus on three specific areas: the caregiving context, the service setting, and the program (Cress 2009). A caregiver assessment gives the care coordinator an opportunity to evaluate the caregiver's needs. It also gives the caregiver a voice and helps acknowledge and affirm the important role they play in the patient's health. Through a trusting caregiver-care coordinator relationship, problems can be identified early and interventions made to protect both the patient and the family member (Cress 2009).

Another benefit of a caregiver assessment is the ability to determine eligibility for support services (e.g., Medicaid). Finally, family caregiver assessment can highlight environmental problems that may interfere with care, such as an unsafe home that presents a major fall risk for the patient (Family Caregiver Alliance 2006). Both the patient and caregiver assessments, combined with a number of other measures, become part of the information necessary to evaluate the effectiveness of a care coordination program.

Guideline development/implementation

Evidence-based guidelines and protocols are incorporated into care coordination programs. Nationally approved guidelines and protocols are accessible from many sources. Care coordination sub-committees review and evaluate guidelines and protocols and establish guidelines for the care coordination team. The care coordination guidelines and protocols address recommendations for medical, nursing, and self-management. Once guidelines and protocols are developed they are reviewed and updated regularly to include the latest advances and recommendations in health care, health promotion, and self-management. The care coordination team is monitored for implementation of guidelines/protocols and the patients are monitored for adherence to agreed upon strategies and recommendations.

Care planning

The care coordinator uses the assessment data to formulate a plan of care that is developed and provided in accordance with evidenced-based practices (EBP). EBP uses the best available evidence in combination with clinical expertise in order to establish guidelines and protocols. Patient preferences are considered to achieve the best possible outcomes. If evidence is unavailable, the care provided should reflect a consensus from expert panels.

The care coordinator helps the patient identify their care preferences, including advance directives. The care coordinator is also in a position to identify undiagnosed co-existing conditions, such as mental health concerns, and refer the patient for additional care interventions. The individualized care plan reflects the patients' and professionals' goals for care, and respects the individual needs and cultural backgrounds of patients. Patient-focused plans also explicitly address and reflect the health literacy levels of the patient and caregivers.

To keep the plan patient-focused, care coordinators use educational strategies that promote self-management and autonomy. For example, in diabetes care, patients identify diet-related changes that they are ready to address, life style changes they will make, and change-related timelines they feel are realistic. The care plans also address educational goals related to wellness, health promotion, and prevention of complications.

Care coordinators use flexible strategies that can accommodate the changing needs of patients and their caregivers. Acceptance and ongoing support for the patient and family, even when decisions may not be what the care coordinator feels are optimal, result in the development of trust and respect. This sets the foundation for long-term, supportive relationships. An ongoing role of the care coordinator is that of patient advocate—not only within the interdisciplinary team, but also in the larger health care system and community agency environments.

Care coordinators are responsible for the actual written plan of care. The plan of care is extremely important because it communicates the plan to everyone involved in the patient's care and promotes continuity and consistency across health care settings while enhancing efficiency and effectiveness of care. Precise and careful planning and the use of evidence based guidelines enable the provision of individualized, efficient, and high-quality care.

The written plan of care identifies potential and actual problem areas, the expected or desired outcomes of care, and the strategies or interventions needed to meet those outcomes. The plan of care is based upon the comprehensive assessment and focuses on techniques that will increase the patient's knowledge base of his/her chronic conditions, enhance self-management strategies, and coordinate services across health care settings while identifying and addressing barriers to care and gaps in care.

Care coordinators individualize the plan of care based on the patient's history, signs and symptoms, preferences, and current therapies. Interventions should enhance the patient's health status, knowledge and self-management skills, teach and monitor medication management and encourage health promotion activities. The care plan intervention should also indicate how to respond to worsening symptoms in order to improve patient outcomes, reduce ED visits and the need for tertiary care. The interventions in the plan of care should facilitate coordination of care across the health care continuum and ensure proactive monitoring and follow up. The interventions are to be specific, realistic, individualized, patient/family centered, cost effective, and focused on patient education, self-management and coordination of care. The roles of individual team members in care planning are outlined in Table 5.3.

Care plan implementation and monitoring

The implementation phase of the process is based on information gathered during the comprehensive assessment and interventions and strategies outlined in the care plan. Proactive monitoring activities are integrated into the plan of care. Using proactive monitoring, the

Table 5.3 Individual Team Member Roles

	Primary Care Provider	Patient	Care Coordinator
Care Plan Interventions	– Diagnoses conditions/problems. – Prescribes medications and procedures as needed. – Recommends review schedule.	– Identifies actions he/she wants to take toward meeting health goals. – Identifies current self-management practices. – Prioritizes health concerns. – Identifies support system to help meet health needs.	– Reviews patient's history. – Determines patient's current status, care regime, and service utilization. – Reviews patient's current level of self-management skills and knowledge base. – Reviews primary care provider recommendations. – Provides education to the patient/family as needed on health conditions and self-management activities. – Coordinates and communicates with all referral sources as necessary and relays pertinent information to the primary care provider. – Coordinates with community service providers.
Health Promotion	– Devises strategies focused on health promotion for their patient panel. – Uses practice guidelines/protocols for immunizations and diagnostic screening procedures for the elderly. – Reviews immunization/health promotion record with the patient annually and as needed. – Counsels patients to adhere to health promotion protocols as pertinent to their condition(s) and preferences.	– Provides accurate information on immunization and health screening history. – Delineates preferences and wishes about aggressiveness of diagnostic screening and immunization plans. – Helps identify realistic expectations for self-management strategies.	– Highlights areas of unmet needs with health promotion behaviors. – Facilitates efficient communication of immunization and health promotion information among team members. – Provides information to patients on community health promotion activities. – Reinforces positive patient efforts toward health promotion. – Devises strategies focused on health promotion for their patient panel. – Uses practice guidelines/protocols for immunizations and diagnostic screening procedures for the elderly.

Patient Education and Self-Management	– Identifies the patient's goals of care. – Provides support for self-management strategies. – Identifies areas where the patient is not meeting or having trouble meeting goals of care. – Follow-up with the patient to ensure their knowledge base has increased and their level of self-management skills has improved.	– Identifies current knowledge level and potential gaps. – Identifies current self-management strategies. – Participates in the development of action plans to enhance and improve self-management strategies.	– Assesses the patient's/family's level of education, learning styles, and readiness for change as needed. – Assesses the patient's current self-management strategies, – Identifies areas where patient/family education and additional self-management strategies are needed. – Ensures patient/family education in areas identified. – Develops with the patient additional self-management activities using patient driven action plans. – Follow-up with the patient/family to ensure their knowledge base has increased and their level of self-management skills has improved.
Referral to Health Providers and Community Services	– Serves as the point of access to other health care providers and may identify the need for community services. – Refers to specialists. – Evaluates the effectiveness of referrals and the ongoing appropriateness of services. – Identifies available community resources and advocates for development of new services when appropriate. – Encourages the patient to coordinate services independently, when appropriate. – Advocates to assure the patient receives the necessary and appropriate services.	– Participates actively in decision-making for understanding the need/purpose for referrals. – Provides feedback to other team members regarding referred care. – Helps team determine the appropriate mix, intensity, and duration of services. – Provides non-professional resources independently when financially able to do so (e.g., transportation).	– Facilitates referrals to community and community providers. – Evaluates care provided and gives feedback to team members. – Ensures follow-up on referrals and communicates to patients/family. – Facilitates information exchange among other providers. – Identifies available community resources and advocates for development of new services when appropriate. – Encourages the patient/family to coordinate services independently, when appropriate. – Advocates to assure the patient receives the necessary and appropriate services.

patient is contacted at predetermined intervals for further assessment, teaching and monitoring of self-management skills, and coordination of care. Patients are encouraged to contact their care coordinator between scheduled contacts if they have questions or need guidance in addressing changes in their condition. Patients and their caregivers/family are asked to report any change in their status or condition, such as a hospitalization or ED visit or if they change their home location. In addition, care conferences may occur with primary care providers and other health care and community providers involved in the patient's care.

The care coordinator initiates contact with other health providers and community agencies involved in the patient's care, or a referral can be made to obtain needed assistance for the patient. If a service is already in place, the care coordinator and representative of the agency review the current status of the service and make changes as needed. For a new referral, a plan is outlined to initiate service. Included in the plan are specific tasks and activities that need to be completed, including the specific duties, time frames, and predetermined dates for further contacts to evaluate the effectiveness and coordination of services. Activities and agency contact names and telephone numbers are added to the patient's plan of care. Future monitoring by the care coordinator assesses the effectiveness of the referral in meeting the patient's needs. The care coordinator has regular contacts with the home care or community agency to make any needed changes in the plan of care.

A monitoring schedule is established for each patient and their caregiver based on the number and type of chronic illnesses and problems, health promotion activities, recommendations from the evidence-based guidelines/protocols, provider feedback, formal and informal support available, type of medications, self-management activities, health utilization history, and patient/family preference. Monitoring contacts occur via telephone, or face-to-face in the patient's home, clinical office, hospital, or other agreed-upon meeting sites. The frequency of these face-to-face contacts is based on the patient's current health status, support system, and plan of care.

During each encounter, the patient should update the care coordinator on current health issues and changes in health status or medications, and results of their self-management activities, such as daily weights, blood sugar monitoring, diet, and exercise/activity level. Teaching/coaching by the care coordinator is included to increase the patient's ability to self-manage and problem solve. Not only does the patient need to know how to monitor their condition, they need to know how to evaluate indicators of change and develop an action plan with which to address the changes.

Monitoring activities are incorporated into the patient's care plan and previously agreed to by the care coordinator, patient/family, and primary care provider. Specific information to be monitored is reflective of the care plan content and addresses any newly identified patient needs. The overall status of the care plan is evaluated during the patient/family monitoring process. Consistent, proactive monitoring allows the care coordinator to obtain information that might signal significant decline in health status. This consistent monitoring enables early intervention by the team, possibly preventing a downward spiral in patient health or functional status. At the completion of the monitoring call or visit, the next monitoring date is set and agreed upon.

Inclusion of primary caregivers and family members in care planning is critical to successful self-management. The unpredictability of complex chronic conditions puts caregivers under tremendous stress. This unpredictability presents major challenges in terms of arranging care, managing symptoms, following care guidelines, preventing and managing crisis, dealing with financial strains and insurance companies, coping with daily changes and intrusions from providers, normalizing relationships, coping with career and job strain, and managing role changes within the home.

Self-management strategies

The importance of patient/family self-management cannot be overstressed (Bodenheimer *et al.* 2002b; Coleman *et al.* 2004; Lorig *et al.* 1999; Lorig *et al.* 2001). Care coordinators will work with patients/families to assess their current level of self-management strategies, assess readiness for change, and teach needed strategies/activities. Interventions will be directed toward empowering them to take ownership of their health care. Patients will be taught problem solving so they can take the data from their self-management activities and act on that information to improve or maintain their current level of health functioning.

In development of a self-management plan, the care coordinator identifies the patient's current level of health literacy, learning style, readiness to change, and performance of self-management activities. Assessment of the patient's knowledge and performance of self-management activities starts during the initial comprehensive assessment. Patients are coached to perform self-management activities and instructed in techniques to increase their problem solving ability so they can act on the results. Patients/families are encouraged to participant in community-based educational and support groups. Educational materials, based on evidence-based guidelines, are provided to the patient/family.

Lifestyle modification is included to improve control of current conditions and decrease the risk of developing other chronic illnesses. Examples include diet to control blood sugar or prevent fluid retention, smoking cessation, and increasing exercise/activity levels. Referrals will be made, if necessary, to assist patients in reaching these goals, such as to a smoking cessation program or pulmonary rehabilitation to learn exercise techniques to improve breathing function.

Instruction is provided to patients/families in health promotion and health maintenance activities. Patients/families are given information on the most recent recommendations regarding what types of health promotion and maintenance activities they should engage in, including those that prevent or detect disease (immunizations, mammograms) and monitor for complications of current disease processes (eye examinations).

End-of-life teaching is an important part of patient/family education. Some disease processes can be slowed but will progress in even the most well controlled person. Patients are encouraged to identify their power of attorney for health care prior to having the need for one. Patients are encouraged to complete a living will so their wishes will be known and the appointed power of attorney will have the essential knowledge to carry out the patient's wishes.

Care coordinators facilitate coordination and education with the goal of no longer needing to intervene in the patient's care. Patients/families are assisted to understand the types of self-management activities they need to do, when to do them, what to do with the information obtained from these activities, and to know what constitutes an emergency. Care coordinators assist patients and families in outlining the signs and symptoms they can manage at home, which ones need a call and/or visit to the primary care provider and which ones constitute a visit to the emergency department.

Care coordinators use a variety of strategies for enhancing self-management skills of the patient/family. Assessment of the patient/family knowledge-base is ongoing. As care coordinators develop a working therapeutic relationship with patients and families, they will be able to identify barriers that may not have otherwise been found.

The patient's ability to change and adopt new health care behaviors/strategies may be influenced by his/her relationship with the care coordinator. In many care coordination models, the care coordinator develops close, and at times, long-term relationships with patients and caregivers. Face-to-face time between the patient and the care coordinator has been shown to be critical in the patient's perception of care; the more face-to-face time, the more satisfied the patient (Dorr *et al.* 2005; Wenger & Young 2007).

Transitional care

The period following discharge from an inpatient setting is a difficult time for patients. They frequently experience a change in medication and self-management needs. According to Kripalani and colleagues (2007), about 19% to 23% of those discharged experience an adverse reaction, typically related to medications. In a study completed by Coleman and colleagues (2004) patients receiving transitional care were only half as likely to return to the hospital setting. In this study, patients had transitional coaches that assisted with medication management, record keeping, identifying emergent or worsening symptoms, and communication with health care providers. The transitional coaches were Master's prepared geriatric nurse practitioners who initiated home visits to the patient during the first 24 to 72 hours after discharge.

The results of a randomized study with high-risk hospitalized older adults conducted by Naylor and colleagues (1999) revealed that transitional care from advance practice nurses reduced expenditures and readmission rates. Care was initiated in the hospital with discharge planning and was continued in the patient's home after discharge. Patients were initially visited in the hospital within the first 48 hours after admission. After discharge, two home visits were conducted. The first was conducted within the first 48 hours after discharge and the second was within the first seven to ten days. The nurses were available seven days a week by telephone and initiated phone calls to the patients at least weekly.

Transitional care is designed to assist patients in smooth transitions from one location or level of care to another. It is defined as a set of activities that ensure coordination and continuity of care (Coleman *et al.* 2005). After discharge from an inpatient setting, older adults with multiple co-morbid conditions are frequently challenged with managing a new medication regime and a new set of self-management activities. It is imperative that they develop these new skills to ensure management of conditions and prevention of rehospitalization. Nurse care coordinators, especially nurse practitioners, are knowledgeable in medications and medication management and can assist with medication reconciliation at admission to an inpatient setting, transition from one setting to another and discharge to home. They are also knowledgeable in needed self-management strategies and can assist patients/families in assimilating these into their daily routines.

Care coordinators not only provide education on medication and self-management techniques, but they can also assist the patient/family in communication strategies to bridge care, identification of needed home care assistance, and identification and management of symptoms. Care coordinators collaborate with physicians and other health care providers to provide optimal home assistance and support to the patient/family. Patient and family are assisted and encouraged to identify their self-care needs and health status changes and communicate these to their primary or attending physician. It is important for patients to be aware of signs and symptoms that signal when their condition is worsening and what level of care they need to seek.

The care coordinators and the patient/family update the plan of care and develop a follow-up schedule that optimizes the patient's ability to self-manage at home. Follow-up post transition includes home visits, office visits and phone calls. The type and location of visit is planned into the plan of care. Initial follow-up includes at least weekly contacts and identification of where patients/families can obtain information and guidance if the care coordinator is not available. The duration of the more intensive and proactive follow up is dependent upon the patient and family and available support systems.

Identification and management of care-related barriers

Patients who use care coordination services tend to be those considered at-risk for both adverse health outcomes and, as a result, in need of expensive care. These individuals also tend to use multiple service providers who cut across numerous service sectors (Mollica *et al.* 2003). For frail elders, the complexity of care coordination needs can become overwhelming. This population tends to use three different provider organizations, with multiple provider visits in each institution (Haggerty *et al.* 2003). Research has also shown that typical Medicare enrollees saw an average of two primary care physicians and five specialists each year. Patients with several chronic conditions visit up to 16 physicians a year (Pham *et al.* 2007).

To safely navigate patients through the complex web of health care institutions and community resources, care coordinators must have excellent interpersonal, organizational, and problem solving skills. For the care coordinator, the goal is to link clients with critical community resources and other specialty providers and agencies in a manner that provides the required services at the most appropriate time.

Effective care coordinators develop strong formal and informal networks with providers and community resources. Usually the care coordinator implements a combination of advocacy strategies that may include: quick access to online resources, knowledge of local community agency resources, disease-specific support groups and educational resources, and federal, state, and county government programs (for example, Social Security Administration, Adult Protective Services, senior centers, and so on).

Care plan evaluation

Evaluation of the implemented plan of care is conducted on an ongoing basis. At each contact, the plan of care is evaluated and adjusted to reflect changes in the patient's status and ability for self-management. Identification of both successful and unsuccessful interventions is noted. Unsuccessful interventions are removed from the care plan and the care coordinator works with the patient/family and primary care provider to determine why the intervention was unsuccessful. New interventions, including those that address any barriers to implementation, are planned, implemented, and evaluated.

All patients are informed of and engage in health promotion activities. Successful plans of care reveal that patients are up-to-date in immunizations and screenings, and they are performing needed health maintenance activities to the best of their abilities.

Plans of care also include guideline/protocol recommendations for management of chronic illnesses. Successful evaluations reveal that patients/families are up-to-date on the guideline/protocol recommendations. The recommended laboratory and diagnostic testing schedules that monitor the condition (that is, Hemoglobin A1c, lipid panels, electrocardiograms), are completed and current, and the patient's medication regimes are those recommended by the guidelines/protocols. As appropriate, the patient's family/caregiver is involved in the plan of care and evaluation.

Care coordinator training

Care coordination requires additional education and training for care coordinators. Education and training programs usually cover a wide range of topics, including chronic disease management for the patient and their caregivers, evidence-based chronic illness guidelines and protocols, comprehensive assessment, action planning, coaching, educating, and empowering patients and their caregivers, monitoring and evaluation, self-management with an emphasis on symptom and medication management, transitional care, collaboration with primary care and community providers, patient and panel management, financing of care, quality and outcome reporting, and principles of adult learning and techniques to facilitate behavior change. For example, the care coordination program developed by Boult and colleagues at Johns Hopkins University (Boyd *et al.* 2007; Sylvia *et al.* 2008) uses RNs to enhance primary care delivery, focusing on disease management and chronic care. These RN care coordinators receive specific program education and training through a 25-module curriculum. The training program areas covered include chronic disease management, geriatric assessment and care planning, transitional care, electronic health records, patient education techniques and motivational interviewing, cultural care, community resources, communicating with physicians, insurance benefits, and ongoing monitoring and follow-up. After training the RNs spend three months in orientation, working with their respective physicians and office staff. Only after integration into the day-to-day routines of the practice environment do they start contacting patients, conducting assessments and planning care.

Although coordinated care interventions have different delivery structures, programs encompasses a variety of traditional and non-traditional techniques to effectively train care coordinators, especially when confronted with the hectic day-to-day "real world" of medicine. These techniques include lecture formats from experts (for example, physicians, advance practice nurses, pharmacists, exercise physiologists, nutritionists, occupational therapists, social workers, an so on), as well as web-based learning technologies, high definition video, simulated practice, pod casts and RSS feeds. In addition, training also usually includes a supervised orientation period before care coordinators begin working with patients directly on their own.

Information technology and quality reporting

Care coordination models use a variety of information technology (IT) tools, such as virtual networks, electronic medical records, patient-focused web sites to provide health promotion materials, disease coordination strategies, and personalized follow-up reminders (Wilcox *et al.* 2005; Dorr *et al.* 2006; The John A. Hartford Foundation 2007b). The use of electronic medical records is considered the basic technology requirement for access to all necessary information at the time patient decisions are made (Reuben 2007). IT tools help organize, prioritize, and track care coordination tasks. They also include decision support reminders for clinicians to provide best practice.

Integrated IT systems compliment the role of the care coordinator and can include such things as a tracking database, a patient summary sheet, and an electronic messaging system (Dorr *et al.* 2006; Vickery *et al.* 2006). These electronic clinical supports improve patient safety and support the development and implementation of quality evaluations. The use of clinical information systems is considered an important strategy in the effective coordination of care management activities. These systems can include real-time electronic clinical alerts, a patient tracking system, time and activity reporting systems, and provider and patient reports. Real-time alerts can be sent automatically via e-mail to the care coordinator to report patient ED visits, hospitalizations, discharges, outpatient procedures, and visits with other providers (Schraeder *et al.* 2005).

Care coordination evaluation

The future success of care coordination interventions will depend on their abilities to show value in terms of benefits to both health and cost. The intervention defined in this chapter is based on the belief that a systematic delivery of key components and services to chronically ill adults will result in improved health status, patient and provider satisfaction, and decreased health care utilization and cost. An evaluation should explain why the intervention fails or succeeds dependent in these key areas.

The design of a coordinated care intervention, including the focus and methods used, must reflect the shared perspectives of the major stakeholders - the funder or funding sources, the sponsoring health care organization, clinical team members, and patients. Identifying the sponsoring organization's primary goals for conducting the intervention is a critical element of the evaluation. Also, designing an evaluation strategy *a priori* is important in maximizing the potential applicability of the intervention as well as the ability to provide ongoing feedback to stakeholders, especially the care management team (Mollica *et al.* 2003) during the intervention.

Evaluation designs typically focus on three primary areas: intervention structure and implementation, quality related care processes, and health care utilization and cost measures. These areas are evaluated within designs that identify treatment compliance measures and behavioral adjustments that are considered accurate indicators of chronic disease out-comes. The approaches are usually standardized and titrated in terms of doses related to the amount of education, support, and monitoring of clinical markers and behavioral patterns related to specific groups of patients (Dorr *et al*. 2006).

We suggest that to properly evaluate the comprehensive care coordination intervention described in this chapter, emphasis must be placed on both a thorough process and impact analysis. The focus of process analysis is on implementation and fidelity assessment. Impact analysis concentrates on quantifying process and quality of care measures, service utilization and cost outcomes, as well as cost savings derived from the intervention. Process analysis examines a number of areas, including a description of the organizational sponsor and the local and regional geographical health care environment; project staffing, including team composition, care coordinator background and training, caseload sizes, pre-existing relationships with physicians, and so on; identification of and recruitment strategies with the target population, as well as the proportion of the target population that is served by the intervention; a description of the intervention components and how they are maintained/modified over time; care-manager patient and provider contact types; how intervention processes are maintained or increased over time; and how efficiencies are maintained to reduce costs and maximize net savings.

Fidelity assessment examines the extent to which the intervention was implemented as designed and intended, barriers encountered in implementation, and how these barriers are overcome. Researchers have indicated that implementation fidelity has a substantial impact on outcomes (Dane & Schneider 1998), yet it is one of the most prominent limi-tations of evidence-based intervention evaluation; there is a difficulty identifying which components are most significant and positively correlated with improved outcomes (Grol *et al*. 1998). Five dimensions have been recommended as important to consider when measuring treatment fidelity (Steckler *et al*. 2002): adherence (is the intervention being delivered as intended?); dose/exposure (how frequently and intensely are services pro-vided?); quality of delivery (how effective is the intervention?); participant responsiveness (are patients active recipients of the intervention?); and enactment (do patients exhibit healthy behaviors in the right situation at the right time?). In tomorrow's health care environment it will be imperative to incorporate fidelity measures into evaluation designs.

The nuts and bolts of most care coordination interventions have centered on process and quality of care and utilization measures. Examples of process of care measures include: adherence to specific medical and nursing clinical guidelines; intensity of alerts of patient deterioration (for example, notification of current hospitalization or ED visit); improve-ment in care transition activities; improvement in patient self-management skills; reduced medication management issues; increased use of preventive services (such as breast and cervical cancer screening, colon cancer screening, prostate cancer screening, vaccines [flu, pneumococcal, hepatitis B]); and increased use of disease specific services (such as fasting blood-glucose tests and eye exams for diabetes, blood tests for elevated lipids for diabetes and CAD). Examples of quality-of-care related outcomes include patient and physician global satisfaction with intervention services; increased patient satisfac-tion with specific services (for example, arranging payment for non-covered services or medications, helping make appointments with specialist physicians or therapy services); increased patient knowledge and adherence to therapeutic regimes; improved physical and mental health and health-related quality of life; and a decrease in all-cause mortality. For additional process and quality of care measures see the USPSTF (U.S. Preventive Services Task Force) guidelines for older adults and Assessing Care of Vulnerable Elders indicators (Wenger *et al.* 2007).

Examples of service utilization outcomes measure the probability of any utilization use (for example, hospital admissions and readmissions, potentially preventable hospital admissions, ED visits with and without hospitalization, skilled nursing facility (SNF) admissions, home health visits) and the amount of each health care service received, including the total days of care for hospital and SNF care. Costs of care include expenses for inpatient and outpatient care and total costs, usually reported in monthly or yearly increments, and projected net savings, with and without intervention costs.

While we have outlined a general approach to evaluating coordinated care interventions, translating quality research findings into practice requires visionary leadership. Even with such leadership, the delivery of care coordination faces many internal and external challenges to its success. Some of these challenges are discussed below.

Ongoing care management coordination challenges

Challenges to care management are not limited to the complexity of medical conditions or to the multifaceted interactions between patients, providers, and caregivers. Effective care management faces both internal and external challenges.

Internal challenges relate to providers who do not understand their patients' needs and do not make appropriate referrals to care management teams. This problem is thought to reflect the lack of education in professional programs that help students prepare for the level of interdisciplinary cooperation needed to care for patients with complex needs (Boult *et al.* 2009; Reuben 2009).

Providers may also believe that the use of evidence-based care takes more time than simply using the status quo. Some also report a belief that the use of guideline-specific care will not result in the desired outcomes (Tabloski 2006; Cress 2007; Reuben 2007).

In addition, many providers have limited knowledge of resources that could help their patients and families. These include community agencies, government programs, and disease-specific support groups that can help patients cope with their illness. Patient and caregiver issues also present challenges due to the complexity of issues they face and variations in their interest in, and ability to, adhere to treatment recommendations. The lack of family resources, either social or economic, can also produce significant challenges to effective care management (Reuben 2007).

Administrative issues can present significant internal challenges. Administrative support is critical and can only occur if administrators are convinced that research-based innovative models make good business sense. Innovations must be simple to understand and compatible with existing values. They must also give a sense of being more advantageous than current practices (Reuben 2009).

Aside from internal challenges, there are also significant external issues related to care management coordination (Bodenheimer 2008). One of these is the current status of the primary care system. Due to a lack of integrated systems of care, the primary care system provides an ineffective and inefficient delivery of care to older adults. In addition to the fragmented system, the future U.S. workforce is not projected to consist of the professional mix needed to staff multidisciplinary teams (Bodenheimer *et al.* 2009).

This primary care crisis is exacerbated by the fact that electronic medical record systems have yet to be systematically implemented. Research into the benefits of electronic medical records is still developing. Initial research results do indicate that electronic medical records have the potential to increase patient safety and reduce costs (Bodenheimer 2007; Bodenheimer 2008).

Reimbursement issues add to the external challenges faced by care management models. Currently, Medicare's reimbursement approach favors acute care situations. This results in minimal reimbursement options for innovative models that focus on wellness and cost-effective health promotion (Weiss *et al.* 2010).

Some researchers believe the best short-term opportunity for reducing costs is improving transitions from hospital to home. Payment reform initiatives could be used to incentivize hospitals and primary care practices to implement these programs. It has been suggested that tying physicians' compensation to quality and efficiency scores may increase the appeal of comprehensive care coordination services. In addition, it has been suggested that Medicare and Medicaid consider a separate reimbursement system for care coordinators implementing proven interventions with targeted, high-risk groups (Schraeder *et al.* 2005).

Evaluation challenges are ongoing in the care coordination arena. While great value is placed on quantitative research designs, cautionary notes are also raised regarding the danger of using standardized measures to such a degree that the diversity of patient needs is missed. Some researchers express concern that reducing chronic disease management to a standard "dose" for diverse patients will unintentionally create systematic inequities and endanger the health system's most vulnerable populations. Some of these vulnerable groups include individuals from diverse cultural backgrounds, people with limited health literacy, and patients in specific age-related cohorts (Yu *et al.* 2008). Qualitative researchers call for a balance that acknowledges the importance of subjective and interpretative data elements that can provide context for quantitatively derived models (Thorne 2008). While data and information on different models and approaches are available, it is not comparable and thus limits the ability to make comparisons across programs (Kodner & Kyriacou 2000).

Conclusion

Effective care coordination bridges the gap between the needs of people with complex chronic health conditions, disease illness, and the fragmented system of care.

Essential components of care coordination include a collaborative, interdisciplinary team, longitudinal care coordination with the patient/caregiver, implementation of the care coordination process, patient/caregiver empowerment and self-management, effective transitional care, identification and management of care-related barriers and facilitators, use of information technology, and consistent, systematic use of evaluation strategies. These components are operationalized through specific care coordination strategies such as team development, training and mentoring care coordinators, targeting appropriate patients, managing barriers, implementing the care management process which includes the use of evidence based guidelines and protocols, and formulating valid and reliable evaluation strategies. The specific functions of care coordinators are central to the care coordination process.

While there is significant potential for coordinated care management to improve the patient's quality of care and decrease system fragmentation, there are also significant challenges to its use. Some of these challenges are internal and relate to the physician's ability to engage in interdisciplinary care, generalizable evaluation strategies, and administrative support. External challenges are found at the system level and reflect a compromised primary care system and the lack of professional workforce mix to meet the changing demographic demands of the aging population. The lack of systematic implementation of clinical information systems and the lack of incentives to use and evaluate creative care management models also presents significant, ongoing barriers.

While the challenges are significant, the pending demographic changes may be the impetus that forces the types of transformations needed to support coordinated care management. Visionary care coordination proposals will include interdisciplinary teams, evidence-based care, creative use of information technology systems, and comprehensive evaluation strategies that result in improved care and quality of life for people with complex, chronic health conditions.

References

Ahmed, A. (2002) Quality and outcomes of heart failure care in older adults: role of multidisciplinary disease-management programs. *Journal of American Geriatrics Society*, 50, 1590–1593.

Anstiss, T. (2009) Motivational interviewing in primary care. *Journal of Clinical Psychology in Medical Settings*, 16(1), 87–93.

Bodenheimer, T., Wagner, E. H., & Grumbach, K. (2002a) Improving primary care for patients with chronic illness. *Journal of the American Medical Association*, 288, 1775–1779.

Bodenheimer, T., Wagner, E. H., & Grumbach, K. (2002b) Improving primary care for patients with chronic illness: the chronic care model, Part 2. *Journal of the American Medical Association*, 288, 1909–1914.

Bodenheimer, T. (2007) Coordinating care: a major (unreimbursed) task of primary care. *Annals of Internal Medicine*, 147, 730–731.

Bodenheimer, T. (2008) Coordinating care – a perilous journey through the health care system. *The New England Journal of Medicine*, 358, 1064–1071.

Bodenheimer, T., & Berry-Millett, R. (2009) *Care Management of Patients with Complex Health Care Needs*. Robert Wood Johnson Foundation, Research Synthesis Report 19, Princeton, NJ.

Bodenheimer, T., Chen, E., & Bennett, H.D. (2009) Confronting the growing burden of chronic disease: can the U.S. health care workforce do the job? *Health Affairs*, 28(1), 64–74.

Boult, C., Pualwan, T.F., Fox, P.D., *et al.* (1998) Identification and assessment of high-risk seniors. *American Journal of Managed Care*, 4, 1137–1146.

Boult, C., Kane, R.L., Pacala, J.T., *et al.* (1999) Innovative healthcare for chronically ill older persons: results of a national survey. *American Journal of Managed Care*, 5, 1162–1172.

Boult, C., Boult, L.B., Morishita, L., *et al.* (2001) A randomized clinical trial of outpatient geriatric evaluation and management. *Journal of the American Geriatrics Society*, 49, 351–359.

Boult, C., Reider, L., Frey, K., *et al.* (2008) Early effects of "guided care" on the quality of health care for multimorbid older persons: a cluster-randomized controlled trial. *Journal of Gerontology: Medical Ssciences*, 63A, 321–327.

Boult, C., Green, A.F., Boult, L.B., *et al.* (2009) Successful models of comprehensive care for older adults with chronic conditions: evidence for the Institute of Medicine's "retooling for an aging America" report. *Journal of American Geriatrics Society*, 57, 2328–2337.

Boyd, C.M., Boult, C., Shadmi, E., *et al.* (2007) Guided care for multimorbid older adults. *The Gerontologist*, 47, 697–704.

Boyd, C.M., Reider, K., Frey, K., *et al.* (2009) The effects of guided care on the perceived quality of health care for multi-morbid older persons: 18-month outcomes from a cluster-randomized controlled trial. *Journal of General Internal Medicine*, 25, 235–242.

Brown, R. (2009) *The Promise of Care Coordination: Models that Decrease Hospitalizations and Improve Outcomes for Medicare Beneficiaries with Chronic Illness*. Mathematica Policy Research, Princeton, N.J. Available at: http://www.socialworkleadership.org/snw/Brown_Executive_Summary.pdf.

Callahan, C.M., Boustani, M.A., Unverzagt, F.W., *et al.* (2006) Effectiveness of collaborative care of older adults with Alzheimer's disease in primary care: a randomized, controlled trial. *Journal of the American Medical Association*, 295, 2148–2157.

Charlson, M., Pompei, P., Ales, K., *et al.* (1987) A new method of classifying prognostic co-morbidity in longitudinal studies: development and validation. *Journal of Chronic Disease*, 40, 373–383.

Charlson, M.E., Charlson, R.E., Peterson, J.C., *et al.* (2008) The Charlson comorbidity index is adapted to predict costs of chronic disease in primary care patients. *Journal of Clinical Epidemiology*, 61, 1234–1240.

Chaudhry, S., Lei, J., & Meltzer, D. (2005) Use of a self-report-generated Charlson comorbodity index for predicting mortality. *Medical Care*, 43, 607–615.

Coleman, E.A., Smith, J.D., Frank, J.C., *et al.* (2004) Preparing patients and caregivers to participate in care delivered across settings: the care transitions intervention. *Journal of the American Geriatrics Society*, 52, 1817–1825.

Coleman, E. A., Mahoney, E., & Parry, C. (2005) Assessing the quality of preparation for posthospital care from the patient's perspective: the care transitions measure. *Medical Care*, 43, 246–255.

Coleman, E.A., Parry, C., Chalmers, S., *et al.* (2006) The care transitions intervention: results of a randomized controlled trial. *Archives of Internal Medicine*, 166, 1822–1828.

Corbin, J., & Strauss, A. (1991) A nursing model for chronic illness management based upon the trajectory framework. *Scholarly Inquiry for Nursing Practice: An International Journal*, 5, 155–174.

Counsell, S.R., Callahan, C.M., Clark, D.O., *et al.* (2007) Geriatric care management for low-income seniors: a randomized controlled trial. *Journal of the American Medical Association*, 298, 2623–2633.

Counsell, S.R., Callahan, C.M., Tu, W., *et al.* (2009) Cost analysis of the geriatric resources for assessment and care of elders care management intervention. *Journal of the American Geriatrics Society*, 57, 1420–1426.

Cress, C.J. (2007) *Handbook of Care Management*, 2nd edn. Jones and Bartlett, Sudbury MA.

Cress, C.J. (2009) *Care Managers: Working with Aging Families*. Jones and Bartlett, Sudbury, MA.

Dane, A., & Schneider, B. (1998) Program integrity in primary and early secondary prevention: are implementation effects out of control? *Clinical Psychology Review*, 18(1), 23–45.

Deyo, R.A., Cherkin, D.C., & Ciol, M.A. (1992) Adapting a clinical comorbidity index for use with ICD-9 administrative databases. *Journal of Clinical Epidemiology*, 37, 773–784.

Dickenson, K.C., Sharma, R., & Duckart, J.P. (2010) VA healthcare costs of a collaborative intervention for chronic pain in primary care. *Medical Care*, 48(1), 38–44.

Dorr, D.A., Wilcox, A., Donnelly, S.S., *et al.* (2005) Impact of generalists care managers on patients with diabetes. *Health Services Research*, 40(5 Pt I), 1400–1421.

Dorr, D.A., Wilcox, A., Burns, L., *et al.* (2006) Implementing a multi-disease chronic care model in primary care using people and technology. *Disease Management*, 9(1), 1–15.

Dorr, D.A., Wilcox, A., McConnell, K.J., *et al.* (2007) Productivity enhancement for primary care providers using multicondition care management. *The American Journal of Managed Care*, 13(1), 22–28.

Dorr, D.A., Wilcox, A.B., Brunker, C.P., *et al.* (2008) The effect of technology-supported, multidisease care management on the mortality and hospitalization of seniors. *Journal of the American Geriatrics Society*, 56, 2195–2202.

Family Caregiver Alliance. (2006) *Assessment of Family Caregivers: A Practice Perspective*. Vol. 1, Report from the Consensus Development Conference. Family Caregiver Alliance, San Francisco, CA.

Grol, R., Dalhuijsen, J., Thomas, S., *et al.* (1998) Attributes of clinical guidelines that influence use of guidelines in general practice: observational study. *British Medical Journal*, 317, 858–861.

Haggerty, J.L., Reid, R.J., Freeman, G.K., *et al.* (2003) Continuity of care: a multidisciplinary review. *British Medical Journal*, 327, 1219–1221.

Idler, E.L., & Benyamini, Y. (1997) Self-rated health and mortality: a review of twenty-seven community studies. *Journal of Health and Social Behavior*, 38(1), 21–37.

Institute of Medicine. (2008) *Retooling for an Aging America: Building the Health Care Workforce*. National Academies Press, Washington, DC.

Kellen, E., Bulens, P., Deckx, L., *et al.* (2010) Identifying an accurate pre-screening tool in geriatric oncology. *Critical Reviews in Oncology/Hematology*, 75, 243–248.

Keogh, M.E., Field, T.S., & Gurwitz, J.H. (2002) A model of community-based interdisciplinary team training in the care of frail elderly. *Academic Medicine*, 77, 936.

Kodner, D.L., & Kyriacou, C.K. (2000) Fully integrated care for frail elderly: two American models. *International Journal of Integrated Care*, 1(1), 1–19.

Kripalani, S., Jackson, A.T., Schnipper, J.L., *et al.* (2007) Promoting effective transitions of care at hospital discharge: a review of key issues for hospitalists. *Journal of Hospital Medicine*, 2, 314–323.

Larsen, A. (2009) *Roles and Responsibilities of Care Managers*. Intermountain Health Care Management Plus Training Workshop, Portland OR.

Leff, B., Reider, L., Frick, K.D., *et al.* (2009) Guided care and the cost of complex healthcare: a preliminary report. *American Journal of Managed Care*, 15, 555–559.

Lorig, K.R., Sobel, A., Stewart, A.L., *et al.* (1999) Evidence suggesting that a chronic disease self-management program can improve health status while reducing hospitalizations. *Medical Care*, 37(1), 5–14.

Lorig, K.R., Ritter, P., Stewart, A.L., *et al.* (2001) Chronic disease self-management program: 2-year health status and health care utilization outcomes. *Medical Care*, 39, 1217–1223.

McGee, H.M., O'Hanlon, A., Barker, M., *et al.* (2008) Vulnerable older people in the community: relationship between the vulnerable elders survey and health service use. *Journal of the American Geriatrics Society*, 56(1), 8–15.

Miller, E.A., & Weissert, W.G. (2000) Predicting elderly people's risk for nursing home placement, hospitalization, functional impairment, and mortality: a synthesis. *Medical Research and Review*, 57, 259–297.

Min, L., Yoon, W., Mariano, J., *et al.* (2009) The vulnerable elders-13 survey predicts 5-year functional decline and mortality outcomes in older ambulatory care patients. *Journal of the American Geriatrics Society*, 57, 2070–2076.

Mollica, R.L., & Gillespie, J. (2003) *Partnership for Solutions: Better Lives for People with Chronic Conditions*. Johns Hopkins University, Baltimore, MD.

Naylor, M.D., Brotten, D., Campbell, R., *et al.* (1999) Comprehensive discharge planning and home follow-up of hospitalized elders: a randomized clinical trial. *Journal of the American Medical Association*, 281, 613–620.

Naylor, M.D., Brooten, D.A., Campbell, R.L., *et al.* (2004) Transitional care of older adults hospitalized with heart failure: a randomized, controlled trial. *Journal of the American Geriatrics Society*, 52, 675–684.

Pacala, J.T., Boult, C., & Boult, L. (1995) Predictive validity of a questionnaire that identified older persons at risk for hospital admission. *Journal of the American Geriatrics Society*, 43, 374–377.

Pacala, J.T., Boult, C., Reed, R.L., *et al.* (1997) Predictive validity of the Pra instrument among older recipients of managed care. *Journal of the American Geriatrics Society*, 45, 614–617.

Peikes, D., Brown, R., Chen, A., *et al.* (2009) Effects of care coordination on hospitalization, quality of care, and health care expenditures among Medicare beneficiaries: 15 randomized trials. *Journal of the American Medical Association*, 301, 603–618.

Peikes, D., Peterson, G., Schore, J., *et al.* (2010) *Effects of Care Coordination on Hospitalization, Quality of Care, and Health Care Expenditures Among Medicare Beneficiaries: 11 Randomized Trials*. Unpublished Report. Mathematica Policy Research, Inc., Princeton, N.J.

Peleg, R., Press, Y., Asher, M., *et al.* (2008) An intervention program to reduce the number of hospitalizations of elderly patients in a primary care clinic. *BMC Health Services Research*, 8(36). Available at: http://www.biomedcentral.com/1472-6963/8/36.

Pham, H.H., Schrag, D., O'Malley, A.S., *et al.* (2007) Care patterns in Medicare and their implications for pay for performance. *New England Journal of Medicine*, 356, 1130–1139.

Pope, G.C., Kautter, J., Ellis, R.P., *et al.* (2004) Risk adjustment of Medicare capitation payments using the CMS-HCC model. *Health Care Financing Review*, 25(4), 119–141.

Prochaska, J.O., & Velicer, W.F. (1997) The transtheoretical model of health behavior change. *American Journal of Health Promotion*, 12(1), 38–48.

Reiss-Brennan, B., Briot, P.C., Savitz, L.A., *et al.* (2010) Cost and quality impact of Intermountain's mental health integration program. *Journal of Healthcare Management*, 55(2), 1–18.

Reuben, D.B., Keeler, E., Seeman, T.E., *et al.* (2003) Identification of risk for high hospital use: cost comparisons of four strategies and performance across subgroups. *Journal of the American Geriatrics Society*, 51, 615–620.

Reuben, D.B. (2007) Better care for older people with chronic diseases: an emerging vision. *Journal of the American Medical Association*, 298, 2673–2674.

Reuben, D.B. (2009) Better ways to care for older persons: is anybody listening? *Journal of American Geriatrics Society*, 57, 2348–2349.

Rollnick, S., Miller, W.R., & Butler, C.C. (2008) *Motivational Interviewing in Health Care: Helping Patients Change Behavior (Applications of Motivational Interviewing)*. The Guilford Press, New York, NY.

Rosen, A.K., Wang, F., Montez, M.E., *et al.* (2005) Identifying future high-healthcare users: exploring the value of diagnostic and prior utilization information. *Disease Management and Health Outcomes*, 13, 117–127.

Saliba, D., Orlando, M., Wenger, N., *et al.* (2000) Identifying a short functional disability screen for older persons. *Journal of Gerontology*, 55, M750–M756.

Saliba, S., Elliott, M., Rubenstein, L.A., *et al.* (2001) The vulnerable elders survey (VES-13): a tool for identifying vulnerable elders in the community. *Journal of the American Geriatric Society*, 49, 1691–1699.

Schraeder, C., Dworak, D., Stoll, J.F., *et al.* (2005) Managing elders with comorbidities. *Journal of Ambulatory Care Management*, 28, 201–209.

Schraeder, C., Fraser, C.W., Clark, I., *et al.* (2008) Evaluation of a primary care nurse management intervention for chronically ill community dwelling older people. *Journal of Nursing and Healthcare of Chronic Illness*, 17, 407–417.

Shortell, S.M., Marsteller, J.A., Lin, M., *et al.* (2004) The role of perceived team effectiveness in improving chronic illness care. *Medical Care*, 42, 1040–1048.

Steckler, A.B., Linnan, L., & Israel, B.A. (2002) *Process Evaluation for Public Health Intervention and Research*. Jossey-Bass, San Francisco, CA.

Sylvia, M.L., Shadmi, E., Hsiao, C.J., *et al.* (2006) Clinical features of high-risk older persons identified by predictive modeling. *Disease Management*, 9(1), 56–62.

Sylvia, M.L., Griswold, M., Dunbar, L., *et al.* (2008) Guided care: cost and utilization outcomes in a pilot study. *Disease Management*, 11(1), 29–36.

Tabloski, P.A. (2006) *Gerontological Nursing*. Prentice Hall, Upper Saddle River, NJ.

The John A. Hartford Foundation. (2007a) *Virtual Integrated Practice Model*. The John A. Hartford Foundation, New York, NY, 50–61.

The John A. Hartford Foundation (2007b) *Geriatric Interdisciplinary Teams in Practice*. Annual Report, The John A. Hartford Foundation, New York, NY, 49–59.

Thorne, S. (2008) Communication in chronic care: confronting the evidence challenge in an era of system reform. *Journal of Nursing and Healthcare of Chronic Illnesses*, 17(11c), 294–97.

Vickery, B.G., Mittman, B.S., Connor, K.I., *et al.* (2006) The effect of disease management intervention on quality and outcomes of dementia care: a randomized, controlled trial. *Annals of Internal Medicine*, 145, 713–726.

U.S. Preventive Services Task Force. *Recommendations for Adults*. U.S. Preventive Services Task Force, Rockville, MD. Available at: http://www.uspreventiveservicestaksforce.org/recommendations.htm

Wagner, E., Davis, C., Schaefer J., *et al.* (1999) A survey of leading chronic disease management programs: are they consistent with the literature? *Managed Care Quarterly*, 7(3), 56–66.

Wagner, E.H. (2000) The role of patient care teams in chronic disease management. *British Medical Journal*, 320, 569–572.

Wagner, E. (2002) Care for chronic diseases. *British Medical Journal*, 325, 913–914.

Weber, J.R. (2008) *Nurse's Handbook of Health Assessment*, 6th edn. Wolters Kluwer, Philadelphia PA.

Weiner J.P., Abrams, C., & Bodycombe, D. (2003) *The Johns Hopkins ACG Case-Mix System Version 6 Release Notes. Section 2. The ACG Predictive Model: Helping to Manage Persons at Risk for High Future Costs*. Johns Hopkins Bloomberg School of Public Health, Baltimore, MD.

Weiss, M., Yakusheva, O., & Bobay, K. (2010) Nurse and patient perceptions of discharge readiness in relation to post discharge utilization. *Medical Care*, 48, 482–486.

Wenger, N.S., Roth, C.P., & Shekelle, P. (2007) Introduction to assessing care of vulnerable elders-3 quality indicator measurement set. *Journal of the American Geriatrics Society*, 55(Supplement 2), S247–S252.

Wenger, N.S., & Young, R.T. (2007) Quality indicators for continuity and coordination of care in vulnerable elders. *Journal of the American Geriatrics Society*, 55(Supplement 2), S247–S252.

Wilcox, A.B., Jones, S.S., Dorr, D.A., *et al.* (2005) *Use and Impact of a Computer-Generated Patient Summary Worksheet for Primary Care*. American Medical Informatics Association Annual Symposium Proceedings, pp. 824–828.

Xyrichis, A., & Ream, E. (2007) Teamwork: a concept analysis. *Journal of Advanced Nursing*, 61, 232–241.

Yu, D.S., Lee, D.T., Kwong, A.N, *et al.* (2008) Living with chronic heart failure: a review of qualitative studies on older people. *Journal of Advanced Nursing*, 61, 474–483.

Chapter 6

Evaluation methods

Robert Newcomer and L. Gail Dobell

Introduction

One purpose of program evaluation is to help provide an evidence basis for clinical practice and policy. In health and long-term care, evidence comes from many sources. These include such things as clinical trials, demonstration projects, accumulated program operational experience, continuous quality improvement efforts, and cost-effectiveness studies. The standards of acceptable evidence depend to some extent on how the information is used (Helfand 2005).

Efficacy has the highest information standards, and is often addressed using an experimental design. Providing guidance for individual patient treatment decision making, or information on program operations and performance, on the other hand, may begin with the assumption of an intervention's effectiveness or comparative benefit. In these studies interest shifts to understanding such things as the causes of practice variation, disparities in access and outcomes like cost and quality of care.

Clarity about the purposes and outcomes desired from care coordination programs is a fundamental starting point for a discussion of evaluation methods. This chapter explores evaluation methods for care coordination by first providing a brief primer on alternative evaluation designs. This is followed by a conceptual look at the continuum of care and the variety of intersections where care coordination plays a potential role. The chapter closes reviewing lessons from care coordination evaluation and how we might improve the approach to and usefulness of such research.

A primer on evaluation designs[1]

Randomized Controlled Trials (RCTs)

Pharmaceutical effects, surgical procedures, and medical device efficacy are areas within health and long-term care where "evidence" most directly influences practice and financing. Discrete interventions such as these, lend themselves to randomized controlled trials (RCTs). These have the characteristic that the "investigator" has control over; both to who receives the innovation, and those with whom the innovation results are compared.

Comprehensive Care Coordination for Chronically Ill Adults, First Edition. Edited by Cheryl Schraeder and Paul Shelton.
© 2011 John Wiley & Sons, Inc. Published 2011 by John Wiley & Sons, Inc.

Randomized assignment of patients/cases into the treatment and control groups is used to assure comparability in these groups. RCTs are the gold standard for determining cause and effect, and are considered such in testing program efficacy.

However, even with randomization there are limitations translating findings into practice (Helfand 2005). Do the findings hold as the program or practice is extended to populations not included in innovation testing? Does efficacy remain when treatment is brought to scale by clinicians and recipients who may not be as well trained, motivated, or monitored for treatment protocols compliance as occurred during the innovation research?

Another potential limitation is that efficacy is relative to the situation used to define *usual care* for the comparison group. This issue is illustrated with medication studies where there may be alternative medications that perform comparably well or better for some groups than others, or those that have lower risk or higher net benefit and lower cost. Not infrequently, such competing alternatives may not be among the options used to define the "comparison" group in the RCT.

Quasi-experimental designs

Random assignment of patients/recipients into treatment and control groups may not be practical at the outset, or may not be possible to sustain over time. A quasi-experimental design may be used when random assignment is not practical. Quasi-experimental designs approximate random assignment using statistical adjustments for recipient and other measured differences. Like RCTs, quasi-experimental designs have a risk of contamination in recipient and provider groups if recipients are allowed to change providers or if providers serve recipients in both groups. One approach for minimizing these risks is to locate treatment and comparison groups in different communities or organizations. This alternative introduces unmeasured differences in recipient and provider preferences and behaviors and adds uncertainty to the study findings.

Whether using a RCT or quasi-experimental design, cause-effect determination is more complicated when multifaceted interventions, like care coordination, are involved. A particular problem is whether it is possible to distinguish the contribution of individual intervention elements from their interactions with other program features like provider practices.

No comparison group designs

A third group of designs relies on pre-post comparisons. As described here, these designs use the treatment, or innovation subjects, as their own controls or comparison group. An example is a study of provider behavior before and after a change in reimbursement rates. Important assumptions are made in pre-post designs. Among these: all outcome differences are explained by the innovative change in practice or policy rather than other concurrent events, and that the recipients and providers groups before and after the change are comparable. These designs are strengthened if they include longitudinal data spanning both periods on recipients and providers. They are weakened if they are drawn from separate samples in each time period. Changes in population characteristics, other than on outcomes, between testing periods weaken the causal attribution of the program or practice changes to the population's outcome. Contextual changes (for example, in financing, services, or providers) during the period further threaten the validity of any cause-effect conclusions.

No comparison group designs are frequently used with naturally occurring experiments such as changes in regulations, reimbursement rates, program eligibility, and operational practices. Comparisons of outcomes and performance could be at the individual level (as with beneficiaries or providers) in the same community or at the organizational or community level.

Performance & effectiveness studies

Evaluation efforts may be applied to refining practice, improving efficiency, and upgrading the program's operational performance, as well as to the effects of practices on recipient outcomes. Using care coordination as an example, consider the question of variation in practice between home and community- based service (HCBS) providers. Variation can have many contributing sources. Among these are the absence of standardized assessments or how they are used; differences in the populations served or the number and mix of available providers; differences in reimbursement levels or treatment incentives; and differences in the training/experience of the care coordinators or providers.

While many differences between providers are outside their control, it may be possible to affect some operational features. Consider the introduction of practice guidelines as an example of an innovation. The assumption is that practice variation can be narrowed and more adherences to efficacious, cost effective, and high-quality treatments can be achieved using a practice guideline. An evaluation of this type of intervention does not necessarily require a comparison group. Comparisons might be against the program targets or standards of practice in the field (such as care coordinators to client ratios; frequency, number, and duration of visits). Emphases on processes rather than outcomes of care could obviate the need for anything other than pre-post or cross sectional observational data. A process of care orientation can also be combined into outcomes of care evaluations.

Continuum of care and the role of care coordination

Figure 6.1 conceptually highlights the levels of care and providers in the health and long-term care continuum. It is organized according to an individual's health status (shown as circles). An illustrative array of services appropriate to that health status is also shown. Overlap between the health status circles represents intersections between the beneficiary status and likely providers.[2]

- Circle 1 represents the absence of health problem(s), treatment emphasis is condition prevention.
- Circle 2 represents the presence of a health condition(s), treatment emphasis is condition management.
- Circle 3 represents the Advance Illness stage, treatment emphasis may shift to palliative and/or end of life care.

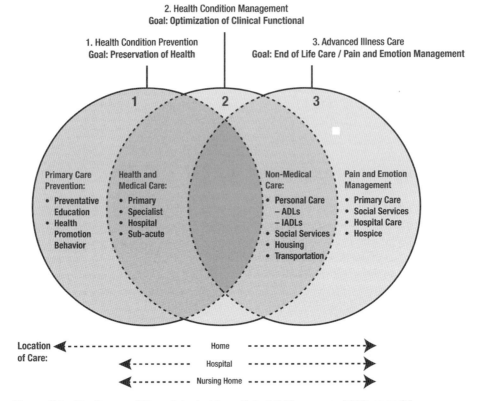

Figure 6.1   Continuum of Care; Adapted from Dobell & Newcomer, 2008, page 27

Provider involvement can occur in more than one level, as represented by the overlap in the diagram's health status level circles. These areas of overlap are the opportunities for care coordination and integration. The bottom of the diagram shows the patient/care recipient's typical location or setting. These settings and the transitions between them add complexity to the involvement of providers and communication between them. The setting may also influence the choice or availability of providers. Changes in setting can be disruptive to continuity of care. The levels and types of care are affected by financing and regulation, the organization, and other environmental contexts. These effects, though present, are not shown.

To illustrate an application of the framework, consider an individual having no notable health problems. The "care" needed might involve a combination of prevention education, self-management, and primary health care. If the individual is diagnosed with a health condition, they progress to Level 2, where condition management becomes a goal. Primary care provision continues as previously, but specialists and episodic acute care may emerge. Within this level, we expect the involvement of two or more medical providers, and others who assist in treatment adherence and self-management. If physical function and/or mental or cognitive limitations are involved, then assistive and various non-medical services may be required to facilitate activities of daily living (ADL), instrumental activities of daily living (IADL), and social needs. For some individuals, communication and treatment adherence, and training and support may begin to involve informal care providers. Most of the Level 2 condition management population resides in community settings, although recipients may be living in congregate or group settings, or nursing homes. Transitioning between these settings and with hospital care is an especially critical time.

As an individual's health status progresses to Level 3, care may shift from active management of the health conditions to one of palliation (for example, symptom management, patient comfort and pain management; and reductions in restorative treatment). Social and other supports to the recipient and the family may intensify. Advanced illness care may continue, but some or all care may be transferred to providers more oriented to supportive assistance. Locations of care might include one's home, hospitals, assisted living, nursing homes, and inpatient hospice settings.

Transitions between levels of care, providers, and/or settings are especially critical occasions. One function of care coordination at these times is assuring communication among providers so as to minimize disruption in the continuity of care. Some information exchange may require physicians coordinating directly with each other, or nurses serving as a communications bridge and coordinator between various medical providers and family members or care recipients. Functions such as social support, accessing community resources, or alternative funding might be best served by social workers.

For any given patient/client, it is likely that multiple elements of care coordination operate concurrently. These may or may not be coordination with each other, and when not, can lead to duplication of effort, contradictory actions, and increase program cost. Another potential complication can occur when there is incentive for cost shifting between payers or organizations, such as when care provision involves transferring or sharing the cost of care. Examples of this include policies in which providers have constrained revenue from the same payer source (for example, hospitals with diagnosis-related or bundled rates for procedures; nursing homes with fixed daily rates; and home health agency maximum days of care). Such payments are at once an incentive for operational efficiency within the care coordinator's organization and a motivation to move the patients to another provider and payer system. Cost shifts are problematic if they reduce the quality of care or if they transfer the cost to systems which do not have sufficient resources to afford this responsibility. Understanding the incentives influencing care coordinator actions is needed when evaluating coordination performance across the continuum of care.

Centers for medicare & medicaid services integration of care demonstration activities

Outcome and operational effectiveness research and its incorporation into policy, program guidelines, and financing is distributed among a number of federal and state government agencies, and other task forces and panels.[3] In this section, discussion is limited to Medicare and Medicaid, programs administered by the Centers for Medicare & Medicaid Services (CMS).[4] Many CMS research and demonstration efforts are mandated by legislation, and consequently offer a window into national policy and programs. Typically, budget neutrality is the CMS focus for new programs or benefits. This means that the innovations cannot cost more than usual care for the same type of recipients. These studies may also be concerned with issues like access to care, beneficiary outcomes, and other aspects of operational performance.

CMS programs finance health and long-term care for some of the most vulnerable populations in the United States (CMS 2005). For example, half of all Medicare spending is attributable to 6% of Medicare beneficiaries and Medicaid pays for more than half of all nursing home care. Given these disproportionate expenditures, identifying those most in need is potentially helpful in achieving budget neutrality. Care coordinators using screening assessments are a common approach to finding these individuals.

Consumer choice is a second perspective influencing CMS practices. This is reflected in such things as data systems that provide consumers with information about the quality of care in hospitals and nursing homes; beneficiary opportunities to change providers and health plans; and consumer directed care, particularly personal care services for persons with disabilities. Care coordination can come into conflict with consumer choice. For many families and individuals, care coordinators may need a balance between being a gatekeeper versus being a coach, educator, and facilitator.

A third characteristic of CMS efforts was noted earlier; they test the efficacy (including budget neutrality and recipient outcomes) of new interventions, and they may document practices and operational efficiencies. These research functions may be distributed between independent evaluators and governmental units that have program oversight.

Programs, such as Medicaid home and community-based service waivers, are generally approved and reauthorized for extended periods. This affords the state and provider the opportunity for incremental operational refinement. Such adjustments and developmental evolution are much rarer in national demonstration projects. We come back to this issue later.

Care coordination tasks and functions

The care coordination innovations and practices of most interest in this book are those attempting to obtain efficiency within levels of care (for example, hospitals, nursing homes, home care), and/or in the transitions between levels of care, providers, or between financing systems. Such work may have goals like improving access to the services offered at one level of care (including primary care, disease management, home care, and so on), minimizing the use of more intensive and/or expensive care (such as hospital care), and reducing practice variation and costs.

Program staffing and practices are basic to operational efficiency. We use this to illustrate delineation of tasks and functions into researchable elements. Each care coordination function has specific staffing considerations such as the number of care coordinators, their professional training, and the average time needed when working with individual clients. Clarity on these specifics and whether care coordinators have multiple functions that combine two or more roles is vital in cross program comparisons. However, many studies and program descriptions compress the issue into staff to client ratios –often without adjustment for full time equivalence in each role.

The complexity of unbundling roles is illustrated by a few of the basic care coordinator functions. We start with the role of gatekeeper into program or benefit eligibility. This function is common in assessing (and reassessing) home care services and nursing home needs. It also applies to disease management and other benefits where enrollment is targeted to specific levels of vulnerability. Assessment may be coupled with care planning, benefit authorization, and recipient training. These functions may also involve consultation with care teams, or other health care providers.

Reductions in cost and practice variation in care coordination have been another program evaluation target. Such efforts have contributed to the adoption of electronic assessment instruments, and algorithms that translate measured needs into care plans, benefit authorizations, and/or dollar allocations. How good are the studies that provided the basis of these procedures? This issue warrants further investigation. To the extent that standardized procedures have been adopted, have the expected efficiency and effectiveness been achieved? How has the saved care coordinator time been reallocated?

Another care coordination function is communication (for example, treatment plans, tests/laboratory results, medications) between the providers responsible for the interfacing levels of care, and between providers and the care recipients. Documentation of these activities is often in the form of recipient care record entries. Activities are likely to be variable based on the particular needs of the recipient and the circumstances relative to providers and other factors. Simple measures are frequently used rather than chart level specifics. These may record the presence or absence of care coordinators (and perhaps their case loads) in specific roles: hospitalists in acute care; teams involved with a patient's transition from hospital to nursing home care; multidisciplinary teams involved with those in nursing homes, community settings, or in advanced illness care; and social service support to physicians in addressing vulnerable populations in community settings.

In these situations, the care coordinator(s) action may be treated as a "black box," in which clients are either exposed to this service or not. This approach to examining the effective components that make up the black box is often sufficient for a first stage answer to the question of whether these programs achieve program goals such as reducing preventable hospital stays/days and emergency room use. Simple refinements to such questions may assess whether the outcomes were associated with the professional background or experience of the care coordinator, and whether the reimbursement methodology provided incentives influencing provider behavior.

A drill down into chart-based processes and intensity of care might be warranted to understand performance differences among individual staff or across programs. Such information might include the number, time taken, and nature of specific encounters; the information transferred and to whom; and whether the information was used. Process of care information is expensive, and usually more appropriate for continuous quality improvement than cross program comparisons.

Training and/or facilitating the patient or care recipients (including family members) in fulfilling their self-care or treatment adherence is another typical care coordinator function. Training might include how to modify personal behaviors (such as smoking, diet, exercise), manage chronic diseases (for example, medication use, symptom monitoring), or help the care recipient gain access to benefits provided by another organization or another unit within the organization.

As in the prior example, the provision of training and facilitation assistance is likely to be implicitly assumed (given a care coordinator's professional training and experience), rather than measured directly. Patient/client outcomes assumed to be attributable to training can be directly measured. In-depth documentation of actions and content would usually be more appropriate for continuous quality improvement purposes, but the introduction of specific training might warrant direct study.

A last consideration in this outline of care coordination functions is the reminder that the effectiveness of care coordination is not isolated from the financial incentives affecting provider behavior. These take a variety of forms: risk-adjusted capitation reimbursement for health plans and providers; fixed payment for hospital stays and selected surgical procedures; other fee-for-service budget caps and bundled payment rates; and recipient co-payments and deductibles.

Capitation and prospective payment have usually been limited to specific levels or types of care, and a single source of payment such as Medicare or Medicaid. Examples include health maintenance organization or managed care plans where Medicare or Medicaid coverage (but not both together) is capitated. Long-term care has usually been excluded from the capitation rates. Among Medicare or Medicaid managed care members, those entering long-term care (especially nursing homes) may be required or encouraged to withdraw from the managed care plan.[5]

The partitioning of Medicare and Medicaid expenditures and service access seems to be changing. CMS, states, and foundations have begun to give increased attention to the expenditures of those dually eligible for Medicare and Medicaid. This includes both studies of those dually eligible and the databases compiling expenditures in each individual program and total expenditures. Among other things, these databases permit consideration of utilization and costs for those entering, and those within long-term care systems.

Looking ahead

The CMS research and demonstration programs highlighted above, and those described elsewhere in this book, are illustrative of state of the art approaches in the development and testing of care coordination policy and practices. These examples address many dimensions of the continuum of care. They also suggest some underlying perspectives likely to be reflected in program and policy design going forward. Key among these are support for consumer choice, the targeting of benefits and strategies to identified vulnerable populations, and an interest in using payment incentives (such as capitation payment) for utilization control and to influence provider behavior. Substantively, disease management, transitional care, and programs that begin to link Medicare and Medicaid financing across the continuum of care for those at risk/or receiving long-term care seem to be enduring or emerging priorities.

Care coordination practices have been operationally transformed and extended by states and provider organizations over the years. This has occurred in spite of a number of negative or ambiguous national evaluation findings that failed to demonstrate cost effectiveness (that is, budget neutrality). Care coordination's face validity for facilitating communication between providers and across levels of care has trumped these studies. This is a good thing, as factors other than ineffective clinical operations have contributed to negative findings.

Some of these involve methodological issues, like failing to prevent the contamination of comparison group samples or provider behavior, or small sample sizes. There are also issues of program maturity, or more precisely, evaluating programs before they have attained steady state performance.

Program maturity

Program maturity has multiple elements. Understanding and addressing these elements is an important next step in attaining an effective and constructive care coordination evaluation program. One problem is illustrated by the lifecycle of national demonstrations in which providers and the program evaluators compete for these time-limited initiatives. Even though the organizations winning these awards have experience in the demonstration topics, they are still challenged to recruit recipients (and comparison groups), build out the intervention, launch it, and begin to immediately test program effects and efficiency. All of this allows very little time for the providers to refine their procedures and practices, even if the evaluation design permitted modification.

The time constraint also truncates the program exposure period for observing program effects. Outcomes measured after just a few months, 12 months, or at most a couple of years in the program, are typical. This limitation, combined with program immaturity, is double jeopardy against the likelihood of observing favorable program effects. A way needs to be found for incremental evaluations of innovations. This would allow for maturation, and protracted intervals for assessing outcomes.

State, community, health plan, and other on-going programs (including Medicaid waiver programs) are existing resources that address many of these limitations. Usually waiver programs do not have tight time constraints affecting operational start-up and performance monitoring. As a consequence, these programs have the opportunity for refinement and revision with experience. However, these opportunities may not be routinely taken. Moreover, these programs may not have a strong, if any evaluation component. Both these factors limit the documentation of the program effects.

Lessons from the field

The dynamic nature of care coordination practices, paradoxically, both complicates the collection of information about clinical and efficiency outcomes and argues for a systematic program to evaluate the operational procedures and tools as they are implemented. The experience of prior care coordination evaluations offers lessons for resolving this paradox and moving the practices forward.

One of these lessons is that evaluations with aims to refine clinical practice, reduce practice variation, and improve operational efficiency are of central importance. These have immediate value to basic operations and budgeting. Moreover, even if a program goal is testing efficacy, understanding how it was implemented is fundamental to determining the circumstances when the program is most effective.

Lesson two is that every operating program makes a determination about the resources committed to the ongoing analyses of program performance and cost effectiveness. These likely total vast sums nationally. Can these be more effectively used or even pooled? Perhaps it is time for a more systematic collaboration among programs. Current ad hoc efforts, such as the 2010 summit[6] of recognized experts in this field convened by the Gerontological Society of America, is illustrative of the recognized value of information sharing. This one-day effort also illustrates the early developmental stage of these collaborative efforts. The proposal made here is to go beyond the "best practice" and informal communications among programs to formulate guidelines and standards relative to evaluation tools and cross-program reporting. Conferences may not be sufficient. An ongoing body or membership collaborative may be required to systematically pursue issues. Examples include:

- Standards for measuring risk, resource use, determining costs, and other outcomes are needed. This will facilitate the understanding of evaluative information from one setting to another.
- Cost-effectiveness analysis also depends on the selection of appropriate programmatic or practice alternatives to which innovations or programmatic changes are being compared. A clearinghouse on operating and conceptual alternatives, and secondary data sets tracking performance of these approaches, are possible resources. Work groups that identify and recommend appropriate comparisons are another possible resource.
- Further, because procedures evolve in clinical practice, evaluations should be revisited periodically after the innovations have been implemented. This notion applies to both individual programs and program models that may be in place in multiple locations. Periodic studies and exchanges of operational procedures, outcomes, and cost effectiveness could provide a helpful feedback loop in refining practice. This work could occur serially within the same programs or as planned variations across programs. Each of these could be in different stages of maturity or operating in different circumstances.
- A collaborative, planned variation approach also allows the experience of programs serving different high-cost, high-prevalence conditions to be compiled and shared in evaluating clinical performance and costs. Similarly, diverse populations of patients from a variety of practice settings can be incorporated into a shared database encompassing a broad range of health outcomes.

Lesson three is that evaluation designs, particularly those involving RCTs, need to be large (and consequently expensive) to have adequate statistical power. Policy makers, payers, and practitioners must decide whether freedom from bias is worth the extra cost. For most work, observational and cost-effectiveness studies that are quasi-experimental or collect pre-post data from the same recipients (or groups of similar recipients) will continue to be popular. Done well, this work can address the efficiency and effectiveness information needs of policy makers and practitioners. Increasing the volume of this work is achievable and could be built into program operations and conducted in collaboration with other states.

Lesson four arises from the organizational changes needed to implement practice innovations – topics frequently ignored in the up-or-down reporting of program outcomes. A key issue is organizational commitment. Organizations participating in a demonstration or any innovation must have a willingness to adapt their communication and service support infrastructure to the service model being implemented. Commitment is evident in a number of ways. Among them:

- Allocation of strong, determined, and consistent administrative leadership for the program; the recruiting and training of critical staff.
- Development and continual refinement of such essential tasks as health-risk screening instruments; electronic data systems that link risk identification, home assessment, program benefits, and care planning with primary care and other providers.
- Continual refinement of communications processes that connect such things as hospital continuity of care, home health care, nursing home care, ambulatory care, and others.
- Another element of commitment is that all critical infrastructure may not be in place at the outset of most innovations. This is especially true when major reengineering of clinical operations is necessary, such as if the organization is accepting financial risk for its operations and outcomes. Building that infrastructure is a major commitment that requires time and continual support throughout the organization. Limited term demonstrations produce little incentive for substantial infrastructure development. Similarly, once the infrastructure is in place, it is disheartening to abandon this with the closing of major demonstrations.

Lesson five is a corollary to the above. Organizational and practice changes do not happen instantaneously. Programs and approaches have to be initiated, phased in, appraised, and refined. This is complicated enough in a single-site program. When multisite programs are involved, time has to be allowed for phasing between sites and the work needed to attain comparable levels of practice. The net result is that it may take more than a year to establish internal operations – even longer among the multiple sites – and it may be very uneven among the network of providers with whom the program interacts.

This lesson loops back to the need to coordinate the innovation's maturity with the evaluation design. One difficult situation is maintaining a comparison sample, especially when treatment and control groups are drawn from the same provider panels or organizations. The risk that sizable proportions of recipients of the comparison sample will move between providers and programs, and/or those providers may adopt some of the innovative practices increases with time. Such shifts contaminate the experiment and risk reducing observed difference with usual care. The failure to identify program effectiveness when it exists is very high in this situation.

These risks can be minimized if creation of comparison groups is deferred until the innovative program has reached an acceptable level of steady state operations. An alternative is to have repeated pre-post comparisons limited to those in the program before and after the introduction of the innovative changes. Another option for maintaining an uncontaminated comparison group across an extended period is to draw them in other communities or organizations. This may be possible only in well-financed evaluations.

Closing thoughts

The importance of having the government and private sectors stimulating experimentation and innovation in care for aged and disabled persons is an underlying assumption of this chapter. The innovations discussed in this book offer examples of the value, challenges, and limitations of the approaches taken to date. The emphasis on most program start-ups, understandably, is on infrastructure development. Fewer resources and much less time is given to incremental refinement in practices as programs gain experience. Public policy would be well served by working to refine, document, and disseminate these experiences and accomplishments. Decisions like this are more easily applied in programs (like Medicaid waivers) that are on-going, but possible with some time limited demonstrations.

Centers of excellence and collaborative networks are common in basic sciences and rehabilitation services. These function with an aim of incremental refinement and repeated testing. Is something analogous possible for care coordination practice?

Natural experiments for collaborations already exist. They include the many state HCBS waiver programs, and other Medicaid long-term care initiatives intended to prevent nursing home placement, or reduce hospital stays. Managed care programs (such as PACE programs, Medicaid and Medicare health maintenance organizations), and the Veterans Administration are other examples.

A third resource are organizations (including current and former care coordination demonstration programs) which are operating care coordination programs and are willing to participate in a collaborative center or consortium. The National Chronic Care Consortium (2001) is one example of this. This voluntary group was formed mainly among managed care providers to share experience and to consider standardization in measures and practice. They have given some attention to care coordination.

CMS (perhaps in collaboration with other federal agencies, private insurance, state governments, and foundations) could likely facilitate the formation of a consortium for care coordination collaboration. These might serve as more than centers for research and program operations dissemination. That function is already available through conferences. What is needed is a think-tank for the development of innovation models and practice refinement, instrument development and standardization, planned variations for program innovations testing, and establishing guidelines of practice. The consortium would likely involve voluntary participation and organizational commitment, but it could provide a resource to expand the evidence-based practice in the field of care coordination.

Notes

1. There is a vast library of readings describing approaches to evaluation research methods. Brinkerhoff (2003), Frechtling (2007), Levin & McElwan (2001), Patton (2001), and Shadish, Cook, & Campbell (2001) are among the authors who have informed our thinking about practical approaches.
2. This framework is adapted from Dobell & Newcomer (2008), p. 27. This work is a synthesis from multiple sources: best-practices in chronic care (Reuben 2002; Wagner *et al.* 2001), disease management (Villagra 2004), integrated care (Stone & Katz 1996), long-term care (Wiener & Stevenson 1998), and Medicare reform (Cassel, Besdine, Siegel 1999; Whitelaw & Warden 1999).
3. Among these are the U.S. Preventive Services Task Force (USPSTF), the American College of Physicians' Clinical Efficacy Assessment Program (CEAP), UL

National Center for Clinical Evidence (NICE), and AHRQ designated Evidence-Based Practice Centers (EPCs; Hefland 2005).

4. This synopsis was derived from the CMS Research Activities: The Active Projects Report. See the CMS web site http://www.hhs.gov/researchers/projects/apr/default/asp for a current listing of projects.

5. The Program of All-Inclusive Care (PACE) is an exception to both the separation of payment source and the exclusion of long-term care liability. This program is targeted to non-institutionalized persons age 55 and over, and operates under capitation payments from both Medicare and Medicaid reimbursement. The PACE provider assumes financial risk for all levels and duration of care across the continuum of care (Eng *et al.* 1997). EverCare is another exception. It is a managed care program for those in nursing homes (Kane *et al.* 2004).

6. Diffusing Care Coordination Models: Translating Research into Policy & Practice held on September 16, 2010, in Washington, DC.

References

Brinkerhoff, R.O. (2003) *The Success Case Method: Find Out Quickly What's Working and What's Not.* Berrett-Koehler Publishers, San Francisco, CA.

Cassel, C.K., Besdine, R.W., & Siegel, L.C. (1999) Restructuring Medicare for the next century: what will beneficiaries really need? *Health Affairs,* 18(1), 118–131.

Centers for Medicare & Medicaid Services. (2005) *CMS Research Activities: The Active Projects Report.* Available at: http://www.cms.hhs.gov/researchers/projects/apr/default.asp.

Dobell, G., & Newcomer, R. (2008) Integrated care: incentives, approaches, and future considerations. *Social Work in Public Health,* 23(4), 25–47.

Eng, C., Pedulla, J., Eleazer, P., *et al.* (1997) Program of All-Inclusive Care for the Elderly: an innovative model of integrated geriatric care and financing. *Journal of the American Geriatrics Society,* 45, 223–232.

Frechtling, J.A. (2007) *Logic Modeling in Program Evaluation.* Jossey-Bass Publications, San Francisco, CA.

Helfand, M. (2005) Using evidence reports: progress and challenges in evidence-based decision making. *Health Affairs,* 24(1), 123–132.

Kane, R.L., Flood, S., Bershadsky, B., *et al.* (2004) Effect of an innovative Medicare managed care program on the quality of nursing home residents. *The Gerontologist,* 44(1), 95–103.

Levin, H.M., & McEwan, P.J. (2001) *Cost-Effectiveness Analysis,* 2nd edn. Sage Publications, Thousand Oaks, CA.

National Chronic Care Consortium. (2001) *Provider Survey Report: Summary of 2000 Survey of MSHO Care Coordinators, Nurse Practitioners, and Physicians.* National Chronic Care Consortium, Washington, DC. Available at: http://www.cnnonline.org/products/M09001.pdf.

Patton, M.Q. (2001) *Qualitative Research and Evaluation Methods,* 3rd edn. Sage Publications, Thousand Oaks, CA.

Reuben, D.B. (2002) Organizational interventions to improve health outcomes of older persons. *Medical Care,* 40, 416–428.

Shadish, W.R., Cook, T.D., & Campbell, D.T. (2001) *Experimental and Quasi-Experimental Designs for Generalized Causal Inference.* Houghton Mifflin, Boston, MA.

Stone, R.I., & Katz, R. (1996) Thoughts on the future of integrating acute and long-term care. In: *Annual Review of Gerontology and Geriatrics*, Volume 16 (eds. R. Newcomer & A. Wilkersin), pp. 217–248. Springer, New York, NY.

Villagra, V.G. (2004) Integrating disease management into the outpatient delivery system during and after managed care. *Health Affairs*, Web Exclusive, May 19, (W4)281–(W4)283.

Wagner, E.H., Austin, B., Davis, C., *et al.* (2001) Improving chronic illness care: translating evidence into action. *Health Affairs*, 20(6), 64–78.

Whitelaw, N.A., & Warden, G.L. (1999) Reexamining the delivery system as part of Medicare reform. *Health Affairs*, 18(1), 132–143.

Wiener, J.M., & Stevenson, D.G. (1998) State policy on long-term care for the elderly. *Health Affairs*, 17(3), 81–100.

Chapter 7

Health information technology

David A. Dorr and Molly M. King

Introduction

Health information technology (HIT) can facilitate significant improvements in the efficiency and effectiveness of health care in the United States (Bates 2002; Chaudhry *et al.* 2006; Blumenthal & Glaser 2007; Marmor *et al.* 2009). Many studies have demonstrated that effective HIT use is associated with improved preventive care (Larsen *et al.* 1989; Litzelman *et al.* 1993; Willson *et al.* 1995; Overhage *et al.* 1996; Cannon & Allen 2000, Demakis *et al.* 2000; Teich *et al.* 2000, Dexter *et al.* 2004), reduced complications (Larsen *et al.* 1989; Kucher *et al.* 2005), fewer adverse events (Evans *et al.* 1992), medical errors (Bates *et al.* 1998; Evans *et al.* 1998), decreased resource utilization (Tierney *et al.* 1993; Bates *et al.* 1999), and lower health care costs (Tierney *et al.* 1993). However, HIT must be implemented carefully and thoughtfully to produce these benefits.

The use of HIT to manage care coordination has received increasing attention because of its capacity to help health care providers and teams meet the complex health care needs of people with chronic conditions. HIT can be used to establish and track care plans and patient goals, to provide resources for patient self-management, to facilitate communication, to manage populations, and to measure and improve quality. This chapter discusses the role of HIT in care coordination, reviews research on the efficacy of HIT systems for care coordination, and outlines specific HIT functions that support care coordination. These critical functions are: clinical summaries; structured, flexible assessments; self-management support; prioritization of clinical tasks and patient needs; and population management. These functions require robust system features that support targeted reminders and facilitate ongoing communication. Existing standards, implementation barriers and facilitators, and opportunities for practices to adopt these functions are also discussed.

Problems addressed through effective HIT use

Fundamental problems

Health information technology is a powerful tool for addressing challenges to the effective delivery of coordinated care, including: complexity of patients' needs; fragmentation of

Comprehensive Care Coordination for Chronically Ill Adults, First Edition. Edited by Cheryl Schraeder and Paul Shelton.
© 2011 John Wiley & Sons, Inc. Published 2011 by John Wiley & Sons, Inc.

the health care system; awareness of patients' needs for such services; and timeliness of appropriate care delivery.

Complexity of need

Complex health care needs require significant, ongoing medical treatment and/or intensive self- or caregiver-management. Patients with such needs include those with multiple chronic illnesses, vulnerable elders, and those with social, economic, or environmental barriers coupled with at least one medical condition. For these groups, the risks of preventable complications and utilization are high.

Patients with chronic illnesses account for approximately 75% of health care expenditures (Hoffman *et al.* 1996), yet they only receive appropriate treatment about 50% of the time (McGlynn *et al.* 2003). These problems are exacerbated for patients with multiple chronic illnesses: a patient with five or more illnesses on Medicare will see 15 different outpatient physicians and fill 50 prescriptions per year (Anderson & Horvath 2002). Patients experience exponential increases in the risk of hospitalizations as the number of conditions rise (Wolff *et al.* 2002). As the number of transitions between providers and settings grows, so does the risk of harm from inadequate information transfer and reconciliation of treatment plans. Such risks are a large part of the reason that 10% of beneficiaries account for a disproportionate 63.5% of Medicare expenditures (Kaiser Family Foundation 2009). These costs could be significantly reduced through better care coordination and primary care (Wolff *et al.* 2002). Health information technology can be used to track both the many interactions with the health care system and the ongoing care plans and risks to patients to avoid unnecessary utilization.

Fragmentation of the health care system

The health care system can be complex and difficult to access. When patients with complex needs seek care from urgent locations (for example, the emergency department [ED] and hospital) for routine care or for conditions that could be more optimally addressed in less expensive settings, health care costs increase without an improvement in quality. Patients, families, and caregivers are challenged by the enormous number of provider communications and medical treatment plan changes that they are expected to follow and track (Dorr 2009). A care coordination team and information system can help patients and caregivers navigate the complex health care system by combining care plans from multiple providers, providing links to community resources, and ensuring that high-risk patients receive timely, recommended care and avoid unnecessary and costly services in the hospital or ED. Care coordinators work with patients to improve self-management skills, to define health care goals and take more ownership of their own care, and to reduce their reliance on acute emergency medical services. The tracking and documentation capabilities provided by a HIT system help maintain updated patient records and allow for health information exchange among different providers and settings. Funding for Health Information Exchanges in the American Recovery and Reinvestment Act of 2009 has led to a flurry of activity; while this will enhance the transfer of accurate, targeted information to various care settings, which should result in improved communication and decreased duplication of services, changing the broader health care system to fill in the gaps will be necessary to see more substantial reductions in fragmentation.

Awareness

The fragmentation of the health care system produces significant challenges to ensuring that all members of a patient's care team are kept fully informed about changes in the patient's status. The development of a reliable coordination system is challenged by the diversity of gaps in communication, including considerations involving local system infrastructure, socioeconomic situations, family or social supports, and patient preferences (Dorr 2009). Communication gaps can be lessened through the use of flexible HIT functions to keep health care team members informed about unique patient situations across spatial and temporal divides.

System fragmentation and communication gaps often encourage a focus primarily on the patient's acute needs, to the detriment of ongoing concerns. Patients with chronic conditions may not receive the care they need if there are no mechanisms to remind them or their care teams about evidence-based care recommendations that are important, but not urgent. Without consistent follow-up with a health care team that addresses chronic as well as acute issues, patients may be unaware of necessary preventative tests or self-management activities. HIT can help remind both clinicians and patients about recommended care processes.

Timeliness

Awareness of the patient's current conditions and of recommended interventions is important, but this information is only useful if acted upon in a timely manner. Advanced HIT systems can support providers in reminding patients about timely preventative care and assessments. Thoughtfully implemented clinical decision support tools "provide the right information, to the right person, in the right format, through the right channel, at the right point in workflow to improve health and health care decisions and outcomes" (Osheroff *et al.* 2007).

These timely reminders and decision supports can be provided through functions such as on-screen alerts, interpretative clinical summaries, protocols with branching logic, or automatic patient reminders. Such reminders can play an important role in ensuring that the limited time in each encounter is used to address chronic as well as acute conditions. One general focus of care coordination is to provide such preventative and proactive services to patients, ensuring awareness of necessary tests and reminding of upcoming encounters.

More advanced problems that HIT may help solve

Aside from addressing the fundamental issues in current health care delivery delineated above, advanced HIT use can also support solutions to a number of other problems.

Patient preferences

Truly patient-centered care delivery demands a number of other transformations in clinical culture beyond implementation of HIT (Berwick 2009). Technical systems can support patient-centered care efforts in a number of ways. Systems can store information for providers about patients' priorities, goals, and family support situations. This can enable members of the care coordination team to tailor their recommendations and communications to what is important to the patient, increasing investment in and satisfaction from the patient-provider relationship. By providing reminders through methods the patient prefers, and communicating with a patient's caregivers or family when the record indicates, care teams can increase the likelihood of patient compliance with care plans.

High level quality and efficiency

Advanced HIT systems provide a clinic-wide view of care quality. Quality measure reports that interface with patient records give care teams an interactive, real-time view of clinic quality and areas for improvement. Systems may provide feedback about prioritization, allow tracking of more complex tasks, and facilitate complex population management in a number of ways. Although performance systems alone may or may not improve clinical quality (Werner & Asch 2005), public reporting on *process improvement* measures is associated with quality improvements in patient outcomes in hospital settings (Werner & Bradlow 2006; Werner & Bradlow 2010).

Equity

Quality reports and resulting clinical improvement processes, together with HIT-supported protocols and decision support, can indirectly improve treatment equity. Such functions can aid the clinic in ensuring that patients in similar situations receive similar recommendations. Additionally, advanced systems can facilitate team management of complex care coordination pathways that might otherwise burden persons with lower health literacy or social support.

The problem HIT can never solve

HIT is a tool that is limited by its programming, implementation and use. Systems of care that are dysfunctional prior to HIT implementation will remain dysfunctional after implementation. In fact, HIT implementation often forces a series of decisions about how to restructure care that may lead to worse outcomes if not done properly. For example, Han *et al.* (2005) found an unexplained increase in mortality in pediatric intensive care units after implementation of an Electronic Health Record system. Though some studies have shown the potential of computerized physician order entry systems to substantially reduce medication errors (Kohn *et al.* 2000; Longhurst *et al.* 2010), they can also pose risks of being ineffective or even causing novel errors (Koppel *et al.* 2005; Reckmann *et al.* 2009). A study of 62 hospitals found that computerized physician order entry detected only half of potentially fatal medication orders and 10% to 82% of orders that would have caused adverse events (Metzger *et al.* 2010), with wide variation between hospitals.

Poor integration of HIT tools into existing workflows or inadequate clinician practice with the new computerized tools can result in neutral or negative outcomes in any of the same areas where HIT offers opportunities for improvement (DesRoches *et al.* 2010). Re-designing delivery to improve care coordination is fundamental to practice improvement, and any HIT implementation should be done as part of a model of care that addresses the broader issues of process, workflow, and patient need. When adopting HIT functions to improve care coordination efforts, system functions must be considered in the overall context of the individual users, the clinical team, and the organizational structure (Callen *et al.* 2008). Processes must be in place for evaluating and negating unintended consequences (Harrison *et al.* 2007). Considerations for effective implementation strategies are discussed in more detail below.

Definitions

Care coordination

In this book, care coordination is defined as a set of activities which assists patients and their families in: self-managing their health conditions and related psychosocial problems more effectively; coordinating their care among multiple health and community providers; bridging gaps in care; and receiving the appropriate level of care. Health information technology should support this set of activities. The following sections describe the HIT functions necessary to successfully implement a care coordination program based in a primary care clinic.

Health information technology systems, models, and benefits

General

Health information technologies, such as electronic health records, computerized provider order entry, clinical decision support alerts, and electronic messaging systems, are widely considered critical to health delivery system transformation (Chaudhry *et al.* 2006). HIT functions and implementation contexts vary widely, but are broadly defined as electronic technologies used to store, view, interpret, and analyze health information for clinical care and health service delivery.

Electronic health record (EHR)

Electronic health records (EHRs) are comprehensive databases for storage of patients' clinical and other health information. EHRs typically include built-in functions for computerized provider order entry, clinical decision support, and other HIT functions that have shown varying levels of benefit (Wears & Berg 2005; Longhurst *et al.* 2010). Clinical decision support systems can improve provider performance, especially when the system automatically prompts users without activation (Garg *et al.* 2005). Though some have debated the efficacy of computerized provider order entry (Han *et al.* 2005; Metzger *et al.* 2010), several studies have demonstrated decreased adverse drug events (Bates *et al.* 1998) and mortality rates (Longhurst *et al.* 2010) when the system is carefully implemented with attention to the context of use.

Personal health record (PHR)

Personal health records provide patient access to individual health data over time and care settings. PHRs may allow access to only limited pieces of patient health information, such as lab tests and upcoming appointments, or they may have more advanced functions, such as secure messaging systems for communication with providers or access to diagnostic imaging results. Some systems also allow the patient to delegate PHR access to other family members or caregivers.

Care management information systems

Specialized HIT systems can be used to support nurse-based care management of patients with complex conditions and/or chronic illness (Dorr *et al.* 2006b; Dorr *et al.* 2007a). A meta-analysis for delivery system redesign for patients with diabetes showed nurse care managers and team reorganization were the changes most successful at improving quality; information technology alone was only moderately successful (Shojania *et al.* 2006). Patients with schizophrenia benefitted from care management supported by HIT (Young *et al.* 2004). Models focused on care management of older adults with complex needs, combined with HIT tools, have shown reductions in hospitalizations and ED visits (Dorr *et al.* 2005; Dorr *et al.* 2007a; Dorr *et al.* 2008). Elements of these systems, as they apply to care coordination, are discussed below.

Telemedicine and telemonitoring

For patients in remote settings, telemedicine may help provide self-management support, personalized care, or other skill-based care coordination elements directly to their homes or to the remote primary care practices in the area. For instance, telemedicine systems can help remote practitioners manage complex protocol-based programs for unusual conditions (Arora *et al.* 2010). Self-management support using peer-support models has been shown to be effective in improving patient-centered outcomes (Lorig *et al.* 2008).

HIT functions to support effective care coordination

Overview

Studies of care coordination models and principles have highlighted the special require-ments and benefits of HIT for the care of patients with complex needs. A review of more than 100 systems identified key elements for the systematic and meaningful use of HIT to bridge some of the health system gaps discussed above (Wilcox *et al.* 2005; Dorr *et al.*

Table 7.1 Summary of IT Functions of Clinical Summaries

Areas of Implementation	IT Functions
Structured Overview of Patient Health Information	Summarize diagnoses, risks, medications, assessments, and labs. Outline care plan, including interventions and recommendations. Allow electronic access by CC, PCP, and/or other specialists. Provide printable format for care conferences and appointments.
Patient Summary Sheet	Provide printable format of the overview for patients and families. Facilitate patient understanding (at appropriate health literacy level). Include lists of diagnoses, medications, reminders for upcoming appointments, and preventative care recommendations.
Care Setting Transitions	Allow electronic access by other care settings. Track admission and discharge dates. Supply structured protocol for post-hospitalization and post-ED follow-up.

2007b). Effective care coordination systems include several critical HIT functions: clinical summaries; structured, flexible assessments and processes; self-management support with follow-up; prioritization; and population management. The system capabilities central to the efficacy of each of these functions are targeted reminders and communication.

Clinical summaries

An electronic clinical summary of a patient provides a snapshot overview of a patient's status, including risk factors, diagnoses, medications, assessments, preventative care recommendations, and reminders of upcoming care actions.

Structured overview of patient health information

The system should provide access to fundamental patient information, such as demographics, diagnoses, medications, assessment, and lab results. Gathering all of this data into one system in a structured, logical interface is critical to efficient access by the care coordinator and medical team. This feature should also include a recorded care plan for the patient's ongoing interventions and assessments, including recommendations, goals set by the patient and provider, and upcoming appointments or other tests.

Patient summary sheet

A printable, patient-friendly version of the clinical summary at the appropriate health literacy level gives the care team a tool for discussing health issues with the patient. A Patient Summary Sheet outlines when a patient should receive appropriate treatment or

Patient Worksheet

Binnes, Harry	PRINT

MRN: 1324234   **Sex:** M   **DOB:** 01/24/1956
Phone: 9874584587   **PCP:** Parnel Fieldman
Care Manager: Susie Example   **Caregiver:**

Next Care Management Encounter

No Records Found

Last Care Management Encounter

Sched Date	Sched Time	Encounter Type
01/06/2010	09:00 AM	CM Office Visit

Diagnoses

Thyroid Disease, Hypertension, Diabetes, Chronic Pain

Medications

Medication	Dosage	PRN	Med Start Date
albuterol		☐	08/07/2008

Goals

Status	Follow Up Date	Goal	Note	score	Set Date
Completed	12/21/2009	Nutrition		10	12/05/2009
Completed	12/21/2009	Activity		5	12/05/2009
Completed	11/13/2009	Activity		6	11/13/2009
Completed	11/13/2009	Nutrition		8	11/13/2009
Pending		Meds			10/06/2009

PHQ

Date	PH2 Score	PHQ9 - Severity	Q9 Suicide	Followup
12/02/2009	6	25	3	
11/05/2009	3	17	3	12/04/2009
07/07/2009		10	2	
07/02/2009			0	

Functional Status

Date	ADL	IADL	MMSE	Pain
07/08/2009			2	9
12/11/2009				

Care Actions

Diabetes	Date/Value	Status
A1c in Last 6 mo	09/30/2009	OK
A1c < 7	7.3	A1c out of Range
LDL Last Year	03/30/2009	OK
LDL < 100	55	OK

Preventative Care	Date/Value	Status
Patient >= 65 need Pneumovax at least once	06/20/2008	NO
Patient > 50 needs flu shot at least once	09/10/2009	NO

Last Doctor's Appointment	Status
02/02/2010	OK

Figure 7.1   A Patient Summary Sheet

monitoring, required lab work, and medications; it contains a problem list, structured medications list, and patient-specific goals and assessments. This record may be given to the patient and family as a printed clinical summary or sent electronically, or both. It provides a valuable self-management tool for the patient to reference for reminders of health promotion activities and preventative care actions such as immunizations, mammograms, prostate exams, nutrition, diet, or exercise classes.

The patient summary sheet provides a solid foundation for behavioral modification, disease- or medication-specific education, and motivational health coaching with the patient, as well as a starting point for effective pre-visit planning in team-based care. Since the amount of information to be reviewed with patients with complex conditions can often be extensive, a patient summary sheet can facilitate discussion of quality metrics, preventive needs, and care planning. In one study, voluntary use of this summary sheet by clinical teams improved process and outcome quality measures by 17% to 30% (Wilcox *et al.* 2005). HIT self-management tools support health improvement goals when embedded in models of patient-centered care that motivate and facilitate their use (Dorr *et al.* 2006b; Dorr *et al.* 2007a); without such models, there is little evidence that clinics can achieve improved outcomes.

Care setting transitions

Clinical summaries are valuable for patient care transitions to another provider or an ED or hospital setting. An electronic or printed summary should be sent with the patient to provide the other setting with the proper background to properly treat the patient and contact information to report results or outcomes back to the primary care coordination team.

In some situations, electronic referrals for specialist consultation may be adequate to answer a patient's or primary care provider's questions. A specialist can sometimes make a recommendation or diagnosis based on descriptions, diagnostic images, and lab results provided via the HIT system. This process improves the efficiency and timeliness of care for all involved (O'Malley *et al.* 2009). Technical specifications, such as the Continuity of Care Record standard, facilitate electronic sharing of information, which supports the reconciliation and continuation of care plans and adherence to patient preferences.

Structured, flexible assessments & processes

A number of medical, psychosocial, and functional assessments provide the foundation for patient-centered care coordination. Protocols should provide structured but flexible guidance for clinical care (Dorr *et al.* 2006a).

Structured encounter form

Given the vast variety of information that must be communicated to and from the patient and recorded during each interaction, a structured encounter form – available during face-to-face and phone encounters – is a core component of an IT system that supports care coordination. The advanced encounter form may function as a checklist for encounters by organizing and prioritizing communication that must be relayed and gathered during interactions between the patient and members of the care coordination team. Important components, such as primary language, preferences, or health literacy, may be tracked in such a way to allow future users to be immediately reminded of them in the next encounter. Advanced functions on the form might include the availability of reminders and feedback about next steps in the care plan, interface for scheduling the next encounter, or health

Table 7.2   Overview of Features for Assessment and Protocol Process Support in an HIT System

Areas of Implementation	IT Functions
Structured Encounter Form	Provide feedback about next steps and recommendations.
	Organize and prioritize information.
	Document communications and visits between any members of care team.
	Fulfill documentation criteria for records and billing.
	Serve as guideline for protocols.
	Track future appointments.
Medication Management	Support medication reconciliation at every encounter.
	Track encounters between CC and pharmacist.
	Provide printable comprehensive medication list.
	Identify and track barriers to medication adherence.
	Track prescription fills.
Assessments for Health, Psychosocial, and Functional Status	Support adherence to evidence-based guidelines.
	Furnish easy-to-fill forms with structured data entry.
	Update easily to document changes in patient status.
	Allow electronic access by CC, PCP, and/or other specialists.
	Provide printable format for flexible use.

promotion protocols. The form should also provide immediate decision support about the completeness of documentation, to aid in the workflow and ensure that documentation requirements are fulfilled for each encounter. High value activities, such as motivational interviewing, education, goal-setting, self-management support, and care conferences, should be tracked individually to see their contribution to the care and health of the person.

The HIT system should also facilitate tracking communication activities with other providers as necessary, either using a flexible encounter form or some other feature. Care conferences and other communication activities between the care coordinator and the primary care provider will be necessary to relay information regarding patient status, goals, and any modifications to protocols or care plans. The care coordinator should also track communications with other care team members, such as pharmacists, mental health providers, community resources, and patient's family members or caregivers.

Medication management

Medication reconciliation and prescribing accuracy are critical to care safety. Having protocols to ensure that clinicians update medication lists with patients and caregivers, document medication discrepancies, and reconcile all relevant records helps reduce the likelihood of adverse events (Lesselroth *et al.* 2009). HIT systems can improve the process dramatically, from querying the patient about current adherence and starting reconciliation to gathering data about medication on-hand from prescription fill records.

Patients with five or more chronic conditions fill nearly 50 prescriptions per year on average (Anderson & Horvath 2002). The HIT system must have the functionality to create and print a comprehensive medication list to ensure that the medication list is accurate and updated regularly. The printable feature allows the medication list to be given to the patient to ensure accurate communication of medication purpose, dosage, and frequency. This medication list should be available to the care coordinator, primary care physician, specialists, hospitals, the patient, and the patient's caregiver or family members (with patient's permission). Transitions between different care settings can be greatly facilitated by ensuring that all parties are provided an accurate medication list. This list is also a tool for the care coordinator to help identify barriers to prescription refills and medication adherence. An advanced system should have the capability of tracking prescription refill dates and coordinate refill dates of all prescriptions to decrease multiple pickup dates and increase adherence. To this end, the system should also be able to track communication between the care coordinator and the pharmacist, whether in the medication information interface of in the encounter form. The advanced system will also be able to track medication reconciliation steps taken and adjustments made.

Assessments for health, psychosocial, and functional status

The HIT system should include built-in forms for assessment of patients' medical, psychosocial, and other needs. Such assessments might include the Patient Health Questionnaire Depression Scale (PHQ9; a nine-item screen used to identify and rate depression severity), mini-mental status examination, or other cognitive evaluations, self-management and medical literacy evaluations, functional assessments such as activities of daily living or instrumental activities of daily living, and forms to record family pattern profile, caregiver contacts, and other social-support information. While data entry of responses should be structured, assessments should also provide a flexible field for extra patient-specific notes. These assessment results should be able to be tracked over time and accessible to all members of the care team. Where applicable, they should also include clinical decision support alerts to ensure that notable results are not overlooked.

Self-management support with follow-up

Care coordinators work with patients to increase their abilities to self-manage their conditions, resulting in healthier behaviors, better medical outcomes, and enhanced quality of life. Self-management skills empower patients to take more ownership of their care and set goals to keep them engaged in health maintenance activities. The benefits of improved self-management may persist beyond the time that the team is involved, accounting for better outcomes even years later.

Table 7.3   Examples of IT Functions to Support Self-Management Training and Follow-Up Activities

Areas of Implementation	IT Functions
Goal-Setting	Facilitate interactive updates and modifications.
	Allow electronic access by CC, PCP, and/or other specialists.
	List recommended self-management activities.
	Track long-term and short-term goals.
Electronic Patient Access	Allow electronic access to clinical summary and goals.
	Facilitate updates and questions to and from patients.
	Remind patients about follow-up appointments, laboratory and other tests, and pending tasks.
Social and Educational Resources	Supply printable educational resources and other materials that can be shared with patients.
	Access availability and requirements of community and social support programs.
	Remind about available health promotion activities.

Goal-setting support

Goal-setting is critical to motivation for health self-maintenance among older patients with multiple challenging illnesses. The IT system must be able to create and track in a structured way both short- and long-term goals. These goals could be related to patient self-management activities, behavior changes, or lifestyle adjustments. The system should provide an interactive goal-setting form that can be modified and updated as the patient's priorities and needs change. The goal record should be accessible by all members of the care team, including the care coordinator, primary care physician, specialists, and pharmacists, social workers, or others, as needed. Ideally, the patient would have electronic access to this goal information, but at minimum, the goal list should be printable to promote patient self-management and enable sharing with caregivers and family members. The ability to share this goal-setting form promotes stronger communication among all members of the care team, enhancing the patient's support system to help achieve these goals.

Electronic patient access

Enabling electronic patient access to the clinical summary will aid in self-management by facilitating reminders and updates to and from the patient. Such access may come in the form of a personal electronic health record populated through the clinic's EHR. The patient interface should allow the patient to view diagnoses, medications, and reminders or updates about recommendation and future encounters. Electronic access to the static patient summary sheet or care plan is a solid starting point. Ideally, the access interface should be more interactive and dynamic, allowing for two-way messaging between the patient and care team members. For instance, it could permit patients to upload test results (such as glucose readings for diabetics) or update goal progress for ongoing clinical monitoring. The system could support a simple workflow for review and integration of patient-supplied data into the primary medical record.

Social and educational resources

The HIT system should provide reminders of and access to information regarding electronic or community-based patient social support and educational resources. This may include links to printable diagnosis fact sheets, contact information for local support groups, or other resources to support the patient's self-management efforts. For example, integrating information about the availability and eligibility requirements of social support programs – such as discounted access to exercise facilities, support groups, or meals-on-wheels programs – into the system would help clinicians offer such services to appropriate patients. To enable such information access, the system must provide a flexible interface for recording local opportunities for easy reference by the care team. The system should record referrals and materials provided to the patient in the care plan, and provide reminders to the care coordinator to follow-up with the patient regarding their efficacy or helpfulness. Some self-management programs are now exclusively online and based on evidence of effectiveness from previous studies (Gremeaux & Coudeyre 2010). Integration of the monitoring and evaluation components of such programs would be an advanced addition to a system.

Prioritization

HIT tools enable providers to break the cycle of fragmented care by regularly identifying and high priority and neglected health care issues. Prioritization of care coordination services must take place on three scales: the clinic level, the panel level, and the individual patient level.

Table 7.4 Overview of Features to Support Prioritization Activities in an HIT System

Areas of Implementation	IT Functions
Risk Stratification List	Support algorithm for selecting high-risk patients.
	Provide a consistent methods to identify and refer patients.
	Generate lists of patients by risk stratification measures, enrollment status, and diagnoses.
Patient-Focused Prioritization	Outline systematic process for working with patients to determine priorities.
	Document priorities, preferences, and goals.
	Furnish adjustable care plans that accommodate patient needs and preferences.

Quality measure selection and improvement cycles

At the broadest level, the clinical team must first delineate priorities for the focus of the care coordination program. The clinic's priorities are embodied in the selection of quality measures, a set of criteria that aide in quantifying improvement of clinical foci through the care coordination program. These choices, along with updated clinical processes and outcomes measures, can be documented and tracked in the HIT system to evaluate longitudinal improvement. Interactive quality measure reports, a population management tool discussed in more detail below, support and reinforce this continuous quality improvement process. Clinical team members should be involved early on in the prioritization of quality improvement areas and measures, as their engagement in and commitment to the quality improvement process is requisite for success. Over time, clinical teams may undertake Plan-Do-Study-Act quality improvement cycles to better their performance on these metrics (Institute for Healthcare Improvement 2010).

Risk stratification list

At the patient population level, prioritization is manifest in risk stratification lists that are based on the quality measures chosen at the clinic level. Assessments of risk level can be done organically in provider meetings with patients or more systematically using a risk stratification algorithm – or, ideally, using a combination of both approaches to address a variety of clinic and patient needs. Using patient records and billing data, HIT systems can use predictive algorithms to establish and maintain a list of patients with great potential to benefit from the care coordination program. Such risk determination can be developed from one or a combination of patient factors, including but not limited to: number and severity of chronic conditions, past hospitalizations, past emergency department utilization, concerning assessment or lab results, family history of certain conditions, or total cost of the patient to the health care system. Based on quality improvement goals, risk stratification helps to select patients to receive focused interventions in the care coordination program and patients to call in first for proactive care improvement. HIT systems should be able to track all assignment methods and planned next steps. The system should also have the capacity to track enrollment status in the care coordination program and the date and source of referrals.

Patient-focused prioritization

Depending on the nature of the program implemented, a care coordinator may provide care for anywhere from 50 to 350 patients. Not only must the care coordinator determine which patients to focus on for interventions, but the coordinator must also determine which issues to focus on first for each patient. The care coordinator must spend time working with the patient (and the patient's family, or caregivers, when applicable) to design and implement a prioritized care plan that focuses on improvement in clinical quality measures and in areas most important to the patient. Developing a care plan involves basic prioritization of health issues, ongoing concerns, and goals, as well as preventative care recommendations and lifestyle changes. This process and resulting care actions can help improve underlying conditions, solidify self-management skills, and enhance overall quality of life for the patient. HIT features to facilitate this process include focused patient protocols, which provide guidance for diagnosis-specific care priorities, and structured forms for establishing and tracking patient goals and preferences. The ability to track the responses to questions such as *What is your biggest concern about your health?* or *What is your most important goal for your health?* is a crucial function of these systems.

Population management

Health Information Technology tools empower the care team to better monitor the statuses and needs of an entire patient population. With so many patients to manage, the ability to identify, categorize, and track tasks and recommended interventions is critical to the care coordinator's daily work flow. Thorough documentation in care plans ensures that all members of the clinical team are current on the patient's status and ensures the accuracy of quality measure reports.

Registries and quality reports

Quality reports are a primary output of advanced HIT systems. As implemented, few EHRs provide quality reports without additional modules and technical support. The creation of population registries is one technique that enables quality reporting from an ambulatory-based HIT. Registries extract data from EHRs and other HIT systems for use in quality reports. A registry reorganizes the data, abstracts it to the correct granularity, and creates a population snapshot that can be used to understand the current performance on a variety of quality measures. Common examples include aggregating all the billing diagnoses for diabetes to create a single list of patients with diabetes, capturing the most recent date and value for all patients with a particular lab test, or creating a list of each primary care provider's patients.

Table 7.5   HIT Functions That Support Population Management Activities

Areas of Implementation	IT Functions
Quality Reports	Track quality measures from evidence-based guidelines.
	Produce specific reports by patient population, provider, care team, and clinic.
Care Coordinator Task Tracking	Identify gaps in completion of tasks.
	Document frequency, duration, mode and outcome of contacts.
Generic Care Plans and Protocols	List specific activities, tasks, goals, and progress on each.
	Generate templates for different diagnoses.
	Remind about pre-planned frequency of encounters.
	Be electronically accessible to CC, PCP, and/or other specialists.

Quality Measures									
Select another Measure									
Selected Measure: HbA1c < 7.0% (18+)									
Total: 1121									Print
Value Adherence Rate: 52.542%				Date Adherence Rate: 56.021%					
Update									Update
No Longer in Practice	Schedule Follow Up Encounter	Patient	Patient Phone	PCP	Quality Item	Result	Date of Result	Exclude from ALL Diabetes Measures	Exclude from this Measure ONLY
☐	☐	Doe, Ally B	6430987543	Cooligan, James	A1C	7.3	09/30/2009	☐	☐
☐	☐	Doe, Helga S	6437661279	Cooligan, James	A1C	8.8	12/07/2009	☐	☐
☐	☐	Doe, Ian A	6438754973	Michum, Karen	A1C	7.0	11/10/2009	☐	☐
☐	☐	Doe, Morgan F	6437750984	Cooligan, James	A1C	6.2	11/20/2009	☐	☐
☐	☐	Doe, Robert P	6433887625	Hariswald, Douglass	A1C	7.2	01/15/2009	☐	☐
☐	☐	Doe, Veronica P	6435487360	Michum, Karen	A1C			☐	☐

Figure 7.2   Example of a Clinical Quality Measure Report

However, registries with static reports may not be adequate for ongoing care improvement initiatives. Interactive quality reports (Figure 7.2) allow members of the care team to easily and quickly generate outreach tasks for high-risk patients. The reports also aid clinicians in continuous and accurate evaluation of clinical quality improvement by allowing exclusions from a particular measure to respect patient preferences and acknowledge unique situations. This built-in flexibility supports the integrity of the quality measure reports for use in quality improvement cycles.

To be effective in improving provider performance, HIT systems must be able to store, make accessible, and translate relevant data into *context-specific* information (Shekelle *et al.* 2006). One example of such a process in care coordination is the capacity of the HIT system to store lab results, display the results in an interactive quality report, give the care coordinator access to that information, and then allow immediate action based on that information, such as scheduling follow-up appointments or sending reminders for patients out of the recommended result range. The ability to generate and use such reports is broadly associated with improvement in outcomes and process (Dorr *et al.* 2007a). An advanced system will provide a quality measure interface that can filter patient populations based on diagnosis, clinical team assignment or care coordination program enrollment. An ideal system would allow the care team to interact with the quality report to note necessary follow-up tasks directly on the report screen. This can be accomplished by checking a box or clicking a button to add a patient from the report to a follow-up call or encounter list.

Care coordinator task tracking

The system must then provide a mechanism for tracking these follow-up tasks, as well as recording encounters scheduled for other reasons. An HIT system should have the ability to track information about each encounters completed by the care coordinator and other team members: with whom the encounter was completed (patient, family member,

Care Manager Encounter Tickler List

Care Manager: ◄— All —► ▾ Start Date: 07/04/2010 End Date: 08/04/2010 Run

Care Manager: All Care Managers
For Time Period: 07/04/2009 to 08/10/2010

Scheduled Date	Scheduled Time	Encounter Type	Reason	EHR ID	First Name	Last Name	Phone	PCP	Notes
2010-08-04		Email/Letter/Fax	Connections to Resources	978253344	Timothy	Hartline	456.235.1125	Carl Generic	
2010-08-03		MD Office Visit	Diabetes	4564444	Jenny	Gibbs	456.235.1499	Carl Generic	
2010-07-20	09:00	CM Office Visit	Goals	0999909999	David	Owen		Carl Generic	Goals Follow-Up: Other: Patient to have an up-to-date Advanced Directive in his medical record;
2010-07-12	10:45	Telephone Contact	Coordination of Care	0999909999	David	Owen		Carl Generic	Follow-up call to discuss the Nutritional Consult Appointment with patient
2010-06-18		Telephone Contact	Clinical Protocol(s)	65748398	Bobby	Cline	987.546.7765	Hillary Caseman	Quality Measure: Diabetes : Lab Date:
2010-06-18		Telephone Contact	Clinical Protocol(s)	8633302	Constance	Desmond	455.635.2536	Carl Generic	Quality Measure: Diabetes : Lab Date:
2010-06-18		Telephone Contact	Clinical Protocol(s)	4987651	Jerry	Montoya	456.2539.8589	Carl Generic	Quality Measure: Diabetes : Lab Date:

Figure 7.3   A Sample "Tickler" List

caregiver, other specialist, social worker, and so on); the location of the encounter (clinic office, hospital, home visit); the duration of various encounter tasks (time spent reviewing charts, meeting with the patient, coordinating resources or specialist care); and outcome or next steps from the encounter. The system should also be able to provide general reports on the frequency, duration, mode, and outcome of contacts. Reports on time spent on various tasks give an overall sense of the resources used to care for the population.

A tickler list (Figure 7.3) is a critical feature in the workflow, allowing the care coordinator to view all encounters for a given time period. This interface should allow the care coordinator or other care team member to track completion of each encounter and to make notes for future reference or appointment documentation. Ideally, a system could identify missed encounters and remind about care plan actions established in past assessments, encounters, or the overall care plan.

Generic care plans and protocols

Flexible, diagnosis-specific protocols and care plans facilitate more efficient and evidence-based care for managing a large population of patients with complex needs. Such features list specific activities, tasks, or goals that are generally recommended for patients with a given diagnosis, providing care coordinators with an interactive template for designing care plans for patients in the program. Such templates could either be available for care coordinators to include in the care plan at their discretion, or automatically populate to a patient's care plan upon diagnosis (with the option for later edits). Decision support features that automatically prompt users are more likely to improve provider performance (Garg *et al.* 2005). Implementation of HIT has a largely positive effect on adherence to guidelines, documentation of diagnostic criteria, and completion of appropriate screening and testing process measures. General reference protocols should be available to all members of the care team within the HIT system, as care plan documentation is a key component of effective collaborative care (Dorr *et al.* 2007b).

Reminders

Timely and appropriate reminders are critical to supporting all of the above functions of the care coordination system. The HIT system should generate reminders for the care coordinator regarding scheduling of future patient encounters, diagnostic and regular lab testing, and specialist or other referral follow-up activities. After population analyses are performed and activities undergo a prioritization process, adding tasks to the encounter tickler provides the care coordinator with a centralized reminder list. This proactive process is crucial to ensure care coordination tasks are completed and patients and families are engaged through the process. Systems should also be able to automatically send reminders to patients about upcoming appointments, labs, prescription refills, or other recommendations.

Health IT can also provide clinical decision support for recommended interventions and the availability of health promotion activities or resources. Clinical decision support reminders can increase the adherence to recommended preventative testing schedules and medication guidelines (Agostini *et al.* 2008; Graber & Mathew 2008). Such alerts should be adaptable to priorities and preferences to avoid user fatigue. As well, for patients with multiple chronic conditions, there may be many potential preventive and chronic care recommended services, and alerts that distract or interrupt the workflow may cause serious distraction and potential harm. For complex needs, "passive" reminders – so called because they do not interrupt workflow – may be far superior to "active" or pop-up alerts.

Communication

Communication facilitation is key to the efficacy of all of the above functions. Communication is both a necessary function of the HIT system to support care coordination and a prerequisite of its successful implementation (Ash 1997). Communications among patients and members of the care team can be facilitated through a number of features, including secure electronic messaging systems, alerts about test results, notification of reviews from other care team members, or patient access to medical records. More and more patients now prefer to use e-mail to communicate with their physicians (Slack 2004), underlining the importance of developing robust electronic messaging systems that fit within the clinical workflow. Timely and accurate communication supports care-team awareness and bridges some of the gaps caused by a fragmented medical delivery system.

Functions as parts of the integrated whole

The ideal HIT system for supporting coordinated care does not merely have each of these functions, compartmentalized into individual screens. Rather, each of these features should be seamlessly integrated to form a comprehensive patient record (for example, with supporting reminder systems and communication mechanisms). One example of these functions in a high-performance HIT care coordination system might be translating stored lab results into an action item in the quality measure interactive report, giving clinical staff prompt and easy access to this information (including specific lab result values) and empowering them to immediately schedule follow-up appointments or reminders with the patients identified in the report, all without ever leaving the screen. The care coordinator can then go back and review a list of these scheduled appointments or view the detail for each individual encounter to see that specific patient's quality measure improvement status. This kind of integration supports a continuous workflow where HIT naturally aides the clinician's care coordination efforts.

HIT system care coordination standards

Many of these HIT functions do already exist in industry standards: the Continuity of Care Document focuses on information summarization to improve the safety of transitions; the Health Level 7 (HL-7) Electronic Health Record System functional model contains many of these functions (Dorr *et al.* 2007b); the Healthcare Information Technology Standards Panel (HITSP) has adopted a set of measures for care coordination in category IS02; and finally, the regulations released by the Office of the National Coordinator for Health Information Technology requires a small subset of these functions for EHR certification (Office of the National Coordinator for Health Information [ONC] 2010). The Standards and Certification final rule establishes standards for required EHR system features (ONC 2010), while another set of regulations outlines requirements to promote the meaningful use of these systems by providers (Centers for Medicare & Medicaid Services 2010). The Continuity of Care Record standard, developed by the American Society for Testing and Materials (ASTM), contains a set of useful categories to more easily transfer information from one setting of care to the next; these recommendations have been harmonized with the Clinical Document Architecture (CDA) standards to form the Continuity of Care Document (CCD) final standard (HL-7 2010). The CCD standard provides one possible framework for ensuring a patient summarization document can be exchanged across sites. Interoperability is fundamental to the efficient and effective use of HIT, and its future development is critical to the widespread success of care coordination efforts (Hersh 2004). Despite this research and the standards of development, adoption and implementation of these IT functions has been slow.

Implementation of HIT systems: facilitators and barriers

Successful HIT implementation is challenged by a number of barriers, including necessary changes in knowledge scope and attitudinal approaches, liability concerns, and institutional structures that may impede the reception of new technologies or workflows (Hersh 2004; Shekelle *et al.* 2006; Koppel & Kreda 2010). The lack of start-up funds, difficulty of system choice, and initial productivity losses can also be barriers in electronic health system implementations (Mostashari *et al.* 2009). HIT must be introduced thoughtfully, keeping in mind not just changes to the technology itself, but supporting adjustments that must be made in clinic workflows, roles, and orientations to primary care provision.

Clinical culture, team-based care and workflow redesign

Health IT can provide great benefits to clinics in supporting care coordination efforts, but only when combined with a systematic approach to broader models of change. In concert with the HIT system and care coordination program implementation, the health care team must acknowledge and embrace a paradigm shift to focus on team-based evaluation and quality improvement.

Success of HIT implementation is largely dependent upon clinical culture (Callen *et al.* 2009), the ways in which the system is introduced, and team members' readiness to change and to work with the new technology. Roles of all team members must be clearly defined to ensure an integrated, efficient workflow and effective, reliable communication (Dorr *et al.* 2006a). Office processes must be standardized, a change that both enables and depends upon HIT system implementation (O'Malley *et al.* 2009). A clear understanding of the appropriate responsibilities and vast potential benefit of the care coordination role(s) will ensure a smooth team transition to a new model of care with increased focus on proactive and patient-focused interventions. This role definition is especially critical when one or a few people in the clinic assume the primary care coordination responsibility.

Technology adoption in the clinical context

The Contextual Implementation Model provides a theoretical framework for understanding HIT adoption by focusing on diversity at the organizational, clinical, and individual levels. The model contends that analyses of the strengths and weaknesses at each level for supporting innovation should be performed prior to implementation attempts. These insights can be used to identify areas where additional training or institutional reorganization may be necessary (Callen *et al.* 2008).

The Model of Information Systems Success conceptualizes implementation factors according to five dimensions: system quality, information quality, use, user satisfaction, and impact. The impact of a system in an organization is directly related to the intentions, use and satisfaction of the users, which is influenced by the quality of the system and information content, as well as its perceived usefulness and ease of use (DeLone & McLean 1992; DeLone & McLean 2003).

Models such as these can inform clinical implementation efforts and lend theoretical understanding to challenges and successes in HIT adoption. HIT implementation failures are often attributable to a lack of understanding of the clinical environment (Leviss *et al.* 2010). Unintended consequences (Ash *et al.* 2004; Ash *et al.* 2007a; Ash *et al.* 2007b; Harrison *et al.* 2007) must be anticipated and mitigated through holistic clinical redesign. One key takeaway lesson is that organizational characteristics, including reward systems for performance, can cause either success or failure in implementing identical HIT systems in otherwise similar contexts. Participatory decision making, strong leaders, and accurate communication must be employed to ensure implementation success (Ash 1997).

Conclusion

Health information technology should include a set of critical functions that support and improve care coordination programs. From providing concise clinical summaries to self-management tools, many current HIT systems need careful modification and implementation to include all of the necessary functions. Facilitating prioritization and population management are particularly important functions that many transaction systems built for billing and documentation lack. Each function must be supported by targeted reminders and robust communication tools. The potential benefits of HIT are especially dramatic for care of patients with complex needs.

Barriers do exist to the successful implementation of these systems, including clinical cultures that resist change, the lack of reimbursement for high-value care coordination activities, the episodic, fragmented nature of health care, and the present focus on extensive, unstructured documentation. These barriers can be mitigated through careful consideration of clinical context in the implementation process, advocacy for new models of payment that support high-level care coordination activities, and HIT with structured documentation and reporting tools to support these processes and quality improvement initiatives. Current HIT can be rewired and new systems developed to fully meet these needs. With thoughtful implementation, HIT holds great potential for supporting the widespread and successful adoption of care coordination programs.

References

Agostini, J.V., Concato, J., & Inouye, S.K. (2008) Improving sedative-hypnotic prescribing in older hospitalized patients: provider-perceived benefits and barriers of a computer-based reminder. *Journal of General Internal Medicine*, 23(Supplement 1), 32–36.

Anderson, G., & Horvath, J. (2002) *Chronic Conditions: Making the Case for Ongoing Care.* Partnership for Solutions, Johns Hopkins University, Baltimore, MD.

Arora, S., Kalishman, S., Thornton, K., *et al.* (2010) Expanding access to hepatitis C virus treatment – extension for community healthcare outcomes (ECHO) project: disruptive innovation in specialty care. *Hepatology*, 52, 1124–1133.

Ash, J. (1997) Organizational factors that influence information technology diffusion in academic health sciences centers. *Journal of the American Medical Informatics Association*, 4, 102–111.

Ash, J.S., Berg, M., & Colera, E. (2004) Some unintended consequences of information technology in health care: the nature of patient care information system-related errors. *Journal of the American Medical Informatics Association*, 11, 104–112.

Ash, J.S., Sittig, D.F., Campbell, E.M., *et al.* (2007a) Some unintended consequences of clinical decision support systems. *American Medical Informatics Association Annual Symposium Proceedings*, 26–30.

Ash, J.S., Sittig, D.F., Dykstra, R., *et al.* (2007b) Exploring the unintended consequences of computerized physician order entry. *Medinfo*, 12, 198–202.

Bates, D.W., Leape, L.L., Cullen, D.J., *et al.* (1998) Effect of computerized physician order entry and a team intervention on prevention of serious medication errors. *Journal of the American Medical Association*, 280, 1311–1316.

Bates, D.W., Kuperman, G.J., Rittenberg, E., *et al.* (1999) A randomized trial of a computer-based intervention to reduce utilization of redundant laboratory tests. *American Journal of Medicine*, 106, 144–150.

Bates, D.W. (2002) The quality case for information technology in healthcare. *BMC Medical Informatics and Decision Making*, 2, 7.

Berwick, D.M. (2009) What "patient-centered" should mean: confessions of an internist. *Health Affairs*, 28, w555–565.

Blumenthal, D., & Glaser, J.P. (2007) Information technology comes to medicine. *New England Journal of Medicine*, 356, 2527–2534.

Callen, J., Braithwaite, J., & Westbrook, J.I. (2008) Contextual implementation model: a framework for assisting clinical information system implementations. *Journal of the American Medical Informatics Association*, 15, 255–262.

Callen, J., Braithwaite, J., & Westbrook, J.I. (2009) The importance of medical and nursing sub-cultures in the implementation of clinical information systems. *Methods of Information in Medicine*, 48, 196–202.

Cannon, D.S., & Allen, S.N. (2000) A comparison of the effects of computer and manual reminders on compliance with a mental health clinical practice guideline. *Journal of the American Medical Informatics Association*, 7, 196–203.

Centers for Medicare & Medicaid Services. (2010) *Medicare and Medicaid Electronic Health Record Incentive Program: Final Rule*. Centers for Medicare & Medicaid Services, Baltimore, MD. Available at: http://www.cms.gov/ehrincentiveprograms/.

Chaudhry, B., Wang, J., Wu, S., *et al.* (2006) Systematic review: impact of health information technology on quality, efficience, and costs of medical care. *Annals of Internal Medicine*, 144, 742–752.

DeLone, W.H., & McLean, E.R. (1992) Information systems success: the quest for the dependent variable. *Information Systems Research*, 3, 60–95.

DeLone, W.H., & McLean, E.R. (2003) The DeLone and McLean model of information systems success: a ten-year update. *Journal of Management Information Systems*, 19(1) 9–30.

Demakis, J.G., Beauchamp, C., Cull, W.L., *et al.* (2000) Improving residents' compliance with standards of ambulatory care: results from the VA cooperative study on computerized reminders. *Journal of the American Medical Association*, 284, 1411–1416.

DesRoches, C.M., Campbell, E.G., Vogeli, C., *et al.* (2010) Electronic health records' limited success suggest more targeted users. *Health Affairs*, 29, 639–646.

Dexter, P.R., Perkins, S.M., Maharry, K.S., *et al.* (2004) Inpatient computer-based standing orders vs physician reminders to increase influenza and pneumococcal vaccination rates: a randomized trial. *Journal of the American Medical Association*, 292, 2366–2371.

Dorr, D.A., Wilcox, A., Donnelly, S.M., *et al.* (2005) Impact of generalist care managers on patients with diabetes. *Health Services Research*, 40, 1400–1421.

Dorr, D.A., Brunker, C.P., Wilcox, A., *et al.* (2006a) *Implementing Protocols is Not Enough: The Need for Flexible, Broad Based Care Management in Primary Care*. Agency for Healthcare Research and Quality, Translating Research Into Practice and Policy (TRIPP) Conference, July 10–12, Washington, DC.

Dorr, D.A., Wilcox, A., Burns, L., *et al.* (2006b) Implementing a multidisease chronic care model in primary care using people and technology. *Disease Management*, 9(1), 1–15.

Dorr, D.A., Bonner, L.M., Cohen, A.N., *et al.* (2007a) Informatics systems to promote improved care for chronic illness: a literature review. *Journal of the American Medical Informatics Association*, 14, 156–163.

Dorr, D.A., Jones, S.S., & Wilcox, A. (2007b) A framework for information system usage in collaborative care. *Journal of Biomedical Informatics*, 40, 282–287.

Dorr, D.A., Wilcox, A.B., Brunker, C.P., *et al.* (2008) The effect of technology-supported, multidisease care management on the mortality and hospitalization of seniors. *Journal of the American Geriatrics Association*, 56, 2195–2202.

Dorr, D.A. (2009) Managing and coordinating health care: creating collaborative, proactive systems. *The Bridge*, 39(4), 21–29. Available at: http://www.nae.edu/File.aspx?id=17673.

Evans, R.S., Pestotnik, S.L., Classen, D.C., *et al.* (1998). A computer-assisted management program for antibiotics and other antiinfective agents. *New England Journal of Medicine*, 338, 232–238.

Evans, R.S., Pestotnik, S.L., Classen, D.C., *et al.* (1992) Prevention of adverse drug events through computerized surveillance. *Proceedings of the Sixteenth Annual Symposium of Computer Applications in Medical Care*, 437–441.

Garg, A.X., Adhikari, N.K., McDonald, H., *et al.* (2005) Effects of computerized clinical decision support systems on practitioner performance and patient outcomes: a systematic review. *Journal of the American Medical Association*, 293, 1223–1238.

Graber, M.L., & Mathew, A. (2008) Performance of a web-based clinical diagnosis support system for internists. *Journal of General Internal Medicine*, 23(Supplement 1), 37–40.

Gremeaux, V., & Coudeyre, E. (2010) The internet and the therapeutic education of patients: a systematic review of the literature. *Annals of Physical and Rehabilitation Medicine*, 53, 669–692.

Han, Y.Y., Carcillo, J.A., Venkataraman, S.T., *et al.* (2005) Unexpected increased mortality after implementation of a commercially sold computerized physician order entry system. *Pediatrics*, 116, 1506–1512.

Harrison, M.I., Koppel, R., & Bar-Lev, S. (2007) Unintended consequences of information technologies in health care: an interactive sociotechnical analysis. *Journal of the American Medical Informatics Association*, 14, 542–549.

Health Level 7 International. (2010) Clinical Document Architecture. Health Level 7 International, Ann Arbor, MI. Available at: http://www.hl7.org/implement/standards/cda/cfm.

Hersh, W. (2004) Health care information technology: progress and barriers. *Journal of the American Medical Association*, 292, 2273–2274.

Hoffman, C., Rice, D., Y Sung, H.-Y. (1996) Persons with chronic conditions: their prevalence and costs. *Journal of the American Medical Association*, 276, 1473–1479.

Institute for Healthcare Improvement. (2010) *Testing Changes: Steps in the PDSA Cycle*. Institute for Healthcare Improvement, Cambridge, MA. Available at: http://www.ihi.org/IHI/Topics/Improvement/ImprovementMethods/HowToImprove/testingchanges.htm.

Kaiser Family Foundation. (2009) *Analysis of the CMS Medicare Current Beneficiary Survey Cost and Use File, 2005: Distribution of Total Medicare Beneficiaries and Spending*. Henry J. Kaiser Family Foundation, Menlo Park, CA.

Kohn, L., Corrigan, J., & Donaldson, M. (eds) (2000) *To Err is Human: Building a Safer Health System*. National Academies Press, Washington, DC.

Koppel, R., & Kreda, D.A. (2010) Healthcare IT usability and suitability for clinical needs: challenges of design, workflow, and contractual relations. *Studies in Health Technology and Informatics*, 157(1), 7–14.

Koppel, R., Metlay, J.P., Cohen, A., *et al.* (2005) Role of computerized physician order entry systems in facilitating medication errors. *Journal of the American Medical Association*, 293, 1197–1203.

Kucher, N., Koo, S., Quiroz, R., *et al.* (2005) Electronic alerts to prevent venous thromboembolism among hospoitalized patients. *New England Journal of Medicine*, 352, 969–977.

Larsen, R.A., Evans, R.S., Burke, J.P., *et al.* (1989) Improved perioperative antibiotic use and reduced surgical wound infections through use of computer decision analysis. *Infection Control and Hospital Epidemiology*, 10, 316–320.

Lesselroth, B., Adams, S., Felder, R., *et al.* (2009) Using consumer-based kiosk technology to improve and standardize medication reconciliation in a specialty care setting. *Joint Commission Journal on Quality and Patient Safety*, 35, 264–271.

Leviss, J., Gugerty, B., Kaplan, B., *et al.* (eds) (2010) *H.I.T. or Miss: Lessons Learned from Health Information Technology Implementations*. American Health Information Management Association, Chicago, IL.

Litzelman, D.K., Dittus, R.S., Miller, M.E., *et al.* (1993) Requiring physicians to respond to computerized reminders improves their compliance with preventive care protocols. *Journal of General Internal Medicine*, 8, 311–317.

Longhurst, C.A., Parast, L., Sandborg, C.I., *et al.* (2010) Decrease in hospital-wide mortality rate after implementation of a commercially sold computerized physician order entry system. *Pediatrics*, 126(1), 14–21.

Lorig, K.R., Ritter, P.L., Dost, A., *et al.* (2008) The expert patients programme online: a 1-year study of an internet-based self-monitoring programme for people with long-term conditions. *Chronic Illness*, 4, 247–256.

Marmor, T., Oberlander, J., & White, J. (2009) The Obama administration's options for health care cost control: hope versus reality. *Annals of Internal Medicine*, 150, 485–489.

McGlynn, E.A., Asch, S.M., Adams, J., *et al.* (2003) The quality of health care delivered to adults in the United States. *New England Journal of Medicine*, 348, 2635–2645.

Metzger, J., Welebob, E., Bates, D.W., *et al.* (2010) Mixed results in the safety performance of computerized physician order entry. *Health Affairs*, 29, 655–663.

Mostashari, F., Tripathi, M., & Kendall, M. (2009) A tale of two large community electronic health record extension projects. *Health Affairs*, 28, 345–356.

O'Malley, A.S., Tynan, A., Cohen, G.R., *et al.* (2009) *Coordination of Care by Primary Care Practices: Strategies, Lessons, and Implications.* Center for Studying Health System Change, Research Brief No. 12, Washington, DC.

Office of the National Coordinator for Health Information Technology. (2010) *Health Information Technology: Initial Set of Standards, Implementation Specifications, and Certification Criteria for Electronic Health Record Technology, Final Rule.* Department of Health and Human Services, Washington, DC. Available at: http://www.HealthIT.hhs.gov/portal/server/pt/community/healthit_hhs_gov_home/1024.

Osheroff, J.A., Teich, J.M., Middleton, B.F., *et al.* (2007) A roadmap for national action on clinical decision support. *Journal of the American Medical Informatics Association*, 14, 141–145.

Overhage, J.M., Tierney, W.M., & McDonald, C.J., *et al.* (1996) Computer reminders to implement preventive care guidelines for hospitalized patients. *Archives of Internal Medicine*, 156, 1551–1556.

Reckmann, M.H., Westbrook, J.I., Koh, Y., *et al.* (2009) Does computerized provider order entry reduce prescribing errors for hospital inpatients? A systematic review. *Journal of the American Medical Informatics Association*, 16, 613–623.

Shekelle, P.G., Morton, S.C., & Keeler, E.B. (2006) Costs and benefits of health information technology. *Evidence Report Technology Assessment (Full Report)*, 132, 1–71.

Shojania, K.G., Ranji, S.R., McDonald, K.M., *et al.* (2006) Effects of quality improvement strategies for type 2 diabetes on glycemic control: a meta-regression analysis. *Journal of the American Medical Association*, 296, 427–440.

Slack, W.V. (2004) A 67-year-old man who e-mails his physician. *Journal of the American Medical Association*, 292, 2255–2261.

Teich, J.M., Merchia, P.R., Schmiz, J.L., *et al.* (2000) Effects of computerized physician order entry on prescribing practices. *Archives of Internal Medicine*, 160, 2741–2747.

Tierney, W.M., Miller, M.E., Overhage, J.M., *et al.* (1993) Physician inpatient order writing on microcomputer workstations: effects on resource utilization. *Journal of the American Medical Association*, 269, 379–383.

Wears, R.L., & Berg, M. (2005) Computer technology and clinical work: still waiting for Godot. *Journal of the American Medical Association*, 293, 1261–1263.

Werner, R.M., & Asch, D.A. (2005) The unintended consequences of publicly reporting quality information. *Journal of the American Medical Association*, 293, 1239–1244.

Werner, R.M., & Bradlow, E.T. (2006) Relationship between Medicare's hospital compare per-formance measures and mortality rates. *Journal of the American Medical Association*, 296, 2694–2702.

Werner, R.M., & Bradlow, E.T. (2010) Public reporting on hospital process improvements is linked to better patient outcomes. *Health Affairs*, 29, 1319–1324.

Wilcox, A.B., Jones, S.S., Dorr, D.A., *et al.* (2005) Use and impact of a computer-generated patient summary worksheet for primary care. *American Medical Informatics Association Annual Symposium Proceedings*, 824–828.

Willson, D., Ashton, C., Wingate, N., *et al.* (1995) Computerized support of pressure ulcer pre-vention and treatment protocols. *Proceedings of the Nineteenth Annual Symposium of Computer Applications in Medical Care*, 646–650.

Wolff, J.L., Starfield, B., & Anderson, G. (2002) Prevalence, expenditures, and complications of multiple chronic conditions in the elderly. *Archives of Internal Medicine*, 162, 2269–2276.

Young, A.S., Mintz, J., Cohen, A.N., *et al.* (2004) A network-based system to improve care for schizophrenia: the medical informatics network tool (MINT). *Journal of the American Medical Informatics Association*, 11, 358–367.

Chapter 8

Financing and payment

Julianne R. Howell, Robert Berenson, and Patricia J. Volland

Overview

This chapter will address both the financing of care management for the chronically ill adult population as well as payment of the providers who deliver the full spectrum of services encompassed within the concept of care management/care coordination. *Financing* addresses the mix of funding from Medicare, Medicaid, and commercial insurance, as well as funding through the Aging Services Network, which is currently required to meet a person's needs across both the "long-term services and supports" and health care dimensions. *Payment* considers how to assure that the appropriate mix of care providers is included and funded. As in the rest of this book, emphasis is placed on both the medical and social/support service dimensions of care management, recognizing that care management for a medically complex and functionally and/or cognitively impaired population requires crossing the current boundaries between acute care and long-term services and supports between Medicare and Medicaid, and between the Centers for Medicare & Medicaid Services (CMS) and the Administration on Aging.

Bodenheimer and Berry-Millett's (2009) definition of "care management" captures the essence and purpose of this function: care management is a set of activities designed to assist patients and their support systems in managing medical conditions and related psychosocial problems more effectively, with the aim of improving patients' health status and reducing the need for medical services. The goals of care management are to improve patients' functional statuses, enhance the coordination of care, eliminate the duplication of services, and reduce the need for expensive medical services. Thus, "care management" encompasses "care coordination" and includes a range of other activities; the broader concept will be the focus of this discussion.

Bodenheimer and Berry-Millett's synthesis notes that care management can occur in a number of settings, each with its own challenges and potentials for success:

- Primary care, although almost half of primary care practices have four or fewer physicians and lack the financial or organizational capacity to implement care management.
- Vendor-sponsored telephonic services, as the commercial disease-management model has begun to evolve from single disease management to more comprehensive care

---

Comprehensive Care Coordination for Chronically Ill Adults, First Edition. Edited by Cheryl Schraeder and Paul Shelton.
© 2011 John Wiley & Sons, Inc. Published 2011 by John Wiley & Sons, Inc.

management; usually offered through health plans that contract with vendor companies that employ nurses working through call centers, these services can be linked to the beneficiary's primary care source or function independent of it.

- Integrated multispecialty groups, located within the primary care practices or in a separate care management department that communicates and coordinates with primary care physicians.
- Hospital-to-home "transitions," a setting with great potential for care management to reduce readmissions and costs for complex patients.
- Home-based, for home-bound patients, offering comprehensive care, rather than traditional short-term home care services.

As other chapters describe, in all of these settings care management can also be effectively implemented through community-based entities, such as in the Vermont Blueprint Program (Vermont Department of Health 2010), and a coaching function that trains patients and their families/other caregivers to manage their own care. Across this array of programs, Bodenheimer and Berry-Millett note seven "keys to success" in improving quality and reducing costs: patient selection; person-to-person encounters; home visits; specially trained care managers with low case loads; multidisciplinary teams, including physicians; presence of informal caregivers; and use of coaching.

As other chapters have demonstrated, the population of chronically ill adults is heterogeneous. The number of co-existing chronic medical conditions, the presence of dementia, socioeconomic status, and the availability of family (and other) caregivers all influence the care management that an individual patient and a particular population may require. "One size does not fit all," for the care management models or for the approaches to financing and payment that support them (Berenson & Howell 2009).

Ideally, financing and payment policies across the public and private sectors would support care management as a key component in assuring patient-centered, high-quality, and cost-effective care for beneficiaries with complex conditions. Unfortunately, current policy in both the public and private sectors has many gaps and inconsistencies, significantly impacting the ability to support effective care management. This chapter focuses primarily on Medicare and Medicaid, the financing sources for the principal populations and models addressed in this volume. Part 2 addresses current financing policies that impact effective care management, with emphasis on Medicare and Medicaid. Part 3 then considers approaches to paying providers, emphasizing limitations for care management inherent in traditional approaches and discussing options that promise to be more supportive of effective chronic disease management. Part 4 provides an overview of the key initiatives regarding financing and payment for care management included in the Patient Protection and Affordable Care Act of 2010 (PPACA) and other recent federal initiatives intended to test significant reforms to current policy. Part 5 presents our conclusions and recommendations, near and longer term.

The challenges (and occasional successes) of financing care management under current policy

Effective care management for the population with multiple chronic conditions, and often functional and/or cognitive impairments as well, requires both medical care and long-term services and supports to address limitations in performing activities of daily living and instrumental activities of daily living. To finance care management under current policy, therefore, often requires linking the acute and post-acute care covered by Medicare and the long-term services and supports covered by Medicaid, and some programs of the Administration on Aging. The major payment policies that impact care management are described below.

Traditional fee-for-service medicare

The traditional Medicare fee-for-service (FFS) benefit structure is designed to cover professional and institutional medical services that are acute and episodic in nature. "Care management" services are not a covered benefit, and the services of many professionals fundamental to care management, including many nurses and social workers, are not billable under current policy. "Discharge planning" is a required component of services covered under an inpatient admission, but the types of in-home and even telephonic follow-up that are essential components of most successful "transitions" models are not covered other than through the grant funding that has supported the development and testing of these models. Further, under current payment policies, hospitals are not penalized for readmissions. Instead, since the dominant hospital business model relies upon keeping beds full, readmissions represent additional revenue. Unless a hospital is running at high occupancy and needs to free up beds for more profitable elective surgical admissions, there is no business case for providing transitions programs that will result in a loss in paid medical admissions (and readmissions).

Beyond specific short-term "post-acute care" services following hospitalization, the kinds of social and support services often required to maintain a beneficiary with multiple chronic conditions functioning effectively at home are not covered by Medicare. Low-income beneficiaries who qualify for Medicaid and who are nursing-home eligible can obtain "home and community-based services" (HCBS), but most higher income beneficiaries lack long-term care insurance that covers such services and often lack the income to pay for such services out-of-pocket.

Since the passage and implementation of the Medicare Prescription Drug, Improvement, and Modernization Act in 2003, Medicare has provided coverage for pharmaceuticals through enrollment in Part D health plans for beneficiaries in the traditional FFS program and as a covered benefit under Medicare Advantage (Part C) plans. Managing a beneficiary's multiple medications is often a key aspect of care management, frequently a challenging endeavor because Part D information is often not readily available and shared with a beneficiary's care providers.

Medicare advantage

As of September 2010, 11.8 million Medicare beneficiaries, nearly one quarter of the Medicare population, was enrolled in a Medicare Advantage (MA; Part C) health plan (Gold *et al*. 2010b). Some of these plans use predictive modeling to identify the beneficiaries likely to require care management and telephonic strategies provided either through in-house staff or on contract to vendors to offer these services. Recent research offers the most positive evidence to date that "enhanced care management" using telephonic interventions targeted to "the people who need them most" can reduce hospital admissions and save medical and pharmacy costs (Wennberg *et al.* 2010). The risk-adjusted monthly payments that a health plan receives for its enrolled Medicare population provide the financial support for these services. The model regulation for calculating the medical loss ratio (MLR) approved by the National Association of Insurance Commissioners in October 2010 includes care management as a medical or quality improvement expense that counts in the 85% required MLR, virtually assuring that care management services will be offered by most MA plans (Care Continuum Alliance 2010).

Medicare advantage/special needs plans

The Medicare Modernization Act authorized the creation of Special Needs Plans (SNPs) to address the care coordination requirements of three categories of Medicare beneficiaries with complex health needs: those living in nursing homes, those dually eligible for Medicare and Medicaid, or those having certain chronic or disabling conditions (Berenson & Howell 2009). SNPs were originally authorized through 2008 and then extended by subsequent legislation, most recently through 2013 by the PPACA. Medicare pays SNPs through the same capitation method used for other MA plans, but risk adjustment for health condition, disability status, and dual eligibility increases the capitation payment compared with other plans in the same region. SNPs that serve beneficiaries dually eligible for Medicaid can also contract with states to receive payments to offer Medicaid benefits, and beginning in 2010, all new and expanding dual-eligible SNPs are required to have contracts with states. Existing dual-eligible SNPs that are not expanding have until January 1, 2013, to establish state contracts. Total SNP enrollment in 2010 was 1.3 million beneficiaries, 800 million of whom were dual eligibles (Gold *et al.* 2010a).

Medicaid

For low-income individuals, Medicaid covers both acute medical care and long-term care, including nursing home care and, through HCBS, a broad range of non-institutional, non-medical supportive services needed by beneficiaries who are nursing-home eligible and have limitations in their capacity for self-care because of a physical, cognitive, or mental disability or condition (O'Shaughnessy 2010). Since the 1980s, state Medicaid programs have been operating primary care case management (PCCM) programs that link beneficiaries to primary care providers and pay providers a small monthly fee (often approximately $3 per beneficiary per month) for basic care management activities. In recent years a number of states have enhanced these basic PCCM programs to include more intensive care management for high-need beneficiaries, to increase the use of performance and quality measures, and to provide the foundation for "accountable systems of care," particularly for beneficiaries with complex needs using non-capitated approaches (Verdier *et al.* 2009).

   Low-income beneficiaries who are dually eligible for Medicare and Medicaid qualify to receive the benefits covered by both programs, but also encounter major obstacles to accessing those benefits. Approximately 8.8 million people in 2006 were dually eligible, representing 21% of the Medicare FFS population but accounting for 36% of Medicare

FFS expenditures. They represented 15% of the Medicaid population but accounted for 40% of Medicaid spending (Kaiser Commission on Medicaid Facts 2009). Medicare is the primary payer for dual-eligible beneficiaries and pays for all Medicare-covered services. Medicaid covers nursing home care, the beneficiary share of Medicare-covered benefits, and home health care for dual-eligible beneficiaries who qualify for nursing home services. States have the option of covering other services, such as HCBS, personal care services, and home health care (for dual-eligibles who do not qualify as needing nursing home services).

In theory, the dually eligible population ought to have the coverage necessary to assure effective care management and coordination. In reality, care coordination is often hampered by the conflicting incentives of Medicare and Medicaid. At the payer level, each often attempts to minimize its own financial liability by avoiding costs through coverage rules, for example, through ambiguity about whether a post-acute care service will restore or improve functional status (covered by Medicare) or simply maintain the status quo (denied by Medicare, but covered by Medicaid). FFS payment methods that limit spending per day or per episode create incentives for post-acute care providers to limit their own costs by hospitalizing patients to make them eligible for higher paid skilled nursing payments when they are rehospitalized, rather than investing in the skilled nursing staff to manage the patient in-house. Care can also be fragmented because beneficiaries are enrolled in a managed care plan under one program, FFS in another, and in yet a separate plan for prescription drug coverage. As a result, no single entity or person has responsibility for the beneficiary's care (Medicare Payment Advisory Commission [MedPAC] 2010a).

Because dual-eligibles are a very high-cost population to both Medicare and Medicaid, innovative "integrated care programs" have been developed in a few states and demonstrate the type of care management/coordinated care that MedPAC recognizes for providing enhanced, patient-centered and coordinated services that target the unique needs of the dual-eligible enrollees (MedPAC 2010a). The basic design of these programs includes: an initial *comprehensive assessment* to identify the patient's level of risk; development of an individualized *care plan* regularly updated; involvement of a *multidisciplinary care team*; assistance in *arranging health care and community services*; *Coordination* of primary care and behavioral health care; and provision of *care transition services* intended to lower total program costs by averting hospitalizations, institutional care, medication mismanagement, and duplicative care.

These fully integrated models of care are financed by bringing together risk-adjusted capitated payments for all Medicare and Medicaid covered services, including some or all long-term care services. The programs using these models are at full financial risk for all (or most) of the services, providing the necessary incentives to coordinate Medicare and Medicaid services and reduce unnecessary utilization or high-cost services. Fully integrated programs are currently found in eight states (Arizona, Massachusetts, Minnesota, New Mexico, New York, Texas, Washington, and Wisconsin). In addition to managing Medicare and Medicaid medical services, care coordinators also address a beneficiary's needs for nonmedical services and supports, such as HCBS, transportation, nutrition, and housing-related supports. Analyses of several programs have demonstrated their ability to reduce nursing home utilization and to lower hospitalization and emergency room use (MedPAC 2010a). To expand the availability of such integrated care approaches, the Accountable Care Act established a new Coordinated Health Care Office (CHCO) within CMS to focus specifically on dual-eligibles (addressed in Part 4).

The aging services network

One important source of "services and supports" available to, at least to some extent, older Americans of all incomes is the "Aging Services Network" comprised of the state and Area Agencies on Aging (Triple AAAs) and a broad array of programs and initiatives funded through the Older Americans Act and, at a state's option, also through Medicaid, the Social Service Block Grant, the State Health Insurance Program (SHIP), Section 398 of the Public Health Service Act, and state and local funds (O'Shaughnessy 2008). Providing convenient access to information and referrals for nutrition services, transportation, home and personal care, preventive services, and family caregiver support are key functions of the Aging Services Network. Linkage to this network is increasingly recognized as an essential component of effective care management, as demonstrated by many of the innovative models described in this volume.

Current approaches to paying providers for care management/care coordination

Under any of these various approaches to financing, payment to providers for services rendered involves two basic options: (1) FFS; or (2) capitation, sometimes called "comprehensive/global payment," since the term capitation has been tainted with the negative experiences of managed care in the 1990s. A "mixed model" that has gained increasing favor in recent years involves providing a per person per month (PPPM) fee to supplement traditional FFS in order to support the infrastructure of staff and information technology required by care management/care coordination. These PPPM fees can be provided to individual physician practices, integrated delivery systems, and/or state/community entities and can be provided by private and/or public sectors payers.

Fee-for-service

The dominant mode of physician payment in the United States is FFS, predominantly for face-to-face office visits. Face-to-face patient encounters have long been a core component of primary care and remain highly valued by patients and physicians. Face-to-face visits are necessary for many clinical problems, while the interaction can help establish a trusting relationship between the patient and their physician and other professionals and staff in the practice.

In the context of chronic care management, the office visit remains a core component and is often necessary to address acute health care problems that chronic care patients may experience – at a higher frequency than patients without chronic conditions. However, the office visit is no longer sufficient as the dominant vehicle by which physicians and patients with chronic conditions interact. The Chronic Care Model, for example, attempts to transform the care for patients with chronic illnesses from acute and reactive to proactive, planned, and population-based (Coleman *et al.* 2009). Evaluations have confirmed that multi-component changes in four categories lead to the greatest improvements in health outcomes: increasing providers' expertise and skill, educating and supporting patients, making care delivery more team-based and planned, and making better use of registry-based information systems (Renders *et al.* 2001).

The classic office visit, as defined by the Common Procedural Terminology (CPT) coding system, does not play prominently in chronic care management, yet it continues to be used by virtually all third party payers, undermining the physician's role in a team-based approach to chronic care management. Physicians are increasingly frustrated by a mode of practice that relies on generating relatively brief patient encounters, and the structure of FFS payments for office visits may be a key contributing factor (Berenson & Rich 2010a).

Most FFS payment approaches were established at a time when the focus of physician attention was responding to patients presenting with acute illnesses. The current definition, or CPT code descriptor, of the commonly used "new" and "established" patient office visit emphasizes the elements of history-taking and physical examination, which are appropriate for patients presenting with symptoms and signs of a new medical illness but not for patients with multiple, established chronic conditions. For patients with chronic conditions, generalized medical history-taking and the general physical examination have already occurred early in the course of the patient-physician relationship and only need to be updated periodically.

Frequent office visits need to focus instead on what the CPT descriptors label "clinical decision-making" and "counseling," but these aspects of the office visit, which are central to patients with chronic conditions, even if the terminology may be outdated, are given insufficient weighting in determining the level of office visit for which payment is requested. Put another way, the code descriptors and the documentation guidelines that assist physicians in coding correctly for payment purposes place too much emphasis on histories and physicals and give too little weight to other physician activities essential to the management of patients with chronic conditions, shared physician-patient clinical decision-making, teaching self-management skills, performing medication reviews, actively coordinating care with other health professionals providing concurrent care, and seeking out evidence of patient depression, a common occurrence in patients with long-standing, debilitating, chronic conditions.

While it would be tempting to codify these other activities and pay FFS for them as well, such an approach is doomed to fail. Consider the relatively simple approach of payment for "non-visit based" communication, including e-mail and phone calls. There is growing recognition that chronic care patients benefit from frequent, short communications with their physicians, for example, in monitoring the effect of an alteration in the patient's medication regimen. Third party payers correctly resist requests to reimburse FFS for e-mails and phone calls (Berenson & Horvath 2003). The transaction costs of submitting and processing legitimate claims could easily exceed the value of the actual reimbursement. Further, verifying that claimed communications actually occurred would pose daunting program integrity concerns (consider the fraud potential for an electronic billing system linked to e-mail generating software; Berenson & Rich 2010a). FFS payment is simply not well equipped to support such activities performed by physicians in the course of providing effective care management.

FFS does even less well in supporting the range of activities conducted by other members of the chronic care management team. Many of these activities involve frequent but short patient interactions or care coordination that occurs without direct patient involvement, all activities not easily paid using the FFS model.

Approaches to payment for primary care practices that support chronic care management

Improving FFS

Given how ubiquitous FFS payment methods are in health care today, particularly for physicians, it is important at least to explore improving the performance of FFS. By far the most important FFS improvement would be to change the CPT code descriptors that over-emphasize history-taking and physical examinations at the expense of a range of chronic care management activities. The current office visit code descriptors and the accompanying documentation guidelines which cause physicians to perform unneeded elements of the history and physical to garner reimbursements should be changed, at least for primary care.

One approach would be to base the level of FFS payment for office visits on time spent by the clinician during the face-to-face encounter, rather than specific activities performed (Lasker & Marquis 1999). The original Harvard work that produced the RBRVS-based (Resource-Based Relative Value Scale) Medicare fee schedule found that intra-service time is a powerful predictor of physicians' perceptions of the work involved in Evaluation and Management (E&M) services (Braun *et al.* 1988). Further research found that the total work did not increase in direct proportion to encounter time, but rather that shorter encounter times were more intense (Lasker & Marquis 1999). The implication is that codes should reflect blocks of encounter time that are meaningful in practice (for example, 5, 15, 20, 30, or 45 minutes). Physicians would determine how best to spend the time available during an office visit, emphasizing activities most applicable to patients with chronic conditions rather than responding to the anachronistic expectations of the current CPT descriptions. This fundamental change to alter how physicians spend time with their chronic care patients would immediately and significantly improve the role of FFS in supporting chronic care management.

In addition, FFS could be altered in two other, potentially complementary ways. One would simply raise the payment rates for office visits in the expectation that physicians would feel less financial pressure to generate more, quick visits, thereby taking more time with patients. Raising office visit payment rates is straightforward administratively, but the strategy assumes that physicians with enhanced revenues would actually cross-subsidize unreimbursed activities. It is likely that some would, whereas others would seek to increase the volume of the now, more highly reimbursed activities. Payers opting for this approach would need to measure performance on some important chronic care activities to assure that the expected cross-subsidization was in fact occurring.

The other FFS approach would involve paying for selected additional chronic care management activities outside of the commonly used office visit codes that would be amenable to concrete description and therefore eligible for specification as reimbursable codes. Examples include payment to clinicians (physicians or other health profession- als) conducting palliative care conferences with patients and families and the activities involved with managing a hospital-to-community transition for patients after discharge from the hospital (Berenson & Rich 2010b).[1]

Per patient per month payments

Other payment approaches deemphasize FFS reimbursement. The approach most com- monly recommended and now being tested by a variety of payers continues FFS payments for office visits, but provides a monthly per capita amount to support the activities less amenable to FFS coding but which together comprise a robust chronic care management approach. As such, the approach is a mixture of FFS and capitation – per patient (or person) per month (PPPM).[2]

Most advocates of this approach assume that FFS reimbursement would continue at current rates with the PPPM supplement for conducting complementary chronic care man- agement activities providing a relatively small add-on payment (Patient-Centered Primary Care Collaborative 2007). An alternative approach worth considering would reduce the fees for standard office visits, freeing up more funds to support the PPPM activities and providing a more even balance between the two fund flows (Merrell & Berenson 2010). This approach would emulate partial capitation,[3] an approach recommended to balance incentives that on the one hand might lead to overuse of services and lack of attention to costs (pure FFS) and on the other hand might lead to stinting on services provided (pure capitation; Newhouse *et al.* 1997).

Capitation

At the opposite end of the spectrum of payment options from FFS is capitation, more commonly now called "comprehensive" or "global" payment to avoid the negative con- notations associated with the use of capitation by managed care in the 1980s and 1990s. In contrast to FFS combined with a PPPM payment for the additional chronic care man- agement services, capitation for all practice activities eliminates FFS payment altogether, allowing practices even broader discretion to determine the appropriate mix of activities to serve the population under care. If FFS payments cannot support the key primary care practice functions that comprise chronic care management, capitation payments arguably should provide the needed flexibility to allow the practice to do so.

Capitation payments can encompass a range of expected activities, from services ex- pected of primary care physician practices only (primary care capitation), to physician and other ambulatory care services (professional capitation) to all services provided under a comprehensive benefits plan, although sometimes excluding particular benefits, such as prescription drugs (global capitation). Whatever the form of capitation involved, risk ad- justment for the underlying health status of each patient for whom payment is made is crucial, yet rarely included as part of health plan-provider contracts. Inadequate risk ad- justment causes payment mismatches (that is, over- or under-payment in relation to disease burden and the corresponding care burden for clinicians; Berenson & Rich 2010a).

If capitation payments to primary care practices caring for patients with greater-than-average need for primary care services are inadequate, practices may choose to offload their professional obligations to others, including specialists, rather than use capitation's inherent flexibility to better manage these patients. In this situation capitation might produce stinting on care, which for patients with chronic care needs would likely be the activities that complement the face-to-face office visit. Paradoxically, then, both FFS and capitation poorly applied can lead to inadequate attention to chronic care management and emphasis instead on acute medical services for which the office visit seems reasonably well suited. For capitation, then, risk adjusting the PPPM payment for patients' underlying health status is essential to provide the needed match of payment and practice requirements. Models are under development that would support such patient-specific risk-adjusted payment although they have not yet been tested (Ash *et al.* 2010).

Performance measurement and pay-for-performance

We have emphasized that basic payment systems can produce untoward effects. Although hybrid payment systems, such as continued FFS for office visits plus a PPPM for care management activities, can attempt to balance incentives, practices instead might choose to respond to each of the incentives separately. For example, the practice might choose to "churn" visits (by seeing patients quickly and often) and accept the PPPM payments without actually performing the expected activities.

Accordingly, payment reform for primary care practices may feature performance measurement and pay-for-performance (paying bonuses or extracting financial penalties based on performance) to complement the basic payment approach that is adopted. There is an extensive literature exploring the potential pros and cons of reliance on measures for assessment of physicians' performance, but scanty evidence on whether employing such measures actually improves performance (Rosenthal & Dudley 2007; Wachter 2006; Pronovost *et al.* 2007). A fundamental problem limiting the potential of performance measurement and pay-for-performance is the current, and likely long-term, paucity of meaningful and valid measures in many areas of interest (Berenson 2010d). For example, an expectation of primary care physicians is the ability to make accurate diagnoses. Yet, diagnostic errors are common and outnumber surgical errors as the leading cause of outpatient malpractice claims and settlements; we lack measures of physicians' rates of diagnosis errors (Wachter 2010).

Even with regard to chronic care management, there are many useful measures of the attention primary care practices pay to primary and secondary prevention for individual chronic diseases, such as diabetes mellitus and congestive heart failure, but very few useful measures for successfully managing patients with chronic conditions in combination, an increasingly common situation (Boyd *et al.* 2005). Nor are there good measures for the quality of the chronic care management process itself.

Nonetheless, when viewed as complementary to the payment incentives contained in new approaches to paying for primary care, current performance measures can play an important role. For example, because an important concern with capitation is that it may lead to underuse (stinting) of needed services, reporting and rewarding performance on primary and secondary prevention measures may help mitigate the perception or reality of physicians' behavior resulting from overzealous response to the capitation incentives. Similarly, for all the payment approaches discussed earlier, patient experience-of-care measures can help assess whether practices have actually adopted some of the important aspects of chronic care management as experienced by patients.

Patient-centered medical homes

Patient-centered medical homes (PCMH), also called "health homes" to remove the implication that only physician practices can qualify, essentially provide a higher level of primary care services than is found in most primary care practices. One of the main objectives of the PCMH is to improve primary care practices' attention to chronic care management while also emphasizing enhanced capacity to serve all patients in more patient-centered ways (Berenson *et al*. 2008).

There is great interest in the medical home concept and, currently, dozens of medical home demonstrations are taking place across the country, with a particular emphasis on Medicaid programs. The various payment approaches that could be used to support primary care practices logically can be extended to medical homes, although the magnitude of payment supplements might have to be increased because the added expectations of the medical home exceed even the Chronic Care Model, which is built on a solid base of primary care. Indeed, all of the various payment models outlined above are being tested in the medical home demonstrations in the field.

One additional payment issue arises in considering requirements for enhanced primary care practices to be able to become patient-centered medical homes – the need for an electronic health record (EHR). Many physician practices require capital to expand their capacity to function as medical homes and are reluctant to borrow even though the enhanced payment models would likely repay them for their medical home investments. To the extent that most of the capital need falls into the health information technology (HIT) category, funding from the 2009 American Recovery and Reinvestment Act (ARRA) HITECH program provides incentives for the "meaningful use" of HIT intended to support needed investment in EHRs. In addition, some payers in demonstrations have provided some up-front dollars for capacity development.

Community entities linked to primary care practices

Anecdotally, larger medical practices and practices that are part of a health care system are better able to become enhanced primary care practices than the more traditional solo or small group practice that remains a dominant form of practice organization. First, larger practices and practices embedded in health systems generally are able to achieve higher payments from commercial insurers to help fund enhanced primary care services. Second, small practices may lack the patient base needed to support the added practice capacity. For example, a solo or small primary care practice may not serve enough patients with multiple chronic conditions to benefit from investment in enhancements to improve chronic care management.

Third, larger organizations can develop the requisite managerial expertise needed to introduce and manage the change inherent in a medical home orientation. Finally, small medical practices are more likely to feel the "hamster on the treadmill" pressure that constrains natural ambition to improve practice performance. They may even reject additional medical home funding because they simply do not want the additional responsibility that extends beyond more narrowly construed physician services.

Given the reality that small practices are less likely to adopt medical home enhancements, a number of states have been working on a delivery model that lodges much of the medical home capacity not in the practice but rather in the community, with the expectation that the community entity would work in collaboration with the practices in "virtual" teams, teams being a hallmark of the patient-centered medical home. Among the leading examples of the community-based approach are the following:

- *Community Care of North Carolina (CCNC)*: one of the best-known and longest standing, CCNC complements the state Medicaid Primary Care Case Management program by supporting 14 regional networks comprising primary care providers, safety net and special care providers, local health and social service departments, and hospitals. Medicaid pays each CCNC network sponsor a monthly fee to hire case managers, care coordinators, and a medical director who works with and supports community physicians. At the state level, CCNC has developed a web-based case management information system that gives all Network participants access to diagnostic and service information on their patients (National Governors Association [NGA] 2010).
- *Vermont Blueprint for Health*: following the prototype of the CCNC, the State of Vermont in 2006 created the Blueprint for Health, a comprehensive state program to improve the health of the overall population and reduce the burden of chronic illness. Local multidisciplinary Community Health Teams (CHTs) that include nurse coordinators, social workers, behavioral specialists, and other health professionals develop community-wide health promotion programs and support people with chronic disease. CHT services are free to all patients and practices. Starting in 2008, three communities were selected to be part of the Blueprint Integrated Pilot Program, a public-private approach that brought together the state Medicaid program, Blue Cross Blue Shield, Cigna, and MVP Health Plan, a not-for-profit health maintenance organization, to align incentives for medical practices to become patient-centered medical homes and support patient self-management. Called the Advanced Primary Care Practice Model (APCP), physicians receive additional payment for attaining national quality standards, coordinating care with CHTs, and monitoring patients' care using health information technology. APCP payments and the costs of the CHTs are supported jointly by all payers. Under legislation enacted in 2010, APCP sites will expand to 14 communities by July 2011 and statewide by October 2013 (NGA 2010).

Financing and payment initiatives in the patient protection and affordable care act of 2010 and other recent federal initiatives

Of the 20 payment and delivery reform models that the PPACA specifies should be priorities to be tested by the Center for Medicare & Medicaid Innovation (CMMI), 15 will be focused on some aspect of "care management" or "care coordination" (Guterman *et al.* 2010). Many of these initiatives are further addressed in specific sections of the Act. Below we highlight provisions likely to be of most interest and impact from the perspective of care management/care coordination.

Practice-based initiatives

As discussed earlier, the medical or health home has received attention largely because of its potential to improve the care for patients with chronic conditions. A number of policy issues related to medical homes remain unresolved and are targets for additional testing that can be facilitated through the CMMI. Indeed, the first "opportunity" listed among models to be tested by the CMMI is "promoting broad payment and practice reform in primary care, including patient-centered medical home models for high-need applicable individuals" (PPACA 2010, Section 3021).

Among the key issues to be addressed is whether specialty practices, such as those of cardiologists and neurologists, which care for patients with chronic conditions on an ongoing basis and adopt most of the practice elements recommended for medical homes, should qualify as a medical-home eligible for a different payment approach – whether or not the practice is formally designated as a patient-centered medical home. Already a debate has begun about this issue as some specialists have adopted medical home elements and seek recognition (Casalino *et al.* 2010).

Another fundamental question on which active debate continues is whether the medical home concept should apply to all patients served by a practice or should instead target patients with chronic conditions, who arguably are best able to be supported by the enhanced medical home capabilities. Currently, most of the activity in pilots and demonstrations has featured "transformation" of the practice for all patients served, but some commercial insurers are resisting the notion that practices need additional payments to serve all of their patients differently when the small number of patients with severe and multiple chronic conditions drive so much of the spending and may uniquely benefit from the elements of the medical home, akin to the Chronic Care Model.

A key implementation issue is whether medical homes should be recognized and thus eligible to receive additional payment primarily through an assessment of their capabilities to provide patient-centered medical home care or through an assessment of their performance as measured through a growing number of quality and utilization metrics. Current demonstrations vary on the balance of upfront assessment of capacity versus monitoring actual performance.

Among models addressed in specific sections of the PPACA (2010) are the following:

Health Homes for Medicaid Beneficiaries with Chronic Conditions (Section 2703): Under this demonstration program, which is supposed to begin January 1, 2011, Medicaid can reimburse a designated provider (such as a physician practice or community health center), team of health professionals working with a provider (for example, a physician, nurse coordinator, nutritionist, or social worker) or a separate health care team (defined in Section 3502 as a "Community Health Team" described below) for six "health home" services for patients with chronic conditions.

Activities eligible for payment include: comprehensive care management, care coordination/health promotion, comprehensive transition care, patient and family support, referrals to community and social services, and use of health information technology to link services. In short, the program is targeted to chronic care but envisions testing multiple varied approaches consistent with the diverse health care delivery systems that serve Medicaid beneficiaries. To increase take-up of this opportunity, the PPACA provides a 90-10 federal-state match for services for the first two years; $25 million is authorized for planning grants.

Community Health Teams (CHTs; Section 3502): to support medical homes, consistent with the approaches used in North Carolina and Vermont described earlier, grants would be provided to establish interdisciplinary CHTs and provide some additional funds to the medical practices as well. A range of professionals might be included on a CHT, including nurses, pharmacists, nutritionists and dieticians, social workers, and behavioral health providers. A set of CHT expectations are delineated, including: supporting medical home practices through disease management, developing patient care plans, and connecting patients with available community prevention and treatment programs. Eligible entities to sponsor the CHTs include states, Indian tribes, and state-designated entities.

Independence at Home (Section 3024): this demonstration, which will test a service delivery model that uses physician- and advanced practice nurse-directed teams to care for frail elderly Medicare beneficiaries (often dually eligible for Medicaid) in their homes, is rarely included in a listing of medical home activities in the PPACA. Participating practices may share in savings if specified quality measures and savings targets are achieved and if other criteria determined by CMS are met. An applicable beneficiary must have two or more chronic illnesses to be designated by CMS, must have had a non-elective hospital admission within the prior 12 months, and must have two or more limitations in Activities of Daily Living requiring the assistance of another person. This demonstration is slated to begin January 1, 2012, and is supposed to run for three years.

Multi-payer Advanced Primary Care Practice Demonstration (MAPCP)

The MAPCP Demonstration will allow FFS Medicare to join Medicaid and private insurers in state-based health reform initiatives aimed at improving the delivery of primary care through use of advanced primary care practices (that is, patient-centered medical homes). CMS will provide an enhanced payment to participating practices for their Medicare patients commensurate with other participating payers in exchange for provision of continuous, comprehensive, coordinated, and patient-centered health care. Implementing a common payment method across multiple participating payers is intended to reduce administrative burden, align economic incentives, and provide participating practices with the resources needed to function in a more integrated fashion. The demonstration will be conducted under state auspices, and as announced by CMS, eight states have been selected: Maine, Vermont, Rhode Island, New York, Pennsylvania, North Carolina, Michigan, and Minnesota.

To be selected, states had to meet certain requirements, including having a state agency responsible for implementing the program, being ready to make payments to participating practices six months after being selected, and having mechanisms in place to connect patients to community-based resources. Ultimately, over 1,200 medical homes are expected to be involved serving almost one million Medicare beneficiaries. The demonstration will last for three years (CMS 2010a; CMS 2010b).

Accountable Care Organizations (ACOs)

The concept of an "accountable care organization" has emerged as one of the most influential delivery and payment innovations included both in PPACA and being pursued in the private sector. As defined by McClellan colleagues (2010), "ACOs consist of providers who are jointly held accountable for achieving measured quality improvements and reductions in the rate of spending growth ... these cost and quality improvements must achieve overall, per capita improvement in quality and cost, and ACOs should have at least limited accountability for achieving these improvements while caring for a defined population of patients" (pp. 982–983). ACOs may involve a variety of provider configurations, ranging from integrated delivery systems to physician group practices to networks of individual practices to hospitals with aligned and/or employed physician practices. All configurations must have a strong primary care base.

The impetus for establishment of ACOs comes from the growing pressure of escalating health care costs combined with evidence that at least some of the spending appears to improve neither quality nor patients' experience with the care they receive. Although experts dispute the exact amount of wasted spending, it is generally thought to be substantial (Fisher *et al.* 2003; Gottlieb *et al.* 2010; Zuckerman *et al.* 2010). ACOs are thought to hold promise for cost containment because responsibility for containing costs (while improving quality and patient experience) is placed directly with clinicians on the front lines of care, who can better target waste and inefficiency if motivated to do so, rather than with distant third-party payers, including managed care plans and Medicare (Berenson 2010c).

Patients with chronic care conditions in need of improved care management and care coordination would be a major focus of ACOs. In one recent accounting, half of Medicare beneficiaries had five or more chronic conditions and were responsible for 76% of Medicare spending (Thorpe & Howard 2006).[4] Patients with chronic conditions, especially those with multiple conditions, often receive suboptimal care despite the fact that individual clinicians may be practicing according to professional standards. In theory, the ACO would address the fragmented care that results from clinicians practicing in silos, producing different diagnoses and treatment plans, prescribing incompatible medications, and delivering redundant, costly care.

Supported by a payment model that rewards high quality, cost-effective care, an ACO would become the entity that organizes chronic care management, consistent with its own culture and delivery characteristics. The payer, whether Medicare or another public or private payer, would not specify models of chronic care management to be used, leaving those decisions up to the ACO. Instead, the payer would establish program specifications and performance measurement related to cost, quality, and patient experience of care to incentivize the ACO to perform well.

Many of the specific approaches described earlier, including various forms of medical homes, are anticipated to be core elements within an ACO structure. However, the ACO, rather than the third party payer, would have flexibility to determine which care models to use and would be responsible for assuring that the specialists and medical home clinicians were coordinating care and that hospitals were working with a medical home to assure a smooth transition of care from hospital to home.

The PPACA includes various models of ACOs and ACO payment. Section 3022 (PPACA 2010) specifies a Shared Savings Program that is based on the Medicare Physician Group Practice (PGP) Demonstration approach, in which FFS payments continue as usual, but the ACO receives a share of savings achieved if total Medicare Parts A and B spending for patients assigned to the ACO is less than a spending target. Proponents of the shared savings approach for ACOs believe that an incremental, nonthreatening program design is the best way to gain initial participation by diverse provider systems across the country and to nudge them in the desired direction of change (Berenson 2010c). Others argue that the shared savings approach is too weak to achieve significant cost containment because it maintains FFS and its inherent incentives to generate unnecessary services. Instead, many advocate the need to move to payment models that involve some degree of financial risk, such as partial or global capitation (Berenson 2010c; MedPAC 2010b). A complete discussion of the merits of different ACO configurations and the various payment models to support them is beyond the scope of this chapter.

Most of the ACO attention has focused on the potential of ACOs in Medicare. However, two sections of the PPACA describe ACO or ACO-like demonstrations in Medicaid. The Medicaid Global Payment System Demonstration (PPACA 2010, Section 2705) would permit up to five states to test a global, capitated payment to a safety net hospital system or network as a replacement for fee-for-service. This demonstration was supposed to have begun in fiscal 2010, and to last three years. The CMMI would be responsible for evaluating the demonstration.

The Pediatric Accountable Care Organization Demonstration (PPACA 2010, Section 2706) would test pediatric ACOs and would be expected to use the payment approach and other design features called for under Section 3022, the Shared Savings Program described above. This demonstration is scheduled to begin on January 1, 2012, coincident with the Shared Savings demonstration in Medicare and conclude Dec 31, 2016, a full five-year demonstration.

Neither demonstration explicitly discusses care for beneficiaries with chronic conditions. Yet, as discussed above, the basic purpose of the shared savings and global capitation payment approaches is to internalize to an organization the incentives to reduce costs while improving quality.

CMS Federal Coordinated Health Care Office (FCHCO)

Section 2602 of PPACA (2010) established a new Federal Coordinated Health Care Office to address the unique problems of the almost 9 million beneficiaries dually eligible for Medicare and Medicaid, more than 7 million of whom still receive fragmented FFS care in both programs (Bella 2010). In two special open-door forums held by CMS leadership in late November 2010, Melanie Bella, the Director of the FCHCO, indicated the new office would pursue two major efforts: (1) improving the alignment between the federal government and the states on benefit structure, eligibility determination, regulations and the array of other program elements that impact beneficiary service; and (2) testing new care models and payment systems. In this latter effort, the FCHCO will work in conjunction with the Center for Medicare and Medicaid Innovation. In the first of these initiatives launched in December 2010, up to 15 state Medicaid agencies will have the opportunity to obtain contracts of up to $1 million to design and implement demonstrations for more integrated care.

Encouraging effective transitions from the hospital to other settings

So far, we have considered approaches to chronic care management, such as medical homes and ACOs, designed to provide patient-centered care that is coordinated across provider silos and provided longitudinally to decrease care fragmentation. The PPACA also includes chronic care management and coordination provisions that are much more targeted to vulnerable periods of time when patients are prone to mishaps because of a lack of care coordination (Coleman & Berenson 2004). In particular, the PPACA focuses attention on the problem of faulty care transitions from hospitals to home or to post-acute care facilities.

This emphasis on improving care transitions is based on research that has demonstrated that Medicare patients were readmitted within 30 days nearly 20% of the time (Jencks *et al.* 2009) and that specific interventions could reliably and substantially reduce the rate of these readmissions (Coleman *et al.* 2006; Naylor *et al.* 2004). Perhaps the most disturbing finding in the research is that more than 50% of the time, the patient, who was sick enough to be in the hospital, was readmitted without seeing a health professional in the interim between discharge and readmission (Jencks *et al.* 2009).

Two different payment approaches are available to try to incentivize hospitals, and through hospitals other providers, to do a better job of ensuring a high quality discharge that provides patients and families with the information (and, ideally, skills) to resume responsibility for their post-hospital care and assures that appropriate follow-up care is provided, whether from the patient's usual source of ambulatory care or by a hospital employee with direct knowledge of the patient's in-hospital care and follow-up needs.

Section 3025 of the PPACA (2010) provides for a "Hospital Readmissions Reduction Program" intended to reduce the rate of avoidable readmissions. An "avoidable or preventable readmission" is considered to be an admission clinically related to the prior admission that could have been prevented by: (1) the provision of quality care in the initial hospitalization; (2) adequate discharge planning; (3) adequate post-discharge follow up; or (4) improved coordination between inpatient and outpatient health care teams (Goldfield *et al.* 2008). Since 2009, CMS has reported quarterly on the Hospital Compare website the rate of readmissions for beneficiaries with the diagnoses of congestive heart failure (CHF), heart attack (AMI), and pneumonia (PNEU). Beginning in Fiscal Year 2013, hospitals will have their base diagnosis related group (DRG) payments reduced for "excess readmission rates," as defined by statute.

An alternative approach would not rely on measuring readmission rates but would change the inherent payment incentives related to readmissions for all hospitals. In what has been called a "warranty" payment approach, the initial hospitalization for a subset of conditions would guarantee that a readmission would not be required within a specified time period, and there would be no (or more likely reduced) additional payment for readmissions within that time. The base payments for these conditions might be increased to make up for the lack of payment for the "warranty" readmissions (Berenson 2010d). This approach has precedent in existing payment policy. For example, in the Medicare in-patient, psychiatric hospital prospective payment system, no additional payments are made for readmissions within the first 72 hours of discharge.

Section 3026 of the PPACA (2010) also provides for a "Community-Based Care Transitions Program" (CCTP) that will assist hospitals with high readmissions rates in improving their transitions for high-risk Medicare beneficiaries. The CCTP builds on the Care Transitions sub-national theme in the 9th Scope of Work through which 14 Quality Improvement Organizations (QIOs) facilitated communities working together to address care transitions. Eligible entities for CCTP are statutorily defined as hospitals with high readmission rates that partner with community-based organizations (CBOs) or CBOs that provide care transition services across the continuum of care and have governing bodies with representation of multiple health care stakeholders, including consumers. In selecting CBOs to participate in the program, CMS will give preference to current Administration on Aging (AoA) grantees that provide care transition interventions with multiple hospitals and practitioners or entities that provide services to medically underserved populations, small communities, and rural areas. CBOs in the CCTP will define their target population and strategies for identifying high-risk patients; specify care transition interventions, including strategies for improving provider communications and patient activation; and specify a budget including a per eligible discharge rate for care transition services. The program will run for five years beginning January 1, 2011 (CMS 2010c).

Conclusions and recommendations, near and longer term

The contributions that effective care management/care coordination can make to improved quality of care at lower costs, particularly for people with multiple chronic conditions, have now been widely demonstrated. Fortunately a number of approaches to financing and paying for care management/care coordination have been and are currently being tested, and the implementation of the many provisions of the PPACA that address various aspects of care management should help to establish the evidence base required to support this essential aspect of health services delivery. Our conclusions at this early point in the transformation of health care payment and delivery system change that the PPACA will hopefully encourage are as follows.

- "One size does not fit all," either in the care management model or the approach to financing and payment. Different models are more effective with different segments of the population and for different purposes. The financing approach will, therefore, differ depending on the purpose.

The diversity in the population with multiple chronic conditions and/or functional limitations, the progression of needs over time for any given individual, and the considerable heterogeneity in market conditions and organizational capacity across the country require that multiple models be available.

The care management model must be targeted to the appropriate population segment (such as high-intensity care management for high-risk beneficiaries, and management of transitions from the hospital to home for most beneficiaries). High-intensity care management can be supported through full or partial risk-adjusted PPPM-capitated fees paid to a variety of different organizational entities. Transitions from the hospital to home or other community-based settings can be encouraged through hospital payment policies that penalize preventable readmissions. The shared savings model for ACOs might encourage adoption of effective transitions models because reduction in hospitalizations is essential for generating savings.

- Effective care management for people with multiple chronic conditions and/or functional limitations requires linkages between medical care and social support services, and under current fee-for-service financing, linkages among fund sources.

The medical dimension of care that works well for people with acute clinical problems is not sufficient to address the needs of many people with multiple chronic conditions and/or functional limitations. Linkages to social service and other state/community-based resources are needed. An interdisciplinary team, including nurses, social workers, pharmacists, and others, is required to provide needed support. This team can be made available and financed in a number of different ways and need not be employed by the same organization that provides medical care, as long as there is a close linkage among all components.

- For the dually eligible population with multiple chronic conditions and/or functional limitations, both Medicare and Medicaid funding sources must be integrated to address care management requirements.

In FFS, the benefit structure of neither program alone covers the spectrum of medical and social support services needed by this population. However, SNPs and integrated programs have demonstrated that dual-eligibles can be provided high-quality, cost-effective care. The requirement that no later than 2013 SNPS must also have contracts with state Medicaid programs should expand the number of beneficiaries receiving effective care management and coordinated services. The new Federal Coordinated Health Care Office at CMS established in 2010 under PPACA should greatly facilitate the SNP and other approaches to serving dual-eligibles.

- Fee-for-service payment is inherently limited in supporting care management activities and providing incentives for effective performance. PPPM fees and risk-based payment models offer greater potential for supporting the team-based care and HIT-supported practices that show promise for improving clinical quality, patient experience, and cost.

As Kane (2009) has noted, "fee-for-service payment is the anathema of effective chronic disease care. Any system that emphasizes production units, especially those based on personal contact, discourages precisely the kinds of activities that lie at the heart of proactive primary care" (p. 2342). Instead, payment approaches, such as a PPPM fee per eligible beneficiary or more comprehensive per capita payment models, can be scaled to the care management model, risk-adjusted for patient complexity, and provide incentives based on the quality of care and care management, patient experience with care, and health spending for a defined population of patients. Such approaches can be used in addition to or in place of FFS payment.

Mixed payment models provide a way to moderate undesirable FFS incentives to permit clinicians to do the right thing. However, because of the possibility that practices may not balance incentives but would instead respond to each incentive separately, it is essential to do risk adjustment in any approach involving a form of capitation and to employ performance measurement. While it is not yet possible to measure overall "value" – quality/cost for a practice or organization, measures are now available for assessing performance on some important aspects of chronic care management, especially those related to patient and family experience with their care.

Notes

1. The latter would specify discrete activities, including at least discussion with the discharging hospital-based physician, review of a discharge summary, non-visit-based communication with the patient shortly after discharge, communication with nurses or other care coordinators assigned to the patient post-discharge, and performance of medication reconciliation if needed, by phone or e-mail.
2. We do not refer to this payment approach as PMPM because in this situation patients are not members of a health plan, which usually involves enrollment and restrictions on patient choice of provider.
3. In health economist Joseph Newhouse's formulation, partial capitation refers to making some payments for FFS, at reduced rates for standard payment schedules and the rest using a PMPM approach. In the context of Accountable Care Organization payment, the term is being used to describe an approach that would provide bonuses and penalties to providers based on whether actual spending is less than or exceeds an expenditure target, with the application of corridors to reduce both upside gain and downside losses. It more properly should be labeled "partial risk," rather than "partial capitation," because the payments remain FFS.
4. This analysis used a liberal definition of a chronic condition. By definition, a chronic condition is supposed to produce some degree of disability, although definitions vary on duration needed to consider a disability chronic (for example, 3 months or 12 months). The study cited considers treatable medical conditions that do not directly produce disabilities, such as hyperlipidemia, to be a chronic condition. Over time, more and more such treatable conditions have been identified, and treated, leading to a significant increase in numbers of chronic conditions per person.

References

Ash, A.S., Ellis, R.P., Kronman, A., *et al.* (2010) *Primary Care Financing Matters: A Roadmap for Reform.* University of Massachusetts Medical School, Department of Quantitative Health Sciences, Worcester, MA.

Bella, M. (2010) *Opportunities to Integrate Care for Dual Eligibles*. National Health Policy Forum, George Washington University, Washington, DC. Available at: http://www.nhpf.org/uploads/Handouts/Bella-slides_07-23-10.pdf.

Berenson, R., & Horvath, J. (2003) Confronting the barriers to chronic care management in Medicare. *Health Affairs*, Web Exclusive, January 22. Available at: http://content.healthaffairs.org/cgi/reprint/gltaff.w3.37v1.

Berenson, R.A., Hammons, T., Gans, D.N., *et al.* (2008) A house is not a home: keeping patients at the center of practice redesign. *Health Affairs*, 27, 1219–1230.

Berenson, R., & Howell, J. (2009) *Structuring, Financing, and Paying for Effective Chronic Care Coordination*. A Report Commissioned by the National Coalition on Care Coordination (N3C). Available at: http://www.urban.org/publications/1001316.html.

Berenson, R.A., & Rich, E.C. (2010a) US approaches to physician payment: the deconstruction of primary care. *Journal of General Internal Medicine*, 25, 613–618.

Berenson, R.A., & Rich, E.C. (2010b) How to buy a medical home? Policy options and practical questions. *Journal of General Internal Medicine*, 25, 619–624.

Berenson, R.A. (2010c) Shared savings program for accountable care organizations: a bridge to nowhere? *American Journal of Managed Care*, 16, 721–726.

Berenson, R.A. (2010d) *Moving Payment From Volume to Value: What Role for Performance Measurement?* Robert Wood Johnson Foundation, Princeton, NJ. Available at: http://www.rwjf.org/files/research/71568full.pdf.

Bodenheimer, T., & Berry-Millett, R. (2009). *Care Management of Patients with Complex Health Care Needs*. Research Synthesis Report 19, Robert Wood Johnson Foundation, Princeton, NJ.

Boyd, C.M., Darer, J., Boult, C., *et al.* (2005) Clinical practice guidelines and quality of care for older patients with multiple comorbid diseases: implications for pay for performance. *Journal of the American Medical Association*, 294, 716–724.

Braun, P., Hsiao, W.C., Becker, E.R., *et al.* (1988) Evaluation and management services in the resource-based relative value scale. *Journal of the American Medical Association*, 260, 2397–2402.

Care Continuum Alliance. (2010) NAIC approves final MLR definition. E-mail alert, October 21, 2010. Care Continuum Alliance, Washington, DC.

Casalino, L.P., Rittenhouse, D.R., Gilles, R.R., *et al.* (2010) Specialist physician practices as patient-centered medical homes. *New England Journal of Medicine*, 362, 1555–1558.

Centers for Medicare & Medicaid Services. (2010a) *CMS Introduces New Center for Medicare and Medicaid Innovation, Initiatives to Better Coordinate Health Care*. Centers for Medicare & Medicaid Services, Press Release, November 16, Baltimore, MD. Available at: http://www.cms.gov/apps.media/press_release.asp.

Centers for Medicare & Medicaid Services. (2010b) *Multi-payer Advanced Primary Care Practice (MAPCP) Demonstration Fact Sheet*. Centers for Medicare & Medicaid Services, Baltimore, MD. Available at: http://www.cms.hhs.gov/DemoProjectsEvalRpts/MD/itemdetail.asp?itemID=CMS1230016.

Centers for Medicare & Medicaid Services. (2010c) *Details for Community Based Care Transition Program*. Centers for Medicare & Medicaid Services, Baltimore, MD. Available at: http://www.cms.gov/DemoProjectsEvalRpts/MD/itemdetail.asp?itemID=CMS1239313.

Coleman, E.A., & Berenson, R.A. (2004) Lost in transition: challenges and opportunities for improving the quality of transitional care. *Annals of Internal Medicine*, 141, 533–536.

Coleman, E.A., Parry, C., Chalmers, S., *et al.* (2006) The care transitions intervention: results of a randomized controlled trial. *Archives of Internal Medicine*, 166, 1822–1828.

Coleman, K., Austin, B.T., Branch, C., *et al.* (2009) Evidence on the chronic care model in the new millennium. *Health Affairs*, 28(1), 75–85.

Fisher, E.S., Wennberg, D.E., Stukel, T.A., *et al.* (2003) The implications of regional variations in Medicare spending. Part 1: the content, quality, and accessibility of care. *Annals of Internal Medicine*, 138, 273–287.

Gold, M., Phelps, D., Jacobson, G., *et al.* (2010a) *Medicare Advantage 2011 Data Spotlight: Plan Enrollment Patterns and Trends.* Kaiser Family Foundation, Menlo Park, CA.

Gold, M., Jacobson, G., Damico, A., *et al.* (2010b) *Medicare Advantage 2011 Data Spotlight: Plan Availability and Premiums.* Kaiser Family Foundation, Menlo Park, CA.

Goldfield, N.I., McCullough, E.C., Hughes, J.S., *et al.* (2008) Identifying potentially preventable readmissions. *Health Care Financing Review*, 30(1), 75–91.

Gottlieb, D.J., Zhou, W., Song, Y., *et al.* (2010) Prices don't drive regional Medicare spending variations. *Health Affairs*, 29, 537–543.

Gutterman, S., Davis, K., Stremikis, K., *et al.* (2010) Innovation in Medicare and Medicaid will be central to health reform's success. *Health Affairs*, 29, 1188–1193.

Jenks, S.F., Williams, M.V., & Coleman, E.A. (2009) Rehospitalizations among patients in the Medicare fee-for-service program. *New England Journal of Medicine*, 360, 1418–1428.

Kaiser Commission on Medicare Facts. (2009) *Dual Eligibles: Meicaid's Role for Low-Income Medicare Beneficiaries.* Kaiser Commission on Medicare Facts, Washington, DC.

Kane, R. (2009) What can improve chronic disease care? *Journal of the American Geriatrics Society*, 57, 2338–2345.

Lasker, R.D., & Marquis, M.S. (1999) The intensity of physicians' work in patient visits: implications for the coding of patient evaluation and management services. *New England Journal of Medicine*, 341, 337–341.

McClellan, M., McKethan, A.N., Lewis, J.L., *et al.* (2010) A national strategy to put accountable care into practice. *Health Affairs*, 29, 982–990.

Medicare Payment Advisory Commission. (2010a) Coordinating care of dual-eligible beneficiaries. In *Report to Congress: Aligning Incentives in Medicare*, pp. 129–157. Medicare Payment Advisory Commission, Washington, DC.

Medicare Payment Advisory Commission. (2010b) *Comment Letter on the Centers for Medicare & Medicaid Services (CMS) Request for Information Regarding Accountable Care Organizations and the Shared Savings Program.* Medicare Payment Advisory Commission, November 22, Washington, DC. Available at: www.medpac.gov/documents/11222010_ACO_COMMENT_MedPAC.pdf.

Merrell, K., & Berenson, R.A. (2010) Structuring payment for medical homes. *Health Affairs*, 29, 852–858.

National Governors Association. (2010) *State Roles in Delivery System Reform.* The National Governors Association, Washington, DC. Available at: http://www.nga.org/Files/pds/1007DELIVERYSYSTEMREFORM.PDF.

Naylor, M.D., Brooten, D.A., Campbell, R.L., *et al.* (2004) Transitional care of older adults hospitalized with heart failure: a randomized, controlled trial. *Journal of the American Geriatrics Society*, 52, 675–684.

Newhouse, J.P., Buntin, M.D., & Chapmen, J.D. (1997) Risk adjustment and Medicare: taking a second look. *Health Affairs*, 16(5), 29–43.

O'Shaughnessy, C.V. (2008) *The Aging Services Network: Accomplishments and Challenges in Serving a Growing Elderly Population.* National Health Policy Forum, George Washington University, Washington, DC. Available at: http://www.nhpf.org/library/details.cfm/2625.

O'Shaughnessy, C.V. (2010) *National Spending for Long-Term Services and Supports (LTSS).* National Health Policy Forum, George Washington University, Washington, DC. Available at: http://www.nhpf.org/library/details.cfm/2783.

Patient-Centered Primary Care Collaborative. (2007) *Proposed Hybrid Blended Reimbursement Model.* Patient-Centered Primary Care Collaborative, Washington, DC. Available at: http://www.pcpcc.net/cee/reimbursement-reform.

Patient Protection and Affordable Care Act. (2010) *P.L. 111-148, Sections 2602, 2703, 2705, 2706, 3021, 3022, 3024, 3025, 3026, 3502.* Available at: http://www.gormanhealthgroup.com/docs/hcr/PL111-148.pds/view.

Pronovost, P.J., Miller, M., & Wachter, R.M. (2007) The GAAP in quality measurement and reporting. *Journal of the American Medical Association*, 298, 1800–1802.

Renders, C.M., Valk, G.D., Griffin, S.J., *et al.* (2001) Intervention to improve the management of diabetes mellitus in primary care, outpatient, and community settings: a systematic review. *Diabetes Care*, 24, 1821–1833.

Rosenthal, M.B., Dudley, A. (2007) Pay for performance: will the latest payment trend improve care? *Journal of the American Medical Association*, 297, 740–744.

Thorpe, K.E., & Howard, D.H. (2006) The rise in spending among Medicare beneficiaries: the role of chronic disease prevalence and changes in treatment intensity. *Health Affairs*, Web Exclusive, August 22. Available at: http://content.healthaffairs.org/cgi/reprint/25/5/w378.

Verdier, J.M., Byrd, V., & Stone, C. (2009) *Enhanced Primary Care Case Management Programs in Medicaid: Issues and Options for States.* Center for Health Care Strategies, Inc., Hamilton, NJ.

Vermont Department of Health. (2010) *Vermont Blueprint for Health: 2009 Annual Report.* Vermont Department of Health, Burlington, VT.

Wachter, R.M. (2006) Expected and unanticipated consequences of the quality and information technology revolutions. *Journal of the American Medical Association*, 295, 2780–2783.

Wachter, R.M. (2010) Why diagnostic errors don't get any respect – and what can be done about them. *Health Affairs*, 29, 1605–1610.

Wennberg, D.E., Marr, A., Lang, L., *et al.* (2010) A randomized trial of telephone care-management strategy. *New England Journal of Medicine*, 363, 1245–1255.

Zuckerman, S., Waidmann, T., Berenson, R., *et al.* (2010) Clarifying sources of geographic differences in Medicare spending. *New England Journal of Medicine*, 363(1), 54–62.

Chapter 9

Education of the interdisciplinary team

Emma Barker, Patricia J. Volland, and Mary E. Wright

Introduction

As the nation's population continues to age at a rapid pace, multiple public and private initiatives are targeting geriatric care by focusing on the education and training of the health care workforce. Many of the educational programs designed to enhance geriatric training for the different health professions use competency-based and interdisciplinary approaches to prepare future clinicians (Mezey *et al.* 2008; Harahan *et al.* 2009; The American Geriatrics Society 2010). By their nature, these educational efforts are meant to reach providers prior to their entry into the "real world" of the health care system and equip these newly minted health care professionals with a grounding in geriatric principles of care and the abilities to function effectively in a team environment. On another front, in the "trenches" of the health care, new models of care coordination are continually being developed and implemented in an effort to overcome the fragmentation and poor quality of care resulting from a system that is currently ill-equipped to serve the chronic care needs of older adults (The New York Academy of Medicine 2008). As efforts to reform the health care system are set in motion, education and training initiatives can and should complement the development of new models of care, because any meaningful progress will not be possible unless these new models are staffed with professionals who have both the training and the spirit of cooperation that fundamental change requires.

The importance of pursuing efforts on both fronts is reflected in the Institute of Medicine's (IOM) seminal report "Retooling for an Aging America," which calls for the enhancement of competence of all members of the health care workforce through changes to educational curricula and training programs, as well as the redesign of models of care to address health care needs both comprehensively and efficiently (IOM 2008). This report underlines that simply expanding the capacity of the current system would be insufficient to meet the needs of older adults; instead health care professionals must be trained to provide care more efficiently, with an associated improvement to quality, by putting their skills to work within a more intelligent, rational approach to care. Ultimately, improving care for older adults through educational programs and care coordination initiatives are the same: bringing together multiple providers through interdisciplinary collaboration, establishing and implementing geriatric competencies, and integrating medical and long-term care needs.

Comprehensive Care Coordination for Chronically Ill Adults, First Edition. Edited by Cheryl Schraeder and Paul Shelton.
© 2011 John Wiley & Sons, Inc. Published 2011 by John Wiley & Sons, Inc.

If educating future professionals in geriatric care and implementing new models of care are necessary steps in responding to the needs of a growing population of older adults with multiple chronic conditions and long-term care needs, then it is also necessary to have a care coordinator to bring all the moving parts together within the care coordination framework. The latter means identifying a specific individual to fulfill the care coordination function, or for the team itself to have designated roles that allow for a genuinely collaborative approach to the development and execution of an ongoing care plan. As care coordination continues its path toward fuller implementation within the context of health care reform, developing a more concrete and detailed understanding of the function of care coordinators themselves, as well as their training and qualifications, will further the goal of attaining quality care.

The aim of this chapter is to provide an overview of the current state of competency-based and interdisciplinary training for the health care professions and its role in the evolution of geriatric care, how these educational movements relate to emerging and established models of care coordination, and the steps currently being taken to develop training and qualification standards for care coordinators. We will also outline what is meant by comprehensive care coordination, which takes into account the broad array of services that may be required by the older adult in addition to medical care, such as long-term care needs, mental health needs, and community-based services. Finally, we will present recommendations on how to best move these initiatives ahead, with a specific focus on the role of the care coordinator and issues pertaining to training, competencies, and licensing or credentialing.

Care coordination, as well as the role of care coordinator, is still coming into its own as a model of care and a professional designation. To date, models of care coordination have come in many shapes and sizes, as they have developed in response to the needs of specific populations in particular settings. In order to single out the most successful programs, experts in the field continue to evaluate the achievements of different models based on clearly defined objectives (Boult *et al.* 2009; Brown 2009). Establishing an evidence base for care coordination helps to identify best practices and find common ground among discrete approaches, while determining which professionals have the basic expertise for performing this role and how they should be further trained. As programs are evaluated and the commonalities are identified, it is anticipated that more clarity will be achieved over time. This will take a concerted effort, but as with the development of any profession or system, it is certainly achievable.

Competency-based educational initiatives and interdisciplinary training

By definition, comprehensive care coordination, which seeks to integrate a full array of health, social support and long-term care services for older adults, requires the involvement of a host of "players," including doctors, dentists, pharmacists, social workers, therapists, direct care workers, caregivers, and, of course, the older adult being cared for. Comprehensive care coordination may be defined as a "client-centered, assessment-based, interdisciplinary approach to integrating health care and psychosocial support services in which a care coordinator develops and implements a comprehensive care plan that addresses the client's needs, strengths, and goals" (National Association of Social Workers 2009). These services are provided by individuals with different levels of training, varying degrees of geriatric competency, and across multiple settings. Given the fiefdoms of different areas of practice, the historical separation of hospital-based acute care from long-term care, and the overall fragmentation of medical care, genuine collaboration can be difficult to achieve (Leipzig *et al.* 2002; Reuben *et al.* 2004). Nevertheless, competency-based training in geriatrics can assist with both the recognition of core competencies across professions and an interdisciplinary approach to providing quality care.

Competencies are measurable professional behaviors composed of knowledge, values, and skills that can be integrated into practice (Council on Social Work Education 2008). Educational models based in competencies that are defined by evidence-based practice with measurable outcomes have been developed by numerous professional organizations. The disciplines of nursing and social work have been particularly active in establishing competencies and guidelines for educational programs (Damron-Rodriguez 2008). Overall, a survey of the literature shows that over the last decade there has been a significant expansion of geriatric competency development in a discipline specific manner for almost all of the professions involved in providing care to older adults.

While it is not our intention to provide a comprehensive analysis of all competency-based training initiatives here, some are worth singling out as representative of the general trend toward reaching consensus on the core elements of knowledge and skills defined as competencies. One of the most recent developments in this area has been the development of a set of competencies for medical school residents that resulted from a systematic, multi-method process to identify and define the minimum geriatrics-specific competencies needed by a new intern to adequately care for older adults (Leipzig *et al.* 2009).

These competencies were finalized during 2007, and part of this process took place at the July 2007 Association of American Medical Colleges (AAMC)/John A. Hartford Foundation (JAHF) Consensus Conference on Competencies in Geriatric Education. The final competencies span across eight domains and are 26 in total, with each domain identifying observable behaviors that medical students must demonstrate to prove competency in the area of geriatric care. The organizers of this project were able to obtain the participation of 450 experts in geriatric medicine, 44% of U.S. medical schools, and several major medical education organizations (Eleazer & Brummel-Smith 2009). Some of this response may stem from the recognition that the woeful lack of geriatric specialization across professions may require the integration of geriatric competencies into academic curricula for all comers, specialists or generalists.

At an earlier point in time, leaders in the field of social work engaged in an iterative process comparable to that described for medical residents, with the development of competencies for both specialists in aging at the graduate level and generalists at the baccalaureate level. The Council on Social Work Education (CSWE) Strengthening Aging in Social Work Education (SAGE-SW), the Geriatric Enrichment in Social Work Education (GeroRich) Project, the Social Work Leadership Institute and the CSWE National Center for Gerontological Social Work Education (Gero-Ed Center) were all engaged at different points in time in the development of these geriatric competencies (Hooyman 2009). The

CSWE curriculum development projects worked to embed gerontological competencies in the foundation curriculum and overall organizational structure of social work programs, where competencies are stated as educational outcomes for students completing required coursework. The Social Work Leadership Institute, through its Hartford Partnership Program in Aging (HPPAE), focused on tailoring competency-based education to prepare MSW students to become specialists in aging, using a rotational model of field education integrated with advanced classroom learning.

Nursing has been singled out as one of the most important professions in geriatric competency development, and as with other fields, a number of organizations have played a role in this process. Of particular note has been the work of the American Association of Colleges of Nursing (AACN) with the Hartford Foundation Institute for Geriatric Nursing to develop competencies as stated in "Older Adults: Recommended Baccalaureate Competencies and Curricular Guidelines for Geriatric Nursing Care" (AACN 2000). These 30 competencies and curricular guidelines are designed to help educators incorporate geriatric content into nursing programs, and have provided a foundation for further efforts to develop competencies for further initiatives, among these the AACN and Hartford Foundation initiative to develop national, consensus-based competencies for advanced practice nurses. Many other professions have followed suit to develop geriatric competencies, as seen with the medical school community most recently. A more comprehensive treatment of this subject can be found in "Examining Competencies for the Long-Term Care Workforce: A Status Report and Next Steps" (Harahan *et al.* 2009).

The development of geriatric competencies has been accompanied by the continued interest in the contributions of interdisciplinary teams that provide quality geriatric care. The benefits of interdisciplinary practice have been recognized and recommended by a number of leading organizations that set standards for the provision of health care services. The Health Resources and Services Administration (HRSA) recommended that competencies for interdisciplinary health care teams cover the areas such as the ability to share knowledge and decision making that transcend individual professional methods and provide client-centered and/or community-based health care needs (U.S. Department of Health and Human Services 2005). The IOM echoed this call for competencies noting that interdisciplinary team training requires competencies founded in evidence-based practice with measurable outcomes and a process of evaluation (IOM 2008), and the American Geriatrics Society has issued a position statement on the importance of interdisciplinary care (American Geriatrics Society 2006).

A comparative study of the competencies developed by five health care professions that include dentistry, medicine, advance practice nursing, social work and pharmacy has documented a high degree of similarity across these competencies (Mezey *et al.* 2008). This study further found that certain competencies were essential to interdisciplinary team work, for example comprehensive assessment, measurable objectives, and communication and collaboration. As such, interdisciplinary collaboration is a lynchpin in the ability of a team to coordinate care, since key elements for the success of an interdisciplinary approach are having a shared purpose and goals, clear roles and responsibilities, coordination of activity, and trust. Not surprising, the competencies developed by individual professions vary in balancing competencies with an interdisciplinary focus versus discipline specific knowledge and skills. At present, none of these competencies explicitly states coordination of care, although many of its elements are included, such as assessment, development and implementation of a care plan, and interdisciplinary collaboration.

With the release in 2010 of a report entitled *Multidisciplinary Competencies in the Care of Older Adults at the Completion of the Entry-level Health Professional Degree*, the Partnership for Health in Aging (PHA) identified "care planning and coordination across the care spectrum" as one of the six competency domains that are relevant to ten different health care disciplines (The American Geriatrics Society 2010). This paper also identifies a domain for "interdisciplinary and team care," or competencies required for collaboration and consultation among health care professionals providing services for the older adult population. Through an iterative process looking at the competencies in the professions of dentistry, medicine, nursing, nutrition, occupational therapy, pharmacy, physical therapy, physician assistants, psychology, and social work, core competencies were defined and endorsed by 28 national organizations. PHA describes the essential skills and approaches these professions should master in order to provide quality care for older adults. The PHA statement of competencies received backing from organizations representing nurses, pharmacists, social workers, occupational therapists, psychiatrists, physicians, physical therapists, national geriatric organizations, and others.

In addition to competency-based training, the movement toward trained interdisciplinary teams providing care coordination for vulnerable populations of older adults has gained momentum and reaches back to initiatives pioneered in the 1970s by the Department of Veteran Affairs (VA). At that time the VA established an educational interdisciplinary team training model for staff and trainees; the Interdisciplinary Team Training Program in Geriatrics (ITTG). In addition the VA funds the Geriatric Research, Education, and Clinical Centers (GRECC) a team-based educational program including social work, nursing, pharmacy, and audiology. The geriatric focused programs (such as the Geriatric Education Centers (GEC), the Geriatric Training Program for Physicians, Dentists, and Behavioral/Mental Health Professions, and the Geriatric Academic Career Award [GACA]), train health care professionals from multiple disciplines. GECs are currently in over 48 states training health care professionals and students in hospitals and university settings from over 35 disciplines.

With funding from the JAHF the Geriatric Interdisciplinary Team Training Program (GITT) has fostered collaboration among medical residents, advanced-practice nursing students, and master's students in social work. The goals of GITT included teaching trainees respect for other disciplines and imparting the skills to work effectively with other health professionals in providing interdisciplinary team care (Reuben 2004). GITT was a substantial program financing eight projects over three years; each program took the form of a partnership between an academic setting and at least one clinical agency (Fulmer *et al.* 2005).

Competencies for care coordinators

Limited information was found from a literature search performed to identify competencies for care coordinators working with the older adult population. However, in work performed for the New York State (NYS) Department of Health in the 2008, The Social

Work Leadership Institute prepared a report entitled "Who is Qualified to Coordinate Care," which identified the knowledge, skills, and attitudes/values needed to perform the essential functions of a care coordinator (The New York Academy of Medicine 2009). In order to distill this information, research was compiled from three major sources: (1) research and analysis of state programs, (2) research and analysis of nationally recognized guidelines, and (3) New York stakeholder perspectives. The methodological approach included information collated from focus groups and stakeholder discussions, surveys of New York State (NYS) care coordination programs, an analysis of the suggested qualifications delineated by national and state programs, and guidelines from prominent national organizations.

As defined by The Social Work Leadership Institute, the essential functions of the care coordinator include seven domains: (1) develop and maintain relationships; (2) train and educate patients, families, and medical and social service providers; (3) goal setting; (4) care planning; (5) coordination of services; (6) ensure cost effectiveness while maintaining quality; and (7) ongoing quality improvement (see Table 9.1). These domains were presented to the NYS Department of Health as recommendations and represent a first step toward delineating the qualifications that might be expected of and individual

Table 9.1 Recommendations for Essential Functions of a Care Coordinator

Develop and Maintain Relationships: Establish effective and respectful relationships with patients, families, professionals, payers, and other relevant parties. One way to do this is to build and maintain trust.
Train and Educate Patients, Families, and Medical and Social Service Providers: When appropriate, use the skills of teaching to ensure understanding by patients, families, and service providers in case management, its goals, skills, and knowledge base, available services, and self-management.
Goal Setting: The care coordinator works with the patient and the family to set appropriate goals to work toward and supports the patient and family in reaching these goals using the skills of coaching and consultation.
Care Planning: Develop an individualized care/service plan with the patient (and family when appropriate) that identified priorities, desired outcomes/goals, and strategies and resources needed to achieve those outcomes. Provide continuous monitoring of the care plan to ensure quality of care/services; and continued appropriateness. Adjust care plan as seen appropriate. Care planning and coordination is done in collaboration with an interdisciplinary team.
Coordination of Services: In order to streamline and integrate the health and social-service delivery systems to prevent delays in receiving care, the care coordinator, depending on the setting, will refer and facilitate access to the services or will directly coordinate the services set out in the care plan. Thereafter, the care coordinator will establish a system for monitoring and subsequently monitor the delivery of the services. On occasion, the care coordinator will act as an advocate if a conflict arises.
Ensure Cost Effectiveness While Maintaining Quality: The care coordinator is mindful of economic cost of services and works to remain within the program's and/or patient's budget while maintaining the quality of care/service.
Ongoing Quality Improvement: The care coordinator participates in evaluating outcomes at the individual level with each patient/client and at the same time participates in agency-wide evaluative efforts to ensure and improve the overall quality of services being delivered.

functioning within an interdisciplinary team of health and social service professionals. This work may provide a starting point for a the development of competencies for care coordinators focused on the older adult population, if organizations representing care coordinators, case managers, and care managers come together to perform a consensus building process as has been seen for nurses, social workers, doctors and others.

Care coordinator qualifications

Care coordination for vulnerable older adults, sometimes referred to as geriatric care management, has evolved as an area of practice within several professions, including social work, nursing, and counseling. There are several types of degrees and licensure within these professions which a geriatric care manager may hold. In social work the most commonly held degrees are LCSW, MSW, and BSW; whereas in nursing the most common are BSN, MSN, and APN. A 2002 AARP survey of members of the National Association of Geriatric Care Managers indicates that more than two-thirds of geriatric care managers are licensed professionals, approximately one-third hold a social work license, and another one-third hold a license in nursing (Stone 2002). In addition, many practitioners also have experience in family work, client advocacy, long-term care and/or psychotherapy. Making the transition from social work or nursing to geriatric care management can be a logical step, particularly if the individual has a background in case management. Many of the credentials offered to geriatric care managers, while they do not always require licensing in another professional domain, in general certainly encourage this.

The practice of care coordination (again, often interchangeably referred to as care or case management) has taken a self-managed approach to regulation that currently substitutes for formal, legal regulation on the state or national level. Through the efforts of voluntary associations that represent geriatric care managers/care coordinators, action has been taken to define and uphold standards of practice, ensure the competency and training of the professionals who practice it through credentialing programs, and enhance consumer protection. However, as noted above, there has not as yet been a movement to identify a set of specific geriatric competencies for this emerging area of practice. Perhaps this is an idea whose time has come, given the increased prevalence of care coordination models as a paradigm of health care delivery for older adults and the increasing number of individuals assigned the role of care coordinator within the context of an interdisciplinary team.

To date, self-regulation has developed in the form of credentialing, which technically is an umbrella term used for licensure, certification, and accreditation, although in the case of geriatric care management it is often used interchangeably with certification. Certification, as part of the self-regulatory process, is distinguishable from licensing, which is typically granted at the state level and provides the state with the legal authority to control various aspects of the practice of a given profession (Rops 2002). Geriatric care management is an unusual case in that it is evolving as a stand-alone area of practice, and yet many who perform this role are already licensed in other professions, primarily social work and nursing. While there is often some degree of indirect oversight via the care manager's primary licensed profession, this does not extend to all practitioners of GCM (Morano & Morano 2006).

In light of the lack of clarity and uniformity surrounding care coordinator qualifications the report prepared for the NYS Department of Health by The Social Work Leadership Institute provided an analysis and recommendations on care coordinator certification, work experience, and continuing education issues, using the research methodology described above to analyze state programs and national guidelines.

Certification and licensure

In 2006, the National Association of Professional Geriatric Care Managers designated four approved certifications for geriatric care managers: Care Manager Certified, offered by the National Academy of Certified Care Managers; Certified Case Manager, offered by the Commission for Case Manager Certification; and Certified Social Worker Case Manager and Certified Advanced Social Worker in Case Management, both offered by the National Association of Social Workers. These programs for certification demonstrate a national movement to professionalize case managers/care coordinators and foster a commitment to work toward uniform standards of eligibility, training, and standards of care coordination/case management practice.

Just over one-third of the care coordination/case management programs researched required certification; of those, most tied this certification to a state-sponsored training program. Of those requiring certification, about half required case managers to pass an exam. Only one program required that professional licensure be maintained (for example, social work) while the person serves in the role of care coordinator. At this time, none of the programs researched required a nationally recognized certification from one of the entities named above.

Work experience

Experience in the field and the community is an important determinant of high-quality care coordination. Many assert that success in care coordination is often based on knowledge, networking, and relationships within the community, all of which take time to build. However, a strict requirement for extensive experience can be a deterrent to filling positions for care coordinators. This problem may be met by embracing a certain amount of flexibility in terms of educational and experience requirements, where strength in one area may compensate for weakness in the other. Experience is always measured in years; and is almost always tied to an educational degree. The eligibility requirements for each of the four accepted certifications by the National Association of Professional Geriatric Case Managers referenced above is instructive in this regard: in general where the candidate for certification has a more general degree at a bachelor's or associate's level, more direct experience is required in terms of supervised experience or working with persons with chronic disabilities.

In-service training and continuing education requirements

An analysis across states showed that pre-service (orientation) and in-service training are both very common practices in state-based care coordination programs. Most programs established set guidelines related to the number of in-service training hours required and the timeframes in which training should occur. Of the programs surveyed, six hours of in-service training per year was the lowest common denominator for ongoing training; at the other end, one program requires eight days of pre-service training with 20 hours of additional in-service training (over a two-year period). It was not uncommon for states to establish guidelines related to the content areas of the training.

It is clear that there is currently no uniform approach to designating care coordinator qualifications and training. However, certain trends have emerged, such as the widespread employment of nurses and social workers as care coordinators, and it has been possible by analyzing different models of care coordination – especially where the evidence supports their efficacy – to determine some of the essential tasks performed by the care coordinator and what knowledge and skills are required to facilitate integrated care across services and settings. The existing situation, namely the practice of self-regulation, the multiplicity of credentials currently offered, different education/training options and the high number of practitioners already licensed in another professional domain, raises important questions regarding the best approach to regulation of this emerging discipline in the future. The larger issues that frame this subject will continue to be the need for consumer protection, universal standards of care, scope of practice, and legislative and regulatory measures that have the potential to impact who can and will provide these services in the future.

Conclusion

Currently our health care system is dominated by a fee-for- service structure that runs contrary to the goal of providing quality care that is integrated across services and settings. The educational initiatives that provide geriatric training based in interdisciplinary, competency-based approaches are needed to equip health and social service professionals with the skills to serve an aging population, but these initiatives will not take root unless there is fundamental reform to the way care is delivered. To date, care coordination programs have been developed and implemented in an episodic fashion, with no significant overhaul of reimbursement structures that support the delivery of acute care services rather than the coordinated treatment of chronic illness. The moderate growth of care coordination initiatives that serve older adults, many of which are targeted toward dual-eligibles, has been primarily achieved through demonstrations and state waiver programs, while the problem of bringing these types of programs to a meaningful scale has yet to be addressed.

The passage of health care reform contains measures that support both workforce development and care coordination initiatives to better serve the needs of an aging population (Patient Protection and Affordable Care Act 2010). Whether these measures will be sufficient to significantly alter our current system remains to be seen, although these measures represent a step in the right direction, for both workforce preparation and the delivery of care to older adults. In order to overcome the fragmentation of care created by gaps in service and poor communication among providers, the ultimate goal will be to have both specialists and generalists from all health and social service disciplines properly trained in geriatric care and the basic precepts of care coordination, with interdisciplinary models of care in place that will support these objectives.

Competency-based training has an important role to play in efforts to improve geriatric care, and it is interesting to note the extent to which geriatric-specific competency development has blossomed over the last decade. The competencies that are focused on interdisciplinary approaches to care are the most closely related to care coordination, while the competencies developed by the Partnership for Health in Aging are the first to explicitly single out coordination across the care spectrum as a competency domain. For those professionals who currently function as care coordinators, there has not yet been a collaborative effort to define the relevant competencies, although there are a number of certification and training programs that have added both legitimacy and an educational/training basis for this role.

The time may be ripe for the development of a set of competencies for individuals or teams who are designated to fulfill the care coordination role. To our knowledge the Social Work Leadership Institute's comprehensive analysis of the skills, knowledge, and attitudes/values of the care coordinator is the first of its type, although as noted there are a number of national certification programs for geriatric care managers. This work could potentially provide a starting point to bring certification and credentialing organizations together in order to identify care coordination competencies and incorporate these at the foundation of their certification programs, as well as continuing education initiatives. The certification process has helped bring an increased number of licensed professionals from areas such as social work and nursing into the care coordination arena. This process has also played an essential role in the education and training of competent, qualified geriatric care coordinators and should continue to evolve toward consumer protection, universal standards of care, and a well-defined scope of practice based in knowledge and skills that are identified as core competencies.

References

American Association of Colleges of Nursing and the John A. Hartford Foundation Institute for Geriatric Nursing. (2000) *Older Adults: Recommended Baccalaureate Competencies and Curricular Guidelines for Geriatric Nursing Care*. American Association of Colleges of Nursing, Washington, DC.

American Geriatrics Society, Partnership for Health in Aging. (2010) *Multidisciplinary Competencies in the Care of Older Adults at the Completion of the Entry-level Health Professional Degree*. American Geriatrics Society, New York, NY. Available at: http://www.americangeriatrics.org/files/documents/health_care_pros/PHA_Multidisc_Competencies.pdf.

American Geriatrics Society, Geriatrics Interdisciplinary Advisory Group. (2006) Interdisciplinary care of older adults with complex needs: American Geriatrics Society position statement. *Journal of the American Geriatrics Society*, 54, 849–852.

Boult, C., Green, A.F., Boult, L.B., *et al.* (2009). Successful models of comprehensive care for older adults with chronic conditions: Evidence from the Institute of Medicine's "Retooling for an Aging America" report. *Journal of the American Geriatrics Society*, 57, 2328–2337.

Brown, R. (2009). *The Promise of Care Coordination: Models that Decrease Hospitalizations and Improve Outcomes for Medicare Beneficiaries with Chronic Illness*. Mathematica Policy Research, Princeton, NJ. Available at http://www.socialworkleadership.org/nsw/Brown_Full_Report.pdf.

Council on Social Work Education, Gerontological Social Work Education Center and the Social Work Leadership Institute. (2008) *Advanced Gero Social Work Practice*. Council on Social Work Education, Gerontological Social Work Education Center and the Social Work Leadership Institute, New York, NY.

Damron-Rodriguez, J. (2008) Developing competencies for nurses and social workers. *American Journal of Nursing*, 108 (Supplement 9), 40–46.

Eleazer, G.P., & Brummel-Smith, K. (2009) Aging America: meeting the needs of older Americans and the crisis in geriatrics. *Academic Medicine*, 84, 542–544.

Fulmer, T., Hyer, K., Flaherty, E., *et al.* (2005) Geriatric interdisciplinary team training program. *Journal of Aging and Health*, 17, 443–470.

Harahan, M., Stone, R.I., & Shah, P. (2009) *Examining Competencies for the Long Term Care Workforce: A Status Report and Next Steps*. Office of the Assistant Secretary for Planning and Evaluation/Office of Disability, Aging and Long-term Care Policy. U.S. Department of Health and Human Services, Washington, DC. Available at: http://www.aspe.hhs.gov/daltcp/reports/2009/examcomp.pdf.

Hooyman, N. (2009) *Transforming Social Work Education: The First Decade of the Hartford Geriatric Social Work Initiative*. Council on Social Work Education Press, Alexandria, VA.

Institute of Medicine. (2008) *Retooling for an Aging America: Building the Health Care Workforce*. National Academies Press, Washington, DC.

Leipzig, R.M., Hyer, K., Ek, K., *et al.* (2002) Attitudes toward working on interdisciplinary healthcare teams: a comparison by discipline. *Journal of the American Geriatrics Society*, 50, 1141–1148.

Leipzig, R.M., Granville, L., Simpson, D., *et al.* (2009) Keeping granny safe on July 1: a consensus on minimum geriatrics competencies for graduating medical students. *Academic Medicine*, 84, 604–610.

National Association of Social Workers. (2009) *Social Work and Care Coordination*. Briefing Paper, National Association of Social Workers, Washington, DC. Available at: http://www.socialworkers.org/advocacy/briefing/CareCoordinationBriefingPaper.pdf.

Patient Protection and Affordable Care Act. (2010) *Sections 5101, 5302, 5305*. Available at: http://democrats.senate.gov/rerform/patient-protection-affordable_care-act-as-passed.pdf.

Mezey, M., Mitty, E., Burger, S.G., *et al.* (2008) Healthcare professional training: a comparison of geriatric competencies. *Journal of the American Geriatrics Society*, 56, 1724–1729.

Morano, C., & Morano, B. (2008) Geriatric care management settings. In: *Handbook on Social Work in Health and Aging* (ed. B. Berkman), pp. 445–455. Oxford University Press, New York, NY.

The New York Academy of Medicine, Social Work Leadership Institute. (2008) *Toward the Development of Care Coordination Standards: An Analysis of Care Coordination in Programs for Older Adults and People with Disabilities*. The New York Academy of Medicine, Social Work Leadership Institute, New York, NY. Available at: http://www.socialworkleadership.org/nsw/resources/NYS_DOH-SOFA_Care_Coordination_Report.pdf.

The New York Academy of Medicine, Social Work Leadership Institute. (2009) *Who is Qualified to Coordinate Care? Recommendations to the New York State Department of Health and the New York State Office for the Aging*. The New York Academy of Medicine, Social Work Leadership Institute, New York, NY.

Reuben, D.B., Levy-Storms, L., Yee, M.N., *et al.* (2004) Disciplinary split: a threat to geriatrics interdisciplinary team training. *Journal of the American Geriatrics Society*, 52, 1000–1006.

Rops, M.S. (2002) Licensure, certification, accreditation, certificates: what's the difference? Available at: http://www.msrops.blogs.com/akac/files/Credentialing_Terminology.pdf.

Stone, R. (2002) *Geriatric Care Managers: Profile of an Emerging Profession.* American
    Association of Retired Persons Public Policy Institute, Washington, DC. Available at:
    http://assets.aarp.org/rgcenter/il/dd82_care.pdf.
U.S. Department of Health and Human Services, Health Resources and Services Administration,
    Advisory Committee on Interdisciplinary, Community-Based Linkages. (2005) *Fifth Annual
    Report to the Secretary of the U.S. Department of Health and Human Services and to Congress:
    Recommendations Interdisciplinary, Community-Based Linkages, Title VII, Part D, Public Health
    Service Act.* U.S. Department of Health and Human Services, Washington, DC. Available at:
    ftp://ftp.hrsa.gov.bhpr/inderdisciplinary/cblreports/rpt5.pdf.

Part 2

Promising practices

Section 1

Primary care models

Chapter 10

Coordination of care by guided care interdisciplinary teams

Chad Boult, Carol Groves, and Tracy Novak

Introduction

More than 125 million Americans have at least one chronic health condition, and 60 million have more than one. These people, many of them elderly, deal with multiple conditions, treatments, medications, and doctors. Primary care doctors often don't have the time, resources, or training needed to manage complex patients properly, so patients and the family members who care for them are often underserved, confused by their treatments and medications, and overwhelmed by high health care costs and other burdens. As the baby boomers retire (beginning in 2011), this problem will grow rapidly. In response, a multi-disciplinary team of experts from the Roger C. Lipitz Center for Integrated Health Care at the Johns Hopkins Bloomberg School of Public Health designed "Guided Care" as a model of comprehensive health care provided by nurse-physician teams for patients with several chronic conditions. Guided Care focuses on the 25% of patients at highest risk for using health services heavily in the future.

In Guided Care, a registered nurse, who is based in a primary care practice, works with three to five physicians to meet the comprehensive needs of 50 to 60 of their most complex, chronically ill patients. Following a comprehensive in-home assessment and an evidence-based planning process, the Guided Care nurse (GCN) monitors the patients monthly, engages patients and families in self-management, and coordinates the efforts of health care professionals, hospitals, and community agencies to eliminate duplication and to ensure that important health-related services do not slip through the cracks.

Preliminary data from a cluster-randomized controlled trial (cRCT) indicate that Guided Care improves the quality of patients' care (Boult *et al.* 2008; Boyd *et al.* 2010), reduces family caregiver strain (Wolff *et al.* 2009; Wolff *et al.* 2010), improves physician satisfaction with chronic care (Marsteller *et al.* 2010), and suggests that Guided Care reduces the use and cost of expensive health services (Leff *et al.* 2009; Boult *et al.* 2011).

Background

The Johns Hopkins Bloomberg School of Public Health facilitated three organizations that provided Guided Care in the cRCT from 2006 to 2009. Kaiser-Permanente Mid-Atlantic

Comprehensive Care Coordination for Chronically Ill Adults, First Edition. Edited by Cheryl Schraeder and Paul Shelton.
© 2011 John Wiley & Sons, Inc. Published 2011 by John Wiley & Sons, Inc.

States, a group-model managed care organization with over 36 medical facilities, operated three community-based primary care practices in the Washington, DC, metropolitan area; Johns Hopkins Community Physicians, a statewide network of community-based practices, operated four community-based primary care practices in the Baltimore metropolitan area; and Medstar Physician Partners, a multi-site group practice, operated one community-based primary care practice in Baltimore.

The study population comprised older people insured by traditional fee-for-service Medicare (34%) or one of two managed care plans: Kaiser-Permanente (45%) or Tricare/USFHP (21%), a federal health insurance program for retired military personnel and their dependents. To recruit participants, researchers screened 12 months of insurance claims generated by older patients (age 65 or older) in the eight practices to identify those at high risk of using health services heavily during the following year, as estimated by the Hierarchical Condition Category (HCC) predictive model (Pope *et al.* 2004). "High risk" was equated with HCC scores of 1.2 or higher, which identifies persons in the highest quartile of risk (Leff *et al.* 2009).

Rationale

To bridge the gap between the growing need for high-quality chronic care and the present fragmented, acute-care-oriented delivery system, researchers have proposed new conceptual models for improving chronic care.

The Chronic Care Model posits that redesign of the delivery system, enhanced decision support, improved clinical information systems, support for self-management, and better access to and communication with community resources would improve clinical and financial outcomes for people with multiple chronic conditions (Bodenheimer *et al.* 2002). In support of the Chronic Care Model, a systematic review has shown that improvements in its individual components can improve clinical outcomes and efficiency in outpatient settings, in the home, and during transitions between sites of care (Bodenheimer 2003).

Several successful community-based innovations in chronic care address individual components of the Chronic Care Model. As summarized in Table 10.1, each of these innovations addresses only a subset of the challenges faced by older people with chronic conditions. Rarely have two or more of these innovations been combined in practice (Eng *et al.* 1997; Newcomer *et al.* 2000).

Guided Care, however, was designed to enhance primary care by infusing the operative principles of all seven chronic care innovations outlined in Table 10.1. Thus, Guided Care seeks to make evidence-based, state-of-the-art, chronic care available continuously from teams of professionals that patients trust.

Intervention

In Guided Care, a registered nurse with a *Certificate in Guided Care Nursing* collaborates with three to five primary care physicians and their office staff to meet the complex needs

Table 10.1 Needs Addressed by Innovation

Model	Comprehensive Patient Evaluation	Individual Care Planning	Promote Adherence with Evidence-Based Guidelines	Empower Patient	Promote Healthy Lifestyle	Coordinate Care of Multiple Conditions	Coordinate Care Across Provider Settings	Caregiver Support and Education	Access to Community Resources
Geriatric Evaluation and Management	XX	XX	X	X	X	X	X	X	X
Disease Management		XX	XX		X		X	X	X
Self-Management				XX	X				XX
Health Enhancement Program	X	X		X	XX			X	XX
Case Management	X	X			X	XX	X		
Transitional Care		X				X	XX		
Caregiver Support								XX	X
Guided Care	XX	XX	XX	XX	XX	XX	XX	XX	XX

Notes: Adapted and Reproduced with permission from Wolff, J.L., Boult, C. (2005) Moving beyond round pegs and square holes: Restructuring Medicare to improve chronic care. *Annals of Internal Medicine* 143, 439–45.
X = addresses need partially; XX = addresses need thoroughly.

of 50 to 60 patients with multiple chronic conditions. The Guided Care nurse (GCN) provides eight essential chronic care services that align scientific evidence with patients' values and preferences (Boyd *et al.* 2007).

1. *Assess the patient at home.* The GCN conducts an initial, two-hour, in-home assessment of each patient. The GCN begins by asking the patient to identify his/her highest priorities for optimizing health and quality of life. Using a standardized questionnaire, the nurse evaluates the patient's medical, functional, cognitive, emotional, psychosocial, nutritional, and environmental status. The GCN inquires about the care the patient receives from family caregiver(s), specialist physicians, and community agencies. The GCN obtains the patient's signature authorizing the release of medical information and gathers supplemental information about the patient's health from the medical records at the primary care office.

2. *Create an evidence-based comprehensive "Care Guide" and "Action Plan."* Back at the office, the GCN uses the practice's health information technology (HIT) to merge the patient's individual assessment data with evidence-based guidelines to create a Preliminary Care Guide (PCG) for managing the patient's chronic conditions. The GCN then meets with the primary care physician for 20 to 25 minutes to personalize the PCG according to the unique circumstances of the individual patient. Later the GCN discusses the PCG with the patient and family caregiver and modifies it further for consistency with their preferences, priorities, and intentions. The GCN then generates the patient's Care Guide (CG), which provides a concise, comprehensive summary of the patient's status, and is a blueprint for the patient's health care for duration of the patient's life. The GCN then converts the information contained in CG into a patient-friendly Action Plan, which is written in lay language and displayed prominently in the patient's home to remind the patient to take prescribed medicines on time, to eat the desired diet, to engage in the recommended physical activities, to self-monitor, to keep appointments with health care providers, and to call the GCN for help when needed.

3. *Monthly monitoring.* Reminded by alerts HIT, the GCN monitors each patient at least monthly, usually by telephone and sometimes in person when patients visit their primary care physicians, to evaluate adherence to the Action Plan and to detect and address emerging problems promptly. During the practice's "business hours," the GCN is also accessible by cell phone to patients and caregivers for problems that emerge between monitoring calls and office visits. When health-related problems arise, the GCN discusses them with the primary care physician, implements appropriate actions, and updates the patient's Care Guide and Action Plan.

4. *Promote patient self-management.* Based on the Action Plan, the GCN teaches self-management skills, promotes the patient's confidence for managing chronic conditions, and encourages the patient to take personal responsibility for his or her health. The GCN uses motivational interviewing to facilitate the patient's engagement in self-care and to reinforce adherence to the Action Plan. When available, the nurse also refers Guided Care patients to local chronic disease self-management programs (CDSMP). Developed and evaluated at Stanford University, these programs are now available for free or at a nominal cost in many communities in the United States (Lorig & Holman 2003).

5. *Coordinate the efforts of all the patient's health care providers.* The GCN coordinates the efforts of the many health care professionals who treat Guided Care patients – in primary care, emergency departments, hospitals, rehabilitation facilities, specialists' offices, nursing homes, and at home. By monitoring the actions of those providers, the GCN keeps the Care Guide current and complete, and shares it with all involved health care providers.
6. *Smooth patient's transitions between sites of care.* The GCN smoothes the patient's transitions between all sites of care while focusing most intensively on transitions through hospitals. The GCN rounds on patients in the hospital, helps design and execute discharge plans, visits patients at home within two days of discharge, and ensures that patients return to their primary care physicians promptly. The GCN also keeps the primary care physician informed of the patient's status and updates the patient's Care Guide and Action Plan to reflect the care received in the hospital.
7. *Assess, educate, and support caregivers.* For the family or other caregivers, the GCN offers individual assistance in the forms of an initial assessment, information about caregiving and their loved ones' health conditions, and ad-hoc telephone consultation to address caregivers' questions and concerns.
8. *Facilitate access to community resources.* The GCN maintains a database of the resources in the local community that may be helpful to people with chronic conditions and facilitates access to these resources to meet the needs of the patient and family caregiver. For example, the GCN may suggest or help a patient or family caregiver contact a transportation service, Meals-on-Wheels, the Area Agency on Aging, a senior center, an adult day care center, or the Alzheimer's Association for additional supportive services.

The primary goal of Guided Care is to improve the quality of life for patients. Identifying patients that are most likely to benefit from Guided Care (that is, those with multimorbidity, complex health care needs, and high health care expenditures) is crucial to the cost-effectiveness of the model. Although clinicians are capable of identifying patients with multimorbidity, electronic predictive models can identify such patients more objectively, consistently, and efficiently (Institute for Health Policy Solutions 2005). As shown in Figure 10.1, the 20% to 25% of older patients on the panel who have the highest estimated need for complex health care in the future are selected for Guided Care. No high-risk patients are excluded because of a condition (for example, dementia) or place of residence (such as a nursing home), although some cognitively impaired patients may be unable to fully participate in chronic disease self-management (Boult *et al.* 2009).

A letter is mailed to eligible patients, notifying them that they are eligible (but not required) to receive Guided Care and that the practice's GCN will follow up by phone. The GCN calls the patient to provide more details about Guided Care, to answer their questions, to ask whether the patient is interested in receiving Guided Care and, if appropriate, to schedule a time for an in-home assessment. The GCN follows the patients for life, unless the patient moves out of the area or changes primary care physicians (to one who does not provide Guided Care). The typical caseload of a GCN is 50 to 60 patients, each of whom has several chronic health conditions (see Table 10.2).

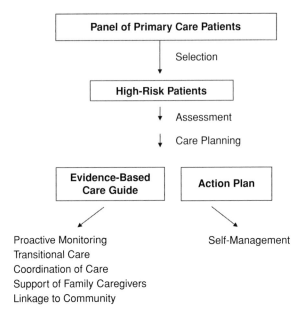

Figure 10.1 Guided Care Flowchart

The GCN interacts with patients both in person and by telephone. The in-home assessment is done in person, and the GCN visits the patient at home within 48 hours following a hospitalization to reconcile medications, to ensure that the patient is following the appropriate regimen, and to address the patient's and the family's questions and concerns. The GCN also meets in person with the patient when he/she visits the primary care office for physician appointments.

The GCN contacts the patient by phone for monthly monitoring and coaching sessions about their health and steps they have taken to achieve their goals. During some of these contacts, the patient may, after learning to trust the GCN, admit to having difficulty adhering to certain activities in the Action Plan. The GCN then uses motivational interviewing to help the patient overcome these obstacles by discussing the desired behavioral change as a method for meeting the *patient's* goals (for example, walking to the shopping center again, attending a granddaughter's graduation, and so on). The GCN is also available by cell phone during business hours to address new symptoms, problems, and questions when they arise.

The average amount of time spent by a GCN on specific activities during a typical forty-hour, five-day week are: three and one-half hours assessing new patients and caregivers, eight hours of scheduled monitoring and coaching, four hours coordinating transitions between sites and providers of care, eight hours documenting activities and updating Care Guides and Action Plans, four hours addressing emerging issues with patients and caregivers, three hours communicating with primary care physicians and other providers, one-half hour accessing community resources, one hour supporting family caregivers, and eight hours on other administrative tasks (that is, meetings, traveling to homes/hospitals, responding to e-mail).

Table 10.2 Characteristics of Guided Care Patients

	Total (n = 904)	Guided Care (n = 485)	Usual Care (n = 419)
Socio-Demographic Factors			
Age, mean years (range)	77.7	77.2	78.1
	(66–106)	(66–106)	(66–96)
Sex (percent female)	54.8	54.2	55.4
Race (percent)			
Caucasian	50.0	51.1	48.9
Black	46.0	45.6	46.3
Other	4.0	3.3	4.8
Ethnicity (percent Hispanic)	1.7	1.9	1.4
Marital status (percent)			
Married	47.3	46.0	48.5
Divorced/separated	11.2	11.6	10.7
Widowed	37.5	37.9	37.0
Never married	4.0	4.5	3.8
Education (percent 12+ years)	45.0	46.4	43.4
Finances at end of month (percent)			
Some money left over	54.5	57.9	51.1
Just enough money left over	33.5	32.8	34.2
Not enough money left over	12.0	9.3	14.7
Habitation status			
(percent living alone)	31.3	32.0	30.6
Type of Medicare (percent)			
HMO-B	44.8	42.1	47.5
Fee-for-service	34.1	31.7	36.5
HMO-A	21.1	26.2	16.0
Health and Functional Status			
Hierarchical Condition Categories (HCC) score,[a] mean	2.1	2.1	2.0
Self-rated health, mean			
Excellent	2.8	2.5	3.1
Very good	16.8	20.0	13.6
Good	37.1	37.7	36.5
Fair	31.2	30.1	32.2
Poor	12.2	9.7	14.6
Mean number of self-reported conditions, mean (range)	4.3 (0–13)	4.3 (0–13)	4.3 (0–12)
Difficulty with 1+ ADL[b] (percent)	30.1	30.9	29.3
Difficulty with 2+ IADL[c] (percent)	23.6	19.6	27.6
Receives help from a person (percent)	50.1	45.2	54.9
Short Form-36 score, mean (range)			
Physical component summary	38.4	38.7	38.1
	(6.7–63.1)	(13.8–63.0)	(6.7–63.1)
Mental component summary	49.5	50.3	48.7
	(6.4–71.9)	(6.4–70.0)	(13.7–71.9)

Source: Reproduced with permission from Boult, C., Giddens, J., Frey, K., *et al.* (2009) Guided Care: A New Nurse-Physician Partnership in Chronic Care. New York: Springer Publishing Company.
Notes:
[a]Hierarchical condition category (HCC) scores indicate the likelihood that Medicare beneficiaries, based on their medical conditions, will use health care services heavily during the coming year. An HCC score of 1.0 indicates that a person has average risk. An HCC score of 2.0 indicates twice the average risk.
[b]ADL = activities of daily living.
[c]IADL = instrumental activities of daily living.

Case studies

Case #1

Mrs. Sheila Johnson is an 86-year-old married woman with a history of hypertension, high cholesterol, osteoporosis, osteoarthritis, and a knee replacement. Mrs. Johnson has two grown children who live out-of-state and an 82-year-old husband who is in good health and acts as her primary caregiver. They live in a small town with limited access to specialty health care services.

During a recent trip to visit their children, Mrs. Johnson was hospitalized for five days with new diagnoses of congestive heart failure and atrial fibrillation. Returning home, she saw her primary care physician who referred her to a cardiologist in a city 25 miles away. She was started on coumadin and, although anxious about the potential side effect of bleeding, was compliant with the medication regime. After eight months on coumadin, she developed severe bruising in her arm and, against the advice of her cardiologist, Mrs. Johnson stopped the coumadin. Three weeks later, she was hospitalized with a minor stroke caused by the atrial fibrillation. Repeat hospitalizations flagged Mrs. Johnson for Guided Care, and she was discharged home on coumadin with a referral to Karen Dobbs, a Guided Care nurse.

On Karen's initial home visit, she discovered Mrs. Johnson having difficulty remembering if and when she had taken her 12 prescribed medications. Always independent, Mrs. Johnson had refused any help from her husband. After Karen introduced a pill box organizer and discussed goals of care, they reached a compromise in which Mr. Johnson was responsible for filling the pill container and Mrs. Johnson took the pills out of the container and self-medicated. Karen contacted the cardiologist and discovered several missed appointments due to the travel distance. After Karen's discussion with the primary care physician, the cardiologist, and the Johnsons, they all agreed the coumadin levels would be drawn at a local laboratory and the results sent to the cardiologist for monitoring. Karen enrolled Mr. and Mrs. Johnson in a chronic disease self-management course, in which they learned how to set goals and create realistic actions to reach their goals. The coumadin had increased Mrs. Johnson's fear of falling and resulted in reduced mobility and altered gait. Mrs. Johnson chose to focus on improving her health through exercise, and she set goals that she now reviews with Karen during monthly coaching calls. Mrs. Johnson has been able to keep her coumadin levels in check with no repeat hospitalization, and she reports enjoying short walks with her husband – something they enjoyed in the past but had given up because of her fear of falling.

Case #2

Mrs. Virginia Adams is an 87-year-old widow with congestive heart failure, coronary artery disease, and diabetes. A patient of Dr. Davidson's for over 16 years, she has steadily declined to the point where she fell recently and bruised her hip while carrying groceries into her home. Meeting the criteria for Guided Care, she received a letter explaining the program and agreed to participate.

Guided Care Nurse Julie Barnes met Mrs. Adams in her home for the initial home visit. The 1890s row house located in Washington, D.C. has street parking and six steps up to enter the two-story home. Mrs. Adams lives alone and she has a daughter in a neighboring city who works full-time and is only available to assist her on the weekends. As Julie completed her initial home assessment, she noted a broken glucometer, smoke detectors that needed batteries, no hand-held shower or grab bars in the bathroom, and carpet spill stains throughout the house. As Julie finalized the Care Guide with Mrs. Adams and Dr. Davidson, they agreed on priorities of obtaining a working glucometer and enrolling in a fall prevention class.

After six months of enrollment in Guided Care, Julie received a phone call from Mrs. Adams who reported swollen legs, shortness of breath, and wheezing. After instructing Mrs. Adams to go immediately to the hospital, Julie met her in the emergency room and provided the emergency physician a copy of the Care Guide, including the results of her most recent echocardiogram. Mrs. Adams was admitted to the hospital, treated for pneumonia, and sent home with a follow-up appointment scheduled for the next day. Unfortunately, on her way to the appointment, she was in a car accident which resulted in hospitalization. In her weakened condition, Mrs. Adams would not be able to return home to recuperate. Julie reached out to her daughter, who agreed to be the primary caregiver and take her mother home when discharged. On Julie's home visit two days post-discharge, she found the daughter overwhelmed with the new responsibility of caring for her mother. The immediate concern was Mrs. Adams wandering the house at night and sleeping during the day. A change in medication by Dr. Davidson along with a pill box organizer provided by Julie helped to stabilize Mrs. Adams' sleeping patterns, reducing her daughter's anxiety and sleep deprivation. In addition, Julie enrolled the daughter in a caregiver support group offered by the community. Mrs. Adams has been able to maintain herself at her daughter's home with the help of her daughter, the GCN, paid aides, and home safety equipment.

Lessons learned

We learned several lessons in six years of testing Guided Care in community primary care practices. Our multi-site randomized trial showed that, compared to usual care, Guided Care improves patients' rating of the quality of their care (Boult *et al.* 2008; Boyd *et al.* 2010), reduces family caregivers' strain (Wolff *et al.* 2009; Wolff *et al.* 2010), improves physicians' satisfaction with chronic care (Boult *et al.* 2008; Marsteller *et al.* 2010), and suggests that Guided Care reduces the use and cost of expensive services (Leff *et al.* 2009).

We also learned that: 1) most patients and their families love Guided Care, saying that Guided Care is "like having a nurse in the family;" 2) it is important to thoroughly orient the primary care physicians and their office staffs to the goals and processes of Guided Care; 3) it is also important to thoroughly integrate the GCN into the many processes of the practice; 4) focused teamwork by the primary care physician and the GCN would be facilitated if each received tangible rewards for attaining the goals of Guided Care.

Practices that are interested in adopting Guided Care need to determine whether they can meet six requirements:

1. Sufficient number of patients with complex conditions: the practice must have a large enough panel of patients so that it includes enough chronically ill patients to constitute a caseload of 50 to 60 patients for the GCN. A practice with at least 300 Medicare patients is usually sufficient. Practices with higher numbers of chronically ill patients may be able to support more than one GCN. Practices with fewer chronically ill patients could share a GCN if they were in close proximity to each other.
2. Office space: a small, private, centrally located office for the GCN. An ideal location is near the physicians' offices with convenient access to the practice's staff, medical records, supplies, and office equipment.
3. Health information technology: the practice must have a system that supports Guided Care by generating and updating evidence-based Care Guides, checking for drug interactions, providing reminders, and documenting contacts.
4. Commitment: the practice's physicians and office staff members need to work collaboratively with the GCN. Integration of a new type of health care provider into a primary care practice is a process that requires careful planning, optimism, open communication, honest feedback, flexibility, perseverance, and patience.
5. Supplemental revenue: Guided Care generates additional costs for the practice: the GCN's salary and benefits, office space, equipment (computer, cell phone), communication services (cell phone service, access to the Internet), and travel costs. To adopt Guided Care, a practice must receive a supplemental stream of revenue to offset these costs, for example, capitated monthly "care management" payments for providing in "medical home" services or for participating in Accountable Care Organizations (ACOs).
6. Patients and families must agree to develop and maintain a partnership with their GCN.

Summary

Guided Care is a practical, interdisciplinary model of health care designed to improve the quality of life and the efficiency of resource use for persons with complex health care needs. The role of the GCN is to work in partnership with the primary care physician, the patient, the patient's caregiver, members of the office staff, and all other involved health care providers to attain the goals of Guided Care. Patients report improved quality of care and family caregivers report reduced strain. Physicians report improved satisfaction with chronic care, and preliminary evidence suggests that Guided Care reduces overall health care costs.

Primary care practices can fully implement Guided Care in six to nine months. Implementation involves hiring a registered nurse who has a Certificate in Guided Care Nursing and integrating the nurse into the practice. Several forms of technical assistance are available to practices that wish to adopt Guided Care, including a detailed implementation manual with many resources and lessons learned (Boult *et al.* 2009), an introductory guide book for patients and families (Grundner 2010), an online course in Guided Care

Nursing (MedHomeInfo 2009a), and an online course for physician and other practice leaders (MedHomeInfo 2009b).

Acknowledgments

The authors acknowledge the Springer Publishing Company for their generosity in allowing some of the information from the book "Guided Care: A New Nurse-Physician Partnership in Chronic Care" to be summarized in this chapter. We also acknowledge the following organizations and government agencies that provided support for the cluster-randomized controlled trial of Guided Care: the John A. Hartford Foundation, the Agency for Healthcare Research and Quality, the National Institute on Aging, the Jacob and Valeria Langeloth Foundation, Kaiser-Permanente Mid-Atlantic States, Johns Hopkins Community Physicians, Johns Hopkins HealthCare, and MedStar Physician Partners.

References

Bodenheimer, T. (2003) Interventions to improve chronic illness care: evaluating their effectiveness. *Disease Management*, 6, 63–71.

Bodenheimer, T., Wagner, E.H., Grumbach, K. (2002) Improving primary care for patients with chronic illness. *Journal of the American Medical Association*, 288, 1775–1779.

Boult, C., Reider, L., Frey, K., *et al.* (2008) Early effects of "Guided Care" on the quality of health care for multimorbid older persons: a cluster-randomized controlled trial. *The Journal of Gerontology: Medical Sciences*, 63A, 321–327.

Boult, C., Giddens, J.F., Frey, K., *et al.* (2009) *Guided Care: A New Nurse-Physician Partnership in Chronic Care.* Springer Publishing Company, New York, NY.

Boult, C., Reider, L., Leff, B., *et al.* (2011) The effect of Guided Care teams on the use of health services: results from a cluster-randomized controlled trial. *Archives of Internal Medicine* (in press).

Boyd, C.M., Boult, C., Shadmi, E., *et al.* (2007) Guided Care for multimorbid older adults. *The Gerontologist*, 47, 697–704.

Boyd, C.M., Reider, L., Frey, K., *et al.* (2010) The effects of Guided Care on the perceived quality of health care for multi-morbid older persons: 18-Month outcomes from a cluster-randomized controlled trial. *The Journal of General Internal Medicine*, 25, 235–242.

Eng, C., Pedulla, J., Eleazer, G.P., *et al.* (1997) Program of All-Inclusive Care for the Elderly (PACE): an innovative model of integrated geriatric care and financing. *Journal of the American Geriatrics Society*, 45, 223–232.

Grundner, T., (2010) *Transformation: A Family's Guide to Chronic Care, Guided Care, and Hope.* Fireship Press, Tuscon, AZ.

Institute for Health Policy Solutions. (2005) *Risk Adjustment Methods and Their Relevance to "Pay-or-Play."* Available at: http://www.ihps.org/pubs/2005_Apr_IHPS_SB2_ESup_Risk_Adj.pdf.

Leff, B., Reider, L., Frick, K.D., *et al.* (2009). Guided Care and the cost of complex health care: a preliminary report. *The American Journal of Managed Care*, 15, 555–559.

Lorig, K.L., Holman, H.R. (2003). Self-management: history, definition, outcomes, and mechanisms. *Annals of Behavioral Medicine*, 26(1), 1–7.

Marsteller, J., Hsu, Y.J., Reider, L., *et al.* (2010). Physician satisfaction with chronic care processes: a cluster-randomized trial of Guided Care. *Annals of Family Medicine*, 8, 308–315.

MedHomeInfo: Your resource to becoming a Medicare Medical Home. (2009a) *"Practice Leaders in Medical Homes" online course.* Retrieved from http://medhomeinfo.org/tools/physiciancourse/index.html.

MedHomeInfo: Your resource to becoming a Medicare Medical Home. (2009b) *Online Nurse Course and Certificate: "Guided Care Nursing."* Retrieved from http://medhomeinfo.org/tools_online_nurse_course.htm.

Newcomer, R., Harrington, C., Kane, R. (2000) Implementing the second generation social health maintenance organization. *Journal of the American Geriatrics Society*, 48, 829–834.

Pope, G.C., Kautter, J., Ellis, R.P., *et al.* (2004) Risk adjustment of Medicare capitation payments using the CMS-HCC model. *Health Care Financing Review*, 25(4),119–141.

Wolff, J.L., Giovannetti, E.R., Palmer, S., *et al.* (2009) Caregiving and chronic care: the Guided Care program for families and friends. *The Journal of Gerontology: Medical Sciences*, 64A, 785–791.

Wolff, J.L., Giovannetti, E.R., Boyd, C.M., *et al.* (2010) Effects of Guided Care on family caregivers. *The Gerontologist*, 50, 459–470.

Chapter 11

Care management plus

Cherie P. Brunker, David A. Dorr, and Adam B. Wilcox

Introduction

More than 130 million Americans live with chronic illness, and two-thirds who are aged 65 and older have chronic conditions, putting them at higher risk of hospitalization, dying, and associated increased health care costs (Anderson 2005; Dorr *et al.* 2006a). Medicare beneficiaries who have one or more of the following characteristics have higher fee-for-service expenditures: multiple chronic conditions, increased hospitalizations, dual eligibility for Medicare and Medicaid, or limited life expectancy (last year of life). Spending is concentrated among beneficiaries; only 25% of beneficiaries account for a disproportionate 83% of expenditures, and of the 20 conditions that are the fastest growing in terms of total spending, 2 are acute and 18 are chronic (Medicare Payment Advisory Commission 2010).

Care Management Plus (CMP) is a model of comprehensive care coordination that addresses the complex issues of patients and their caregivers, and includes the following process areas: identification of the individuals who may benefit from care coordination, assessment, care planning, use of disease management guidelines, teaching/coaching patient and family self-management skills, attention to care transitions, coordination of providers, proactive monitoring, and providing ongoing guidance and support. With multiple chronic illnesses and health care needs, care coordination programs must address the holistic needs of a person. CMP is a program that intends to address a broad set of needs for people at risk to reduce disability, improve health, reduce hospitalizations, and reduce mortality.

Care management plus in primary care

CMP is a primary care based interdisciplinary team model from Intermountain Healthcare and Oregon Health and Science University. CMP includes specially trained care managers, most often registered nurses (RNs) or social workers, and information technology (IT) tools to help clinicians better care for patients with complex chronic illness. The model helps the clinical team prioritize health care needs and prevent complications through structured protocols, and provides tools to assist patients and caregivers to self-manage chronic diseases. Specialized IT includes the care manager tracking database, the patient summary sheet, and messaging systems. These tools allow clinicians to access care

Comprehensive Care Coordination for Chronically Ill Adults, First Edition. Edited by Cheryl Schraeder and Paul Shelton.
© 2011 John Wiley & Sons, Inc. Published 2011 by John Wiley & Sons, Inc.

plans and receive reminders about best practices, and the tools facilitate communication among the health care team and with other providers such as subspecialists. Evaluation studies from implementing CMP were highly positive, and reflected improved clinical and economic outcomes. The initial seven sites for testing CMP were urban practices, each comprised of six to ten clinicians. These clinics employed full-time RN care managers who worked with a panel of about 150 active patients.

The development of CMP was funded by the John A. Hartford Foundation. Researchers worked with the care managers to create tools and training materials to help the primary care team manage patients more effectively and efficiently. They also studied various care manager tasks to determine which were the most important in helping patients, as well as how the care managers interacted with physicians and patients (The John A. Hartford Foundation 2007).

About 3% to 5% of patients in a primary care clinic receive care coordination. CMP is not a rigidly prescribed model of care. There is flexibility in identifying patients who may benefit, a variety of services provided, and adjustment of time and length of care (dosage) for patients and their caregivers. Optimally, the adoption of CMP should occur in settings which include disease management guidelines, health information technology (HIT) with electronic health records (EHRs), secure electronic communications, and decision support tools to facilitate proactive, coordinated care which is integrated with other health care providers such as subspecialists and with other providers and community resources.

Outcomes and dissemination

The clinical and cost outcomes of the CMP approach in its initial testing were significant and positive. Care managers in seven clinics cared for more than 23,000 patients over five years, rendering more than 100,000 services (Dorr *et al.* 2006b). In the initial evaluation, patients with diabetes had better control of their blood sugars and were more likely to be tested, which would be expected to result in 15% to 25% fewer long-term complications (Dorr *et al.* 2005). This translates into significant savings in medical and social service costs, and allows patients with chronic illness to live independently far longer. Seniors with diabetes had a 20% reduction in mortality and a 24% reduction in hospitalizations, potentially saving Medicare up to $75,000 per clinic (Dorr *et al.* 2006c; Dorr *et al.* 2008).

CMP focuses on two primary areas: (1) well-trained care managers within the practice, and (2) technology to help them manage patients with chronic illnesses. Figure 11.1 describes the primary aspects of the CMP program. Patients with complex needs are referred by their provider. The care manager then co-creates a care plan with the patient, acts as a catalyst and guide to help the patient/family meet their goals, and facilitates access to necessary resources when they need assistance. The role and information needs of care managers highlight the specific elements of care coordination, collaboration, and communication needed to be successful in caring for patients with complex needs (Wilcox *et al.* 2007). More than 50% of the information seeking of care managers does not fit into standard typologies for primary care practice (Dorr *et al.* 2006d).

One of the primary discoveries we made was that clinics already had many of these functions, and that IT use could be successfully enhanced through addition of a small set

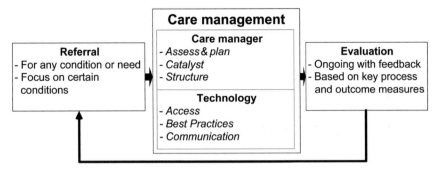

Figure 11.1   Components of the Care Management Plus Program

of functions. These functions can be separated into two categories: quality and care coordination. The amount of information related to measures of disease management, assessed in decision making, and discussed and reviewed with patients was extensive. The patient summary sheet, a succinct report that includes decision support information, facilitated discussion of disease management measures, preventive needs, and care planning, and as well as helping plan and direct the visit, could be given to the patient to take from the appointment. Voluntary use of this summary sheet improved process and outcomes measures for quality by 17% to 30% (Wilcox *et al.* 2005).

Additionally, software was created for the care manager that tracks self-management goals and care plans, provides reminders about best practices, and facilitates many elements of provider and patient communication. Detailed information about the tools is available at the CMP website (www.caremanagementplus.org). Use of the tracking system was a crucial component to the positive outcomes described above, as it allowed the care managers to facilitate multiple different population management and care planning components simultaneously. The system was created separately from the internally developed EHR at Intermountain Healthcare because the population management and care management tasks required a different information model and functions.

Due to the successful CMP outcomes and the overwhelming need for redesign of chronic care services, the Hartford Foundation has supported program dissemination during the past four years. An implementation process was developed for interested health care organizations (Figure 11.2) and the original care manager training curriculum was augmented and updated, still keeping the key elements of case-based learning, emphasis on geriatrics training, and identification and utilization of community resources. In addition to educating health care leaders, physicians, clinic managers, and care managers, foundation support allowed providing assessment of existing EHR functions and adoption of IT. To date, over 150 clinical teams in 15 states have implemented CMP.

With additional support from the Agency for Healthcare Research and Quality we developed the Integrated Care Coordination Information System (ICCIS) which has enhanced CMP-proven HIT functions that can interface with a health care organization's current computer systems (including EHRs, standards, and workflow). The ICCIS is a web-based application that meets Healthcare Information Technology Standards Panel (HITSP) and Health Insurance Portability and Accountability Act (HIPAA) privacy and security requirements. The ICCIS also includes additional caregiver information, designated patient goals, improved tracking of workflow, and a dashboard of specific quality measures.

To implement provisions of the American Recovery and Reinvestment Act of 2009, the Centers for Medicare & Medicaid Services announced rulemaking provisions to include incentive payments to providers for the "meaningful use" of EHR functions for improving quality and safety, providing care coordination, examining population management, and engaging patients and their families (DesRoches & Rosenbaum 2010). CMP has identified best practices in the coordination of care and care management techniques and incorporated them into HIT. Many of these components are similar to those suggested for medical home accreditation (such as through the National Committee for Quality Assurance 2008). The medical home accreditation, however, does not include identification of patients with complex illnesses. For care coordination, the first step is to refer a patient for ongoing care management.

The analysis of CMP also included optimal "dosage" which identified a number of care coordination patterns that worked well for patients with complex illness (Dorr *et al.* 2007a). In all, 22,899 services were completed for 4,735 patients. Care managers spent an average of 230.5 ($\pm$ 268.2) minutes working with patients and their families per year, seeing them, on average, 4.8 times and providing 2.6 different types of services. Patterns of care management that emerged included active coordination, active disease management, or brief, intense interactions (Table 11.1). These patterns contributed to a 10% to 25%

Table 11.1 Example Patterns and Elements of Coordinated Care Found Through CMP
($N = 4,735$)

Coordination of Care Pattern	Coordination Element	% of Pts with Service	Similar Medical Home Concepts
Referral	Referral to Case Management	100%	Communication
Engagement	Explaining and sharing summaries*	82%	Communication
	Assessing for activation and readiness to change	86%	Patient Preference
Brief, Intense	Education (self-management, chronic illness, other)	77%	Self-Management
	Goal setting and follow-up	82%**	Care Management
Active Disease Management	Care management assessment	98%	Care Management
	Following protocols*	95%	Protocols
	Motivational interviewing/coaching	71%/51%+	Care Management
Active Coordination	Communication with other providers/ community resources	77%	Coordination
	Patient/family assessment for barriers, preferences	93%	Assessment
	Care conferences	24%	Coordination

Notes:
*Also closely related to quality
**From team-based EHR Use
+71% for one, 51% for two or more coaching encounters per protocol.

absolute increase in the accomplishment of process measures of care. The active disease management and brief intense patterns also improved the odds of achieving positive outcomes in patients with diabetes and cardiovascular disease by reducing HbA1c and LDL levels.

Curriculum

Education and acquiring skills are important to implementing new models of care. As part of implementing CMP, following the clinic or health care system's readiness assessment and enrollment (see Figure 11.2), care managers, health care leaders, physicians, and clinic managers attend in-person training sessions (Widmier *et al.* 2010). CMP care managers also complete online training. After successful completion, care managers receive 30 hours of American Nurses Credentialing Center credits. Their learning starts with eight to twelve hours of in-person training for an intensive jumpstart in gaining skills in assessment of patients and families, functional, cognitive, and depression screening, and motivational interviewing (Larsen 2009). These skills are reinforced and complemented by a series of online learning modules that cover the fundamentals of care management, special issues in geriatric syndromes and concepts, chronic disease management with related assignments, case-based learning, discussions, and expert calls, and they rely heavily on resources such as the John A. Hartford Geriatric Nursing Initiative.

The CMP curriculum objectives include the following: (1) Empower patients with multiple chronic diseases to organize, prioritize, and implement suggested self-management strategies; (2) Identify barriers to care and intervene to overcome or eliminate these when possible; (3) Coordinate resources to ensure that necessary services are provided at the most appropriate time and level of care; (4) Identify patient situations at risk for destabilization and intervene to eliminate the risk when possible; and (5) Gather, interpret, and

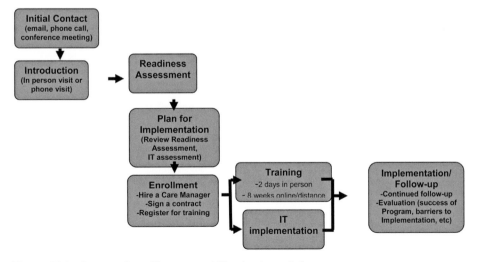

Figure 11.2   Steps to Care Management Plus Implementation

use data to identify problems and trends and to demonstrate clinical outcomes and cost-effectiveness. Faculty and mentors include instructors from Intermountain Healthcare, Oregon Health & Science University, University of Utah, and other institutions.

Case discussion

Ms. Viera is a 75-year-old woman who has Diabetes Type 2, systolic hypertension, Class B congestive heart failure, osteoarthritis, and recently diagnosed mild to moderate dementia. Ms. Viera and her daughter, who is her caregiver, come to clinic with several problems, including hip and knee pain, trouble taking all of her current 12 medicines, dizziness when she gets up at night, low blood sugars in the morning, and a recent fall. Her daughter also mentions that she is concerned about her mother being alone during the day when she is at work. These multiple medical and psychosocial issues can overwhelm a busy primary care practitioner. The addition of the care manager can help prioritize and address these complex issues.

The physician addresses the low blood sugars, the recent fall and the medication issues, and is able to decrease or discontinue four of the 12 medications. The patient summary sheet, with the medication updates, is given to Ms. Viera and her daughter to remind them of the changes made. Referral to the care manager results in a personal introduction in the clinic and referral to county aging resources and the Alzheimer's Association to address the options for daytime assistance and caregiver support.

The care manager completes documentation in the Care Manager Tracking Tool and schedules a phone call in two days and a return appointment in the next week. These tasks appear on the "tickler" list to remind the care manager. The reminders remain until completed. On return to the clinic, Ms. Viera and her daughter meet with the care manager during which patient and caregiver assessments are completed and coaching and follow-up to earlier discussions occur. The care manager also prints a patient summary sheet to review with them. The care manager has lab work completed per standing order by the physician after prompted by the patient summary sheet reminders for laboratory tests which are due for diabetes management and medication monitoring. The care manager completes a brief progress note and sends a message to the physician regarding the patient's progress.

At Intermountain Healthcare Medical Group, physicians who work with care managers are more productive compared with matched physicians who do not (Dorr *et al.* 2007b). In addition, physicians perceive that working with care managers increases their productivity, improves quality of care, produces a better understanding of patient status, and helps them have higher satisfaction in their work. They also recognize and appreciate the additional skill and expertise that the care manager brings to the team (Wilcox *et al.* 2007).

Summary

Care Management Plus is an innovative, evidence-based care model for older adults with complex needs and for others with chronic conditions. It features a unique blend of specialized care management and information technology support. It has been shown to improve outcomes, reduce costs, increase teamwork, and streamline workflow associated with caring for older patients with challenging issues. At the heart of CMP is a care manager (usually a nurse or social worker), who teams with primary care physicians, advanced practice nurses or physician assistants in primary care. CMP is a proven model of interdisciplinary team care to help meet the complex needs of people with multiple conditions, to address the high prevalence of geriatric syndromes such as falls, cognitive loss, and frailty, and to attend to the complicated psychosocial needs of patients and their caregivers. High cost of care and a need to increase efficiency are prime motivators for innovations in care. Goals of CMP include improved patient outcomes, increased coordination of care and decreased health care costs all in the context of the individual patient's preferences and goals.

References

Anderson, G. (2005) Medicare and chronic conditions. *New England Journal of Medicine*, 353, 305–309.

DesRoches, C.M., & Rosenbaum, S.J. (2010) Meaningful use of health information technology in U.S. hospitals. *New England Journal of Medicine*, 362, 1153–1155.

Dorr, D.A., Wilcox, A., Donnelly, S.S., *et al.* (2005) Impact of generalist care managers on patients with diabetes. *Health Services Research*, 40(5 Pt I), 1400–1421.

Dorr, D.A., Jones, S.S., Burns L., *et al.* (2006a) Use of health-related, quality-of-life metrics to predict mortality and hospitalizations in community-dwelling seniors. *Journal of the American Geriatrics Society*, 54, 667–673.

Dorr, D.A., Brunker, C.P., Wilcox, A., *et al.* (2006b) *Implementing Protocols is Not Enough: The Need for Flexible, Broad Based Care Management in Primary Care.* Agency for Healthcare Research and Quality, Translating Research Into Practice and Policy (TRIPP) Conference, July 10–12, Washington, DC.

Dorr, D.A., Wilcox, A., Burns, L., *et al.* (2006c) Implementing a multi-disease chronic care model in primary care using people and technology. *Disease Management*, 9(1), 1–15.

Dorr, D.A., Tran, H., Gorman, P., *et al.* (2006d) Information needs of nurse care managers. *American Medical Informatics Association Annual Symposium Proceedings*, 913.

Dorr, D.A., Wilcox, A., Jones, S., Burns L, *et al.* (2007a) Care management dosage. *Journal of General Internal Medicine*, 22, 736–741.

Dorr, D.A., Wilcox, A., McConnell, K.J., *et al.* (2007b) Productivity enhancement for primary care providers using multicondition care management. *The American Journal of Managed Care*, 13(1), 22–28.

Dorr D.A., Wilcox A.B., Brunker C.P., *et al.* (2008) The effect of technology supported, multidisease care management on the mortality and hospitalization of seniors. *Journal of the American Geriatrics Society*, 56, 2195–2202.

Larsen, A. (2009) *Roles and Responsibilities of Care Managers.* Care Management Plus Training Workshop, Portland OR.

Medicare Payment Advisory Commission. (2010) *A Data Book: Healthcare Spending and the Medicare Program.* Medicare Payment Advisory Commission, Washington, DC.

National Committee for Quality Assurance. (2008) *Physician Practice-Connections Patient-Centered Medical Home.* National Committee for Quality Assurance, Washington, DC. Available at: http://www.ncqa.org/tabid/631/Default.aspx.

The John A. Hartford Foundation (2007) *Geriatric Interdisciplinary Teams in Practice*. Annual Report, The John A. Hartford Foundation, New York, NY, 28–40.

Widmier, L., Brunker, C., Dorr, D. (2010) *Comprehensive Curriculum for Care Managers: Expanding Geriatrics Skill Sets with Care Management Plus*. Unpublished Report. Oregon Health & Sciences University, Portland, OR.

Wilcox, A.B., Jones, S.S., Dorr, D.A., *et al.* (2005) Use and impact of a computer-generated patient summary worksheet for primary care, *American Medical Informatics Association Annual Symposium Proceedings*, 824–828.

Wilcox, A.B., Dorr, D.A., Burns, L., *et al.* (2007) Physician perspectives of nurse care management located in primary care clinics. *Care Management Journal*, 8(2), 58–63.

Chapter 12

Medicare coordinated care

Angela M. Gerolamo, Jennifer Schore,
Randall S. Brown, and Cheryl Schraeder

Introduction

Coordinating care for individuals with multiple chronic conditions is challenging because they frequently see numerous providers with no one integrating treatment (Pham *et al.* 2007). In addition, providers often do not routinely communicate with each other, in large part because fee-for-service systems do not provide reimbursement for such coordination. Designating one provider (or organization) responsible for coordinating care and facilitating patient self-management has intuitive appeal as an approach to improving care; however, even among studies with strong research designs, the effects of such interventions to date have been mixed (Brown 2009; Mattke *et al.* 2007; Gravelle *et al.* 2007; Smith *et al.* 2005; DeBusk *et al.* 2004; Galbreath *et al.* 2004; Congressional Budget Office [CBO] 2004). The lack of clear-cut findings has resulted in the inability of program payers and policymakers to identify promising practices in coordinated care that would be cost effective to fund.

A key question that emerges from these mixed findings is "Why are some coordinated care interventions effective while others are not, when they appear to include similar components such as assessment, care planning, monitoring, and patient education?"[1] The answer may be that although the interventions are similar in design, they differ in how intensively and by whom they are implemented, how they are refined over time, the environmental context in which they are set, and the population that is targeted (Mahoney 2010).

This chapter addresses this question using, as a basis, the 15 programs that were part of the Medicare Coordinated Care Demonstration (MCCD) sponsored by the Centers for Medicare & Medicaid Services (CMS) from 2002 to 2006.[2] Only 2 of the 15 programs reduced hospitalizations overall (Peikes *et al.* 2008), and for both, the effects were concentrated in a subgroup of high-risk beneficiaries.[3] For the high-risk group, only 4 of the 12 programs with enough cases to examine subgroup effects significantly reduced hospitalizations by 8% to 33%.[4] The disparity in impacts between these 4 programs and the other 8 programs points to the need to examine critically how the interventions were implemented by the 4 programs. This chapter draws on findings from the impact and implementation analyses conducted during the original and extended evaluations of the

Comprehensive Care Coordination for Chronically Ill Adults, First Edition. Edited by Cheryl Schraeder and Paul Shelton.
© 2011 John Wiley & Sons, Inc. Published 2011 by John Wiley & Sons, Inc.

MCCD as well as additional qualitative data collection from 7 of the 11 programs that continued to operate through 2008.[5] The interventions implemented by the 4 programs that reduced hospitalizations among high-risk Medicare beneficiaries, Health Quality Partners (HQP), Hospice of the Valley, Mercy Medical Center (Mercy), and Washington University (Washington U), are the focus of this chapter.

This chapter begins with a description of the programs' target-patient populations and settings and the similarities and differences in how they implemented basic coordinated care components. The chapter then highlights promising practices that were consistently present across the 4 programs and likely contributed to their effectiveness in reducing hospitalizations. Emphasis is placed on the characteristics of these programs that were not prevalent among the programs that did not reduce hospitalizations. The chapter concludes by describing the extent to which the literature supports or refutes these practices and discusses implications for practice and policy.

Similarities and differences across program interventions

Setting and target population

Although the four programs shared many features, they were implemented in four disparate settings: (1) a hospital that is part of an integrated delivery system in rural Iowa (Mercy Medical Center in Mason City), (2) a safety-net academic hospital in a major city (Washington University in St. Louis), (3) a hospice with expanded program services (Hospice of the Valley in greater Phoenix), and (4) a quality improvement services provider that acts as an adjunct to primary care (HQP in suburban and rural Pennsylvania). The positive effects in these varied settings suggest that care coordination, if targeted to the appropriate populations and including essential intervention features, can be effective in diverse settings throughout the country. Table 12.1 illustrates the setting, service area, populations targeted, and exclusion criteria for each program.

All programs had to apply the CMS demonstration-wide eligibility criteria for participating beneficiaries who were enrolled in Medicare Parts A and B, had Medicare as primary payer, and not enrolled in a Medicare managed care plan. Programs could then develop their own selection criteria. Although all four programs targeted Medicare beneficiaries with a wide range of medical diagnoses and complex conditions, they each targeted different patient populations (See Table 12.1). The HQP program used a formal assessment tool to classify patients into four risk levels. HQP chose not to enroll patients in the lowest of its four risk groups from the inception of demonstration, and it also stopped enrolling moderate-risk patients in 2006 (those in its second-lowest risk group). Two programs, Hospice of the Valley and Mercy, required its enrollees to have at least one hospital admission in the year prior to enrollment. At the start of the demonstration, Washington U identified patients using the proprietary algorithm of a commercial disease management (DM) vendor. After dissolving its partnership with the DM vendor, Washington U targeted beneficiaries with risk of hospitalization over the following year and it relied on referrals from providers to identify potential enrollees.[6] Table 12.2 shows the baseline characteristics of the Medicare beneficiaries randomized through December 2006.

Table 12.1 Program Setting, Service Area, and Target Population

	HQP	Hospice of the Valley	Mercy	Washington U
Program Setting	Quality improvement services provider	Hospice with expanded program services	Integrated Delivery System (Mercy Health Network)	Academic medical center partnered with commercial disease management provider[a]
Service Area	Eastern Pennsylvania; mix of rural, suburban, and urban areas	Maricopa County, Arizona (greater Phoenix); urban	14-county service area in central Iowa and centered in Mason City; rural	St. Louis city; eight counties in Missouri and three counties in Illinois; urban and suburban
Target Population[b]	Chronic heart and lung conditions, diabetes, and uncontrolled hyperlipidemia or hypertension	Advanced CHF, COPD, cancer, and neurological conditions and at least one hospital admission in the year prior to enrollment	CHF, chronic lung disease, liver disease, stroke, other vascular diseases, or renal failure and a hospital admission or emergency room visit in the year prior to enrollment	At least one chronic medical condition and at high risk of incurring substantial medical costs within the next year (prior to 2006 based on proprietary screening algorithm)
Exclusion Criteria	Learning difficulties due to psychosis or dementia, under age 65, organ transplant candidates, cancer, or long-term nursing home residents	Under age 65, have end-stage renal disease, or receive Medicare hospice benefits	Long-term nursing home residents, receiving Medicare hospice benefit, or end-stage renal disease	Receiving hospice services, organ transplant candidates

Source: Site visit notes and documents from original and extended MCCD evaluations (Peikes et al. 2008; Schore et al. 2009).
Notes:
[a]The collaboration with the disease management provider was dissolved in January 2006.
[b]Target population for original demonstration was not cost-effective. These four programs were only cost effective for identified high risk patients as defined by Peikes et al. 2009; Peikes et al. 2010).
CHF = Congestive heart failure; COPD = chronic obstructive pulmonary disease.

231

Table 12.2 Characteristics of Medicare Beneficiaries*

		Treatment and Control Group Members Enrolled Through December			
Characteristics of Beneficiaries at Enrollment	HQP (N = 1613)	Hospice of the Valley (N = 1597)	Mercy Medical Center (N = 1144)	Washington U (N = 2780)	Medicare Total in 2003 (N = 42.3 million)
Age					
< 65	0	0	4.6	27.2	14.4
≥ 85	7.3	27.6	16.9	10.5	11.1
Male	40.3	41.1	54.3	44.8	44.0
Race/Ethnicity					
Nonwhite, Non-Hispanic	0.7	1.3	0.3	38.4	9.5
Hispanic	0.0	1.0	0.1	0.2	7.8
Medicaid	2.2	12.3	11.6	20.3	19.3
Less than High School Education	10.6	18.5	30.5	25.6	30.4
Diagnosis					
CAD	38.3	63.1	69.1	62.9	40.5
CHF	12.3	51.8	64.2	46.2	40.5
Diabetes	23.4	27.3	32.9	40.8	20.6
COPD	7.6	38.4	46.5	25.5	15.3
Cancer	9.6	21.3	14.8	26.7	17.3
Stroke	4.0	16.4	12.1	10.0	12.1
Depression	7.0	22.1	21.9	24.3	NA
Dementia	1.8	24.1	4.5	10.5	5.2
Number of 12 Possible Chronic Conditions	1.6	3.6	3.4	3.3	NA
Number of Annualized Hospital-izations	0.3	1.4	1.4	1.8	0.3
Number of Enrollees in High-Risk Subgroup (% of All Program Enrollees)	273 (17)	1,138 (71)	904 (79)	1,975 (71)	NA
Monthly Expenditures, $	484	2,230	1,509	2,496	552

Source: Peikes *et al.* 2010
Notes:
*All figures are percentages unless otherwise noted.
CAD = coronary artery disease; CHF = Congestive heart failure; COPD = chronic obstructive pulmonary disease; NA = not applicable.

Program structural features

Program structural features include staffing and training (for example, types and number of professionals hired), caseloads, electronic recordkeeping, quality management, and physician relations. These features, in turn, affect the nature, mode, and intensity of care coordinator contacts with patients as well as availability of other clinical and support staff. Table 12.3 illustrates structural features for each program.

Program staffing and training

All programs required care coordinators to be experienced registered nurses. Washington U also required certification by the Commission for Case Manager Certification. Overall, the programs' staffing was stable, with very low (or no) turnover among care coordinators over the five years of the demonstration. Mercy, Washington U, and Hospice of the Valley also employed a social worker either full-time or part-time during the demonstration, whereas HQP relied on nurse care coordinators to arrange for social services or to refer patients with complex mental health problems to a psychiatric clinical nurse specialist. Although HQP did not have a dedicated social worker, the project manager was a clinical social worker and served as a resource to care coordinators as needed.

The programs had administrative and/or other clinical staff to support the nurse care coordinators. Mercy had a full-time office manager throughout the demonstration and HQP had either a part-time or full-time administrative assistant throughout the demonstration. HQP also employed a chart abstractor until August 2007, to abstract patients' clinical measures from physician practice records; it had to eliminate the position due to cost concerns. Washington U had an operations director and augmented its staff with three care assistants who verified program eligibility and assumed clinical responsibility over time as caseloads increased (for example, contacting patients by telephone). Hospice of the Valley also employed an administrative assistant in addition to having a recruiter/data manager and a part-time marketer.

All four programs provided orientation to newly hired care coordinators; however, they each varied in structure, content, and duration. HQP's care coordinator orientation lasted the longest and included the most in-depth supervision. The three- to six-month orientation used role-playing and shadowing of supervisors; its content included training in behavior change theory and in the provision of group education. Hospice of the Valley's orientation included one week of formal training covering disease processes, pain management, advance directives, policies and procedures, and community resources, among other topics. It included a field training period of two to six weeks depending on each care coordinator's educational level and needs. Mercy's orientation was a four- to six-week, self-guided, competency-based training overseen by another, more experienced care coordinator. Washington U's orientation included instruction on assessment, care planning, the data management system, and Medicare guidelines and coverage and provided ongoing learning opportunities through team conferences. After separating from the DM vendor, Washington U's care coordinators also attended continuing education through the local chapter of Case Management Society of America (CMSA).

Table 12.3 Program Structural Features

	HQP	Hospice of the Valley	Mercy	Washington U[a]
Program Staffing and Training				
Number of Care Coordinators	9 (7 full-time/2 supervisors)	8	5 (4 full-time/1 supervisor)	9
Care Coordinator Case Load (average per FTE)	108 35 per Supervisor	45	75 60 per Supervisor	90
Type of Care Coordinator Training	Didactic, structured teaching, and ongoing clinical supervision	Didactic, structured teaching, and initial clinical supervision	Self-directed competency-based training with preceptor oversight	Didactic, structured teaching, and case management certification
Other Staff to Provide Direct Care	Psychiatric clinical nurse specialist	Social worker Pharmacist	Social worker Pastor	Social worker Care manager assistants
Support Staff	Administrative assistant Chart abstractor[b]	Administrative assistant Marketer[c] Recruiter/data manager[c]	Office manager	Operations director
Information and Quality Management				
Information Management System(s)	Microsoft Access database; chart review database	HomeWorks for Hospice™	Case Management Information System[d]	Care Coordination Information System[e]
Access to External Electronic Health Records	Yes	No	Yes	Yes
Reports Clinical Indicators	Yes	No	No	Yes
Monitors and Reports ED Visits and Hospitalizations	Yes	Yes	Yes	Yes
Monitors and Reports Care Coordinator Performance	Yes	Yes	Yes	Yes

Sources: Site visit notes from original and extended MCCD evaluations (Peikes *et al.* 2008; Schore *et al.* 2009).
Notes:
[a] Descriptions are based on program redesign after separation from the disease management vendor.
[b] This position was eliminated in August 2007, due to cost constraints.
[c] These staff members assisted with marketing to physician practices and recruiting beneficiaries.
[d] The case management information system was developed for use during the demonstration.
[e] The care coordination information system was developed by the University of Scranton. Washington U purchased the system and modified it for use in the demonstration after the program separated from the disease management vendor.

234

Caseload size

Staff size, availability of other resources, and most importantly, patient characteristics influenced the size of care coordinator caseloads. HQP care coordinators had larger caseloads than their Hospice of the Valley, Mercy, and Washington U counterparts. Six to seven years into the demonstration, HQP had nine care coordinators: seven with an average of 108 patients, and two supervisors with 35 patients each. However, HQP's patients were far healthier than those in the other three programs. Hospice of the Valley had eight care co-ordinators with 45 patients each. Mercy had five care coordinators, four with an average of 75 patients, and one supervisor with 60 patients.[7] Washington U had nine care coordinators with up to 90 patients each, although the intention was to maintain a caseload of 70 patients. Based on impacts observed and the cost of employing full-time nurses, it appears that caseloads of 80 to 100 would be necessary to achieve cost neutrality (Brown 2009).

Electronic recordkeeping

Hospice of the Valley used HomeWorks for Hospice case management software that stored assessment, care planning, and monitoring information; however, care coordinators did not have direct access to the system. After its separation from the DM vendor in 2006, Washington U modified a care coordination information system developed by the University of Scranton. The system maintained assessment and preventive screening data, contact dates, reassessment dates, medication lists, hospitalizations and ED visits, and care plans with outcome indicators. The program used these data to monitor program outcomes and care-coordinator performance.

HQP and Mercy developed information management systems to track recruitment, eligibility, enrollment, demographics, emergency contact information, referring physician, and (as required for the evaluation) information on program contacts with patients. Both programs also used paper records to maintain information from the initial and ongoing assessments and to keep detailed notes from contacts. In 2006, HQP began analyzing patient data from its Microsoft Access-based system (which included information abstracted from physician practice records, patient self-reports, and clinical measures – such as blood pressure – that care coordinators obtained directly) using a web-enabled platform, Statit e-QC. This new analytic capability allowed coordinators to generate reports and graphs; a drill-down feature allowed analyses that ranged from program-wide statistics (for example, on the percentage of patients who had flu shots over time), to individual care coordinator caseload statistics, to individual patient data (such as specific patients who had not had flu shots). The reports often compared the outcomes with program- or patient-level goals or national benchmarks. Other reports showed the extent to which needed tests were overdue.

Although none of the programs had a full electronic health records system that linked directly to other providers, HQP, Mercy, and Washington U care coordinators had access to the electronic databases of the hospitals that served the majority (60% to 95%) of their patients.[8] These hospital databases included information about hospitalizations, emergency department (ED) encounters, diagnostic testing results, clinic visits with physicians that were part of the hospital system, and medications. The three programs scanned these databases to identify program patients who were hospitalized or had recently visited the ED. Hospice of the Valley had no link to hospital data, thus, there was no consistent access to primary or specialty care physicians' medical records.

Quality management

Quality management includes ongoing monitoring of the intervention over time to identify opportunities for process improvement and to ensure program effectiveness. This involves systematic data collection and monitoring, evaluating findings, and making changes based on those findings. HQP collected and analyzed data to assess program effectiveness from the beginning of the MCCD, and its capability to perform these functions became more sophisticated over time. Unlike the other programs, HQP care coordinators used reports to track whether their patients as a group were meeting goals and to guide specific behavioral interventions. For example, they used individual patient graphs over time to show patients how they were doing and to link improvements or declines in outcomes (such as weight, blood glucose level, blood pressure) to behavior change or life events. At the program level, managers and care coordinators used reports on program processes and patient outcomes to determine whether the program was meeting its goals concerning patient health and to ensure adherence to standard operating procedures, guidelines, and protocols. The program made decisions to change or add to interventions based on these data and on research suggesting the intervention would be effective for its target population.

After Washington U switched to a different data management system in April 2006 (following its separation from the DM vendor), the program began conducting internal monitoring to assess program effectiveness and care coordinator performance. For example, program directors assessed the timeliness of contacts with patients and providers to ensure adherence to program protocols. They also monitored hospital and ED admissions and other clinical indicators. Findings were shared with individuals' care coordinators informally; however, if a widespread performance issue was identified, they were all retrained.

Mercy's quality improvement efforts consisted primarily of the routine assessments of staff competencies conducted for all staff affiliated with Mercy Medical Center, including the Mercy coordinated care program. These assessments focused on two areas of improvement each year. Topics included, for example, increasing rates of influenza vaccination, increasing use of advance directives, and maintaining patient privacy. Mercy also conducted a study in 2006, to determine the effects of reducing in-person contacts on outcomes for established patients and discovered that the reduction resulted in no increase in adverse patient outcomes (for example, hospitalizations). As a result, Mercy care coordinators began to contact patients with whom they had already developed good working relationships more frequently by telephone instead of in person. Although the decision to alter contact mode was based on these data, Mercy's approach to implementing change more generally tended to be relatively informal and driven by a consensus among care coordinators and other staff that a particular change was needed.

At Hospice of the Valley, quality improvement planning for the coordinated care program was conducted in conjunction with the Hospice of the Valley Quality Improvement Committee. The program monitored the following indicators on a quarterly basis: average number of patient referrals to the program, patient contacts, rates of hospital and ED admissions, and other patient outcomes such as falls. Patient satisfaction was monitored annually.

These data were discussed with care coordinators during team meetings, and the group developed a plan if a change was needed, an approach similar to the one used by Mercy.

Programs' relationships with physicians

Since it can be difficult for a care coordination program external to physicians' practices to get physicians' attention, let alone their full participation, all of the programs promoted their care coordinators to physicians as "their eyes and ears" with patients between office visits. To foster care coordinator-physician relationships, HQP, Hospice of the Valley, and Mercy tried to assign patients so that each physician only worked with one care coordinator; however, this did not always happen as geography and the need to balance patient-illness severity level within coordinators' caseloads usually took precedence. Programs tailored their communications to each physician's preferences and minimized the amount of paperwork sent.

The two Mercy care coordinators based in the hospital clinics saw physicians more frequently than their HQP, Hospice of the Valley, and Washington U counterparts. Mercy care coordinators in general had strong and collaborative relationships with physicians, due in large part to the care coordinators and many physicians sharing the same employer (Mercy Health Network), and all residing in the same close-knit rural communities. Many had known each other professionally, and sometimes as neighbors, for many years. As a result, physicians and their office staff trusted the care coordinators to triage patient problems. If a care coordinator requested that the physician see a patient immediately, they knew the situation was truly urgent.

Although Washington U care coordinators were not co-located with physicians, they shared an employer with a majority of patients' physicians. Washington U still had limited contact with physicians even though they shared the same employer. The care coordinators attended physician appointments with some patients and used these opportunities to establish themselves as credible clinicians, and demonstrate their value to physicians. Over time, physicians occasionally contacted care coordinators to see if they were able to attend upcoming appointments and to share patient information. In addition, the Washington U program further strengthened its relations with its patients' physicians through a physician advisory board that provided input to the programs operating procedures. Members of this board were compensated for their contribution.

Unlike Mercy, the HQP and Hospice of the Valley programs were unable to capitalize on strong pre-existing organizational and physical ties to physician practices. Although some HQP care coordinators had space in physicians' offices early in the demonstration, these arrangements were terminated as practices grew, eliminating opportunities for informal communication between care coordinators and physicians. HQP also worked with more than 70 different physician practices, which precluded the degree of care coordinator-physician familiarity and communication enjoyed by Mercy. Similarly, although Hospice of the Valley attempted to build care coordinator-physician relationships by having care coordinators attend physician visits and sending patient updates to physicians every six months, they worked with too many physicians' practices spread over a large geographic region with whom they did not have previous close operational and organizational relationships to establish truly close connections.

Programs' process features

Programs' process features are the specific actions performed by the care coordinators, such as assessment, care planning, monitoring, education, and facilitating communication with and among providers. Programs conducted comprehensive assessments, provided self-management education, served as a liaison between providers and patients, and used a comprehensive approach to medication management. HQP and Washington U were distinguished, however, by their use of structured protocols to standardize the management of care transitions across all care coordinators. For example, both programs used protocols that specified when and how to contact hospitalized patients and when to follow up during the post-acute care period. Both HQP and Washington U also received timely notification of hospital admissions for a majority of their patients. Mercy and Hospice of the Valley relied much more on their care coordinators' discretion to determine the details of their interventions (for example, when a care coordinator contacted a patient after discharge from the hospital).

Assessment

The assessment process provided care coordinators with a picture of the patient's health, functional status, and resources for self-management, from which the care coordinator identified problems appropriate for the program to address. All four programs' care coordinators performed initial assessments within two weeks after a patient's enrollment and also conducted periodic reassessments. HQP, Hospice of the Valley, and Mercy performed the initial assessment in person at the patient's home and/or physician's office, whereas Washington U conducted initial assessments by telephone.

The programs' assessment tools varied widely. Following its pre-random-assignment assessment with the Sutter Health Questionnaire, the tool used to determine level of severity, HQPs highest-risk patients were further divided into those with and without geriatric frailty.[9] (High-risk patients with geriatric frailty typically have multiple medical, social, and functional problems that require significant caregiver and social supports.) Those without geriatric frailty then received an in-person disease-specific assessment, and those with geriatric frailty received an in-home geriatric assessment. The in-home assessment covered physical, cognitive, and nutritional status; depression; violence screening; home safety; pain and sleep rating; incontinence; and caregiver ability. As part of the initial assessment for all patients, and periodically thereafter, the care coordinators also conducted physician chart reviews.[10] In 2009, HQP began conducting a formal annual reassessment using the Sutter tool.

Hospice of the Valley's initial assessment was always conducted in the patient's home and included four tools based on the Outcome and Assessment Information Set (OASIS): (1) patient history form, (2) comprehensive care coordinator's assessment form, (3) management of medications form, and (4) Short Portable Mental Status Questionnaire. In addition, the program used the Missoula-Vitas Quality of Life Index and the *Medi*Caring[TM] Physician Report. These tools cover medical and surgical history, functional status, nutrition, psychosocial status, availability of social support, caregiver grief, home safety, medications, and a physical and pain management assessment. The initial

Table 12.4 Initial Assessment and Problem Identification

	HQP	Hospice of the Valley	Mercy	Washington U[a]
		Initial Assessment		
Initial Assessment in Person	Yes	Yes	Yes	No
Patient Stratification Based on Severity Level	Yes; Sutter Health Questionnaire	Yes; no formal tool	No; although did so initially to balance caseload by acuity	Yes; Life Indicators Tool (began in 2006)
Assessment Tools Used	Disease-specific initial assessment; In-home Comprehensive Geriatric Assessment (for high-risk patients with geriatric frailty)[b]	Patient History Form; Nursing Assessment Form; Management of Medications Form; Short Portable Mental Status Questionnaire[c]	Nursing assessment; Spiritual assessment; Social services assessment; Morse Fall Scale[d]	Initial Health Screen; Nursing assessment; SF-36; Life Indicators tool[e]
Formal Reassessment	Annual reassessment with Sutter Risk Assessment and depression screening	Six month reassessment	Six months after enrollment and annual reassessment	Depression screening every three months; Six month reassessment with SF-36 and Life Indicators tool

(*Continued*)

Table 12.4 (*Continued*)

	HQP	Hospice of the Valley	Mercy	Washington U[a]
	Problem Identification and Planning			
Use of Nursing Classification System[f]	No	No	Yes; NANDA, NIC, NOC	Yes; NANDA, NIC, NOC
Sharing of Care Plan with Physicians	Initial assessment summary is sent to physician.	Care plan is faxed to physician after six month reassessment.	Physician is asked to sign care plan annually.	No; patients encouraged to discuss with physician.
Care Plan Updated with each Contact	Yes	Yes	Yes	Yes

Source: Site visit notes from original and extended MCCD evaluations (Peikes *et al.* 2008; Schore *et al.* 2009).

Notes:

[a] Descriptions are based on program redesign after separation from the disease management vendor.

[b] Assessment tools are multidimensional and include validated instruments as well as questions developed by HQP regarding physical assessment, violence screening, behavioral and caregiver assessment, prevention, psychosocial assessment, home safety, sleep, and incontinence. Instruments embedded in the assessment tools include: Mini-Mental Status Exam (Folstein *et al.* 1975); the Clock Drawing Test (Heinik *et al.* 1997); CAGE Questionnaire (Ewing 1984); Geriatric Depression Scale Short Form (Yesavage *et al.* 1983) Nutritional Risk Assessment (Nutrition Screening Initiative, 1991); Numeric Rating Scale (Jacox *et al.* 1994).

[c] The Patient History Form and the Nursing Assessment Form Management of Medications Form was developed by Hospice of the Valley for use in the demonstration; the assessment also used the Short Portable Mental Status Questionnaire (Pfeiffer 1975).

[d] The nursing, spiritual, and social services assessments were developed by Mercy for the demonstration; the assessment also included the Morse Fall Scale (Morse 1985)

[e] Washington University's assessment included Initial Health Screen which was developed by StautsOne, a nursing assessment, the Medical Outcomes Study Short Form SF-36 (Ware and Sherbourne 1992); and the Life Indicators Tool which was developed by Washington University.

[f] Nursing classification systems provide a standard taxonomy for classifying nursing diagnoses, interventions, and outcomes. The North American Nursing Diagnoses Association (NANDA), Nursing Intervention Classification (NIC), and the Nursing Outcomes Classification (NOC) are recognized as the official nursing languages by the American Nurses' Association.

assessment emphasized end-of-life care and advance directives. For almost all patients, the program also requested medical records information from patients' physicians and typically received information back on about 85% of these requests. Hospice of the Valley care coordinators performed a formal reassessment using a reassessment tool that includes items from the initial assessment tools. Reassessment occurred every six months or when there was a change in health status or an admission to the hospital or ED.

Mercy's initial assessment tool was modeled on Mercy Health Network's home care assessment; it covered medical and surgical history, review of body systems, functional status, nutrition, psychosocial status, availability of social support, home safety, medications, and a social services and spiritual assessment. In 2005, the Morse Fall Scale was added to the initial assessment due to high fall-risk among patients. For the approximately 65% of patients who were part of the Mercy system, care coordinators also drew information for their assessments from the network's electronic health records system, Cerner Power-Chart, which was implemented in 2005. Mercy care coordinators reassessed patients six months after enrollment and annually thereafter using the same initial assessment tools.

At the beginning of the demonstration, Washington U's initial assessment included the Initial Health Screen (IHS), which was used to identify current conditions, medications, and treatments; recently used health services; activities of daily living; and support needed. This information was used to develop an acuity score that determined the frequency of patient contact with care coordinators. During the next contact, care managers then completed an initial comprehensive nursing assessment and a baseline functional status assessment using the Health Assessment Questionnaire, developed by the DM vendor and modeled after the SF-36. After the program separated from the DM vendor and delivered all services locally, the program developed and used the Life Indicators tool to standardize acuity scoring done by care managers. Washington U also implemented the SF-36, which measured physical functioning, role limitations due to physical health and emotional well-being, pain, general health perceptions, and mental health. Patients were screened for depression routinely every three months and were formally reassessed using the SF-36 and the Life Indicators tool every six months.

Care planning

Care planning is an ongoing and dynamic process for developing measureable goals, prioritizing problems identified during assessments, determining the most appropriate approaches to address them, and deciding when they have been resolved. Care plans focus on illness prevention, health promotion and maintenance, patient education, and required support services. Mercy and Washington U care coordinators developed formal nursing care plans using the North American Nursing Diagnoses Association (NANDA) classification system and used the Nursing Intervention Classification (NIC) and the Nursing Outcomes Classification (NOC) systems, which include a taxonomy of standard nursing interventions and patient/family responses to them. Although Mercy sent the care plan to the patient's primary physician each year to review, add to (if desired), and sign, Washington U did not. As in Washington U's program, Hospice of the Valley did not share a written care plan with patients' physicians, but its care coordinators faxed patients' six-month reassessments to their physicians, noting any changes in condition and new medications. Washington U care coordinators gave patients a written summary of the care document and encouraged them to discuss it with their providers. Although HQP did not use a formal nursing care plan, it did use assessment summaries; these summaries were shared with the patient's primary provider. In 2009, HQP developed an electronic problem list to prioritize patients' needs because staff felt they sometimes lost track of less urgent patient problems over time. All programs updated their care plans during each patient contact.

Monitoring

Monitoring includes assessing patient status and responding quickly to physiological, behavioral, and other changes that could lead to a hospitalization or an ED visit. All program care coordinators monitored their patients through regular contacts. These contacts typically included addressing patients' ongoing needs, identifying new needs, and following up on progress toward care plan goals. Other specific topics covered were whether the patient had an ED visit or hospitalization since the last contact, and if so, why, as well as how a repeat event could be avoided – and a discussion of physician visits, both planned and unplanned, since the last contact. Medication management was also an important focus during contacts. Care coordinators asked patients at every contact about changes in medications since the last contact, whether medications were having the desired effect, adverse reactions, whether they were being taken as prescribed, and difficulty obtaining or affording medications. If necessary, the programs helped patients apply for financial assistance to purchase medications or discussed less costly generic alternatives with their physicians. During home visits, HQP, Hospice of the Valley, and Mercy care coordinators also reviewed patients' medication bottles to ensure the patient understood why he or she was taking the medications, if medications were taken as prescribed, and to identify redundant or expired medications and over-the-counter products that could interfere with prescribed medications.

Because patients may only discuss prescriptions they have filled and omit those prescribed but not filled, all of the programs collected information about patients' medications beyond patients' self-reports and medication bottles. Thus, the programs abstracted information from physician charts (HQP), required information from patients' physicians and pharmacists (Hospice of the Valley and Washington U), or pulled data from electronic health records (Mercy). In addition, Hospice of the Valley required that a pharmacist review all medications for potential drug-drug interactions for patients taking 10 or more medications at a time. If any discrepancies were identified between information sources, care coordinators instructed patients to call their physicians or did so on their behalf.

All programs felt that in-person contacts were critical to establishing trusting relationships in which patients were comfortable telling the care coordinators about new problems and concerns. In particular, visiting patients in their homes allowed care coordinators to observe them in their environment and assess its impact on health status (for example, by evaluating neighborhood and home safety). However, in order to manage their caseloads, care coordinators used a combination of in-person and telephone contacts. According to data collected for the original evaluation (Peikes *et al.* 2008), during the early years of the demonstration, HQP care coordinators averaged 2.2 contacts per month with their patients

(0.92 per month for in-person contacts); Hospice of the Valley averaged 2.5 contacts per month (0.93 in person); Mercy averaged 1.4 contacts per month (0.97 in person); and Washington U averaged 1.2 contacts per month (0.06 in person).[11]

HQP care coordinators' in-person contacts took place in the patient's home, during group education in the program's main office, at the patient's physician's office, or in community locations rented by the program (for example, community centers and a wellness center). Hospice, Washington U's, and Mercy's in-person visits took place in the patient's home, at the patient's physician's office and hospital. Hospice of the Valley in-person visits took place in the home.

The Hospice of the Valley program did not use guidelines to specify the frequency of visits, rather, the frequency of a patient's in-person visits depended on how long the patient was enrolled in the program. During the first six months after enrollment, patients were visited as frequently as needed based on the care coordinators' judgment. If a patient avoided hospitalization or an ED visit during that time and was making progress toward his or her goals, the visit frequency then became monthly, and the care coordinator decided whether these would be in person or by telephone. As mentioned earlier, Washington U used the Life Indicators tool to develop an acuity score which then guided the *minimum* frequency of contacts. For example, acuity scores range from 1 to 5, with 1 reflecting the

Table 12.5 Ongoing Monitoring

	HQP	Hospice of the Valley	Mercy	Washington U[a]
Ongoing Monitoring				
Mean Number of Contacts per Month[b]	2.2	2.5	1.4	1.2
Mean Number of In-Person Contacts per Month	0.92	0.93	0.97	0.06
Contacts Based on Level of Severity	Yes	Yes	Yes	Yes
Location of In-Person Contacts	Home, physician office, community space, program office	Home, physician office	Home, physician office	Home, physician office
Care Coordinator Availability	Regular office hours only	Regular office hours but may telephone triage nurses or care coordinators 24/7	On call 24/7	On call 24/7

Source: Program contact data and site visit notes from original and extended MCCD evaluations (Peikes *et al.* 2008; Schore *et al.* 2009).
Notes:
[a]Descriptions are based on program redesign after separation from the disease management vendor.
[b]Contact data were collected during patients' first year of enrollment in the program.

highest level of acuity. Patients with acuity scores of 1 or 2 were contacted at least every one to two weeks, whereas patients with acuity scores of 5 were contacted at least every four to six weeks. In contrast to the other three programs that only used care coordinators, Washington U used care manager assistants, who were under the supervision of care coordinators, to contact patients with lower levels of acuity.

Patient education

All care coordinators educated patients on signs and symptoms of disease and problem-solving skills patients needed to confidently manage their chronic conditions. They also taught patients when to call their physicians and coached them on how to communicate more effectively (for example, by reminding patients to prepare lists of questions in advance of physician visits and to always carry current medication lists). They sometimes used role-play to teach patients how to advocate for themselves. Rather than merely conveying factual information, the care coordinators based their education on the transtheoretical behavior change model[12] and used the techniques of motivational interviewing.[13] However, the programs' education interventions differed in how consistently they used the transtheoretical behavior change model and how extensively care coordinators were trained in its application. HQP and Washington U care coordinators received formal training in the use of behavior change theory during orientation, whereas Hospice of the Valley provided ongoing guidance on the approach during monthly patient conferences. Unlike the Washington U and Mercy care coordinators, the HQP and Hospice of the Valley care coordinators formally assessed readiness to change during contacts, tailored each educational activity accordingly, and routinely addressed relapse (which, according to the transtheoretical model, is a normal part of the change process). In 2006, HQP also began to use graphs of patients' clinical data (for example, a graph of weight over time) as educational tools; this allowed patients to make the connection between changes in personal behaviors and changes in outcomes and to see that they had some control over their health.[14]

HQP care coordinators were the only ones providing group education classes (for patients able and willing to attend).[15] The HQP care coordinators were trained to provide cardiovascular education (Heart Healthy workshop); weight loss (LEARN Program) and weight maintenance; physical activity (Active Living Every Day, chair exercise classes, and walking groups); and balance and mobility training (FallProof). HQPs staff added various group education classes after they recognized the need and were able to identify effective programs; the LEARN and Active Living Every Day classes were added in 2004, and FallProof was added in 2005.

Facilitating communication and coordination

One of the challenges facing people with chronic illness is that the communication between their many providers is often poor. Making sure that all providers have key information at the right time and that patients understand the self-care that their providers have prescribed for them is likely to be especially important for high-risk patients who see more physicians, require more diagnostic testing, and take more medications. Patients and their caregivers can take on some of the responsibility of improving communication and coordination, and self-management education in all of the programs included teaching patients (or their caregivers) to coordinate their care across providers, to the extent that they were able to do so. For example, care coordinators emphasized the importance of keeping all providers apprised of any new medications prescribed. Care coordinators also took on the communication facilitator role; that is, they served as a link between patients, physicians, and other providers when problems were identified. The programs differed, however, in that Mercy care coordinators took on the role as part of their routine, day-to-day practice, whereas HQP, Washington U, and Hospice of the Valley care coordinators only did so around specific events or practice issues, such as hospital admissions or urgent patient problems (for example, serious symptoms or significantly out-of-range laboratory values). This role typically included making sure patients got preventive care and diagnostic tests recommended by evidence-based guidelines for their conditions, managing medications (previously described), and helping with care setting transitions (discussed further on). Moreover, Mercy's two care coordinators who were based in the Mercy Health Network's internal medicine and family practice clinics had particularly strong opportunities for enhancing communication and coordination. Their frequent informal contact enabled them to routinely share patient information (for example, the results of patients' visits with specialists since care coordinators attended the visits and diagnostic information from the Cerner system) with their patients' primary care physicians.

Table 12.6 Communication and Coordination with Physicians

	HQP	Hospice of the Valley	Mercy	Washington U[a]
Communication and Coordination				
Formal Communication with Physicians	Summary of initial assessment form	Care plan	Communique Form	Quarterly meetings with physician advisors[b]
Common Mode of Interactions Between Care Coordinators and Physicians	Telephone	Telephone, fax	Telephone, In-person for two care coordinators co-located in office	Telephone, fax
Opportunities for Informal Communication	Accompany some patients to physician appointments	Accompany some patients to physician appointments	Accompany some patients to physician appointments, Co-location in office	Accompany some patients to physician appointments

Source: Site visit notes from original and extended MCCD evaluations (Peikes *et al.* 2008; Schore *et al.* 2009).

Notes:
[a]Descriptions are based on program re-design after separation from the disease management vendor.
[b]Many program patients' physicians participated in the Physician Advisory Committee (PAC) which provided input to the program's protocols and procedures.

Managing care transitions

Over 20% of chronically ill Medicare patients are readmitted to the hospital shortly after discharge (Jencks *et al.* 2003); these readmissions are often the result of well-documented failures in communication with patients and coordination among providers that typically occur when patients' transition from hospital to home (Bodenheimer & Berry-Millett 2009; Coleman *et al.* 2005a; 2005b; 2006; Flacker *et al.* 2007; Naylor 2003; Naylor *et al.*, 2004). Patients often leave the hospital with several new medications, some of which are redundant with existing regimens or even contraindicated. Patients' acute illnesses are improved but still not completely stable, and they frequently go home with an incomplete understanding of what signs and symptoms to look for as warnings of deterioration in their condition, and what to do if problems arise. Once home, they do not fully understand medication and other discharge instructions and may feel too ill to make needed follow-up doctors' appointments or do not keep them because they do not fully understand their importance. Unfortunately, patients' primary physicians are frequently unaware that their patients have been hospitalized because they were admitted by a specialist or through the ED (this was, in fact, the repeated experience in the four programs).

In order to intervene in and improve their patients' care transitions, the care coordination programs had to learn of patients' hospitalizations in a timely way. As described above, the HQP, Mercy, and Washington U care coordinators had access to the electronic health records of the hospitals that serve most of their patients and thus could scan daily inpatient rosters to see if any of them had been admitted. The Hospice of the Valley care coordinators did not have such access, however, and relied on patients or patients' families to notify them of any hospitalizations.

The HQP and Washington U care coordinators followed a structured protocol for hospitalized patients to ensure consistent completion of necessary interventions. In HQPs protocol, care coordinators were required to contact the hospital case manager upon admission and every four days thereafter. They also contacted the patient within one working day after discharge from the hospital and arranged to visit the patient at home within one week. Washington U's care coordinators were required to contact the patient by phone within 24 to 48 hours after discharge from the hospital and used their discretion to determine the timing of an in-person home visit. In both programs, the focus of these post-discharge contacts, whether in-person or telephone, was to reconcile medications, review signs and symptoms of the precipitating illness, identify strategies to avoid a repeat event, and ensure that patients understand discharge instructions and had scheduled follow-up appointments with their physicians. In contrast, although the Mercy care coordinators communicated with hospital care managers and sometimes visited hospitalized patients, they did not follow an explicit protocol in doing so, relying instead on their experience and judgment. The Mercy program encouraged its care coordinators to make an in-home visit within one week after discharge, with the same goals as the HQP and Washington U's post-discharge contacts.

The Hospice of the Valley program did not always know about patients' hospitalizations. However, program management estimated that they knew about hospitalizations for 40% of patients and further determined that care coordinators conducted in-home visits for 80% of these cases within seven days of hospital discharge. Features of Hospice of the

Table 12.7 Care Transition Management

	HQP	Hospice of the Valley	Mercy	Washington U[a]
		Care Transition Management		
Use of Formal Protocol for Managing Care Transitions	Yes	No	No	Yes
Process for Identifying Whether Patients had ED Visits and Hospitalizations	Inpatient and ED reports from main hospital received daily and reviewed by supervisor	Patients and their caregivers expected to notify care coordinators	Office manager reviews; Cerner (Mercy hospital's electronic medical record system) for inpatient and ED reports	Inpatient and ED reports received from main hospital daily
Provides Relevant Information to Hospital Staff	Yes	If informed of admission	Yes	Yes
Hospital Visits	Occasionally	If informed of admission	Occasionally	At least one visit while patient is hospitalized
Frequency of Contact with Hospital Discharge Planners	Telephone call upon admission and every 4 days thereafter	Varies	Varies	Varies
Post-Discharge Care	Telephone call to patient within 1 working day after discharge; arranges visit within 1 week; Increased monitoring	If informed of admission, care coordinator visits within 1 week after discharge; reconciles medications and assess home safety	Usually visits within 1 week after discharge; reconciles medications and ensures follow-up care	Contacts patients within 2 days after discharge; reconciles medications; visits to patients based on care coordinator discretion

Source: Site visit notes from original and extended MCCD evaluations (Peikes *et al.* 2008; Schore *et al.* 2009).

Note:

[a] Descriptions are based on program redesign after separation from the disease management vendor.

Valley's post-discharge interventions were similar to the other three programs and included identification of the causes of hospitalization, assessing home safety, and reconciling medications.

Improving access to support and counseling services

As noted earlier, the Washington U, Hospice of the Valley, and Mercy programs employed social workers (though Mercy's was only dedicated part-time to the program, and the social worker employed by Washington U's program had a dual function as a care coordinator but was available to assist all patients). HQP care coordinators referred patients who needed support services to local Area Agencies on Aging and consulted with a clinical nurse specialist for patients with complex psychiatric problems including personality disorders and cognitive deficits. In addition, HQPs project manager had a background in clinical social work and was available to provide social work input on specific cases as needed. Mercy also had a chaplain affiliated with Mercy Medical Center who counseled program patients if care coordinators determined that they would benefit from pastoral care. None of the programs used a formal procedure to assess the effectiveness of support services to which they have referred patients; rather, they asked patients about their satisfaction with the services during routine contacts.

Summary of promising practices

Although the four programs that reduced hospitalizations among high-risk beneficiaries differed in how they implemented their interventions, six features were consistently present in the programs and could be considered promising practices for adoption by others who seek to deliver effective care coordination. In addition to these practices, other well-intentioned features were used by either all or most of the programs in the original demonstration including: (1) implementation of mutual goals and action plans monitored frequently through patient/family contacts with adjustments made as needed; and (2) use of evidence-based guidelines and protocols for chronic illnesses and geriatric problems. Although these features did not necessarily distinguish programs with impacts from those without, evidence suggests that they are important for delivering individualized care to patients with complex chronic conditions.

The following section first discusses the extent to which the literature supports or refutes targeting high-risk populations, because that is the subgroup that demonstrated favorable outcomes. Then, the section describes the literature related to the six features consistently present in the four programs. In addition to targeting the right population, the promising practices featured:

(1) *in-person contact with patients* approximately monthly (three of four programs also perform the initial patient assessment in-person rather than by telephone[16]);
(2) *behavioral change theory and motivational interviewing* to guide patient education, coaching and support effective self care;
(3) *collaborative and interdisciplinary approach* to medication management;

Table 12.8 Promising Practices in Coordinated Care

Target Population: High-Risk Patients[a] with Multiple Chronic Conditions
In-person contact with patients approximately monthly
Use of behavior change theory and motivational interviewing to guide patient education and self-management; coach and mentor patients
Collaborative and interdisciplinary approach to medication management
Facilitator of communications with health and community providers when problems arise, telephoning about change in patient status, updating other health and community providers on change in status
Comprehensive approach to managing transitions across care settings (for example, after hospitalization)
Opportunities for face-to-face contact with patients' physicians such as attending physician visits and rounds

Note: The identification of promising practices is based on qualitative comparisons between four programs with favorable outcomes versus five programs in the original MCCD evaluation that did not achieve similar outcomes. These structural and process features were consistently present in all of most of the four programs with positive outcomes.
[a]Patients with chronic obstructive pulmonary disease (COPD), congestive heart failure (CHF), or coronary artery disease (CAD) and at least one hospitalization in the prior year or any of 12 chronic conditions and two or more hospitalizations in the prior 2 years.

(4) *facilitator of communication* with health and community providers when problems arose;
(5) comprehensive approach to *managing care transitions* (three of the four programs also received timely notification of hospital admissions); and
(6) *opportunities for face-to-face contact with patients' physicians* through, for example, care coordinators attending office visits, co-location with physicians, or regular contact during hospital rounds.[17]

Although all four programs did not set out to target high-risk beneficiaries, this subgroup of patients benefited most from the programs' interventions, suggesting that targeting high-risk patients may be necessary to reduce hospitalizations and achieve cost savings. Other studies of care management programs targeting complex or high-risk patients have generally shown positive results, whereas studies of interventions in patients at lesser risk have shown more mixed results. The Geriatric Resources for Assessment and Care of Elders (GRACE) (Counsell et al. 2007; Counsell et al. 2009) and a multi-disease care management program employing nurse care managers supported by specialized information technology (Dorr et al. 2008) had statistically significant effects on costs for a subgroup comprised of high-risk patients but not for the full set of patients served by the program. In addition, quasi-experimental evaluations of a primary care based disease management and chronic care intervention in high-risk, chronically ill older adults in the community found that it improved physician-patient communications, lowered health expenditures, and reduced hospitalizations and emergency room visits, although the differences were not statistically significant (the Guided Care intervention; Boyd et al. 2008; Sylvia et al. 2008). In their literature synthesis, Bodenheimer and Berry-Millett

(2009) concluded that care management programs are more likely to reduce costs when they target patients with multiple disease conditions who are at high risk for undergoing expensive care. The results from these four programs are consistent with the literature.

In-person contact with patients

Sharing an underlying belief that some form of regular in-person contact is key to establishing trusting relationships with patients, the programs ensured approximately monthly in-person contact that included visiting patients in their homes or a community center, accompanying patients to physician appointments, and in some cases, visiting patients during hospitalization. Furthermore, to enable meaningful and sufficiently frequent face-to-face contacts, the programs' caseloads ranged between 45 and 108 patients. It should be noted, however, that demonstration programs with caseloads lower than 80 patients were not cost neutral. The literature supports the need to design interventions that include at least some face-to-face contact with patients. Periodic contact with patients that is almost exclusively by telephone is not sufficient to detect early warning signs and prevent hospitalization (Bott *et al.* 2009; Brown 2009). Moreover, Sochalski and colleagues (2009) found that, among 10 care coordination programs for patients with heart failure evaluated with randomized designs, those with in-person contacts reduced hospital readmissions. Similarly, multiple in-person nurse visits to older adults with disabilities were associated with positive outcomes (Liebel *et al.* 2007).

Behavioral change theory and motivational interviewing

There is ample empirical evidence to support the usefulness of several behavioral change theories in designing interventions to change peoples' health behaviors, such as quitting smoking, increasing exercise, following a healthy diet, and of greatest relevance, chronic illness self-management (Bandura 1977; Prochaska & DiClemente 1983). Self-management education supports patients to live with the highest quality of life with their chronic conditions by teaching problem-solving skills and self-efficacy to change behaviors (Bodenheimer *et al.* 2002). The four programs all reported use of one the most popular and well known of such theories, and care coordinators were trained to apply behavior change theory when providing education on self-management. It should be noted, however, that although managers and care coordinators in the four programs cited the use of the transtheoretical model and motivational interviewing techniques as a key to their success, the evaluation did not examine how well care coordinators' educational efforts actually adhered to behavioral change theory or applied motivational interviewing techniques.

HQP offered group education interventions while the other three programs did not. There is some evidence for the effectiveness of the use of group education and group interventions to promote self-management of chronic conditions. Coleman and colleagues (2001) demonstrated the effectiveness of such an intervention delivered in a primary care setting by a multidisciplinary team (a nurse, a pharmacist, and a physician) to older adults with multiple chronic conditions. Although the intervention focused on self-management education, it also included peer and professional support and health-promotion activities. Patients receiving the intervention were significantly less likely to visit the emergency room than members of a control group during the two-year intervention period. An intervention featuring seven peer-led weekly training sessions that focused on exercise, diet, guided relaxation, and managing emotions also reduced hospitalizations (Lorig *et al.* 1999). Similarly, a randomized study showed that older women with heart disease who received three months of self-management education in a group setting had fewer heart-related hospital days and costs over a two-year period (Wheeler 2003). Group education, however, may not be practical or feasible in many health care settings or for some patient populations.

Collaborative and interdisciplinary approach to medication management

Elderly patients with chronic illnesses tend to take many medications prescribed by several physicians, many of whom are often unaware of all the other medications taken by the patient. These patients are thus at high-risk for polypharmacy, redundant medications, and drug-drug interactions. In addition, patients may not always fill prescribed medications. Supplementing patient self-reports of prescribed medications with reviews of patients' medical records and augmenting care coordinator knowledge with input by pharmacists and physicians could reduce these medication risks.

The programs thus did not rely solely on patient self-reports of prescribed medications; each sought information on patients' prescriptions from other sources such as patients' records. Care coordinators in all four programs addressed medication management during each patient contact by assessing changes in medications since the last contact, their perceived effectiveness of medications, adverse medication reactions, their adherence to medications, and their difficulty obtaining or affording medications. Care coordinators in all four programs also consulted with pharmacists and physicians to discuss potential medication problems and identify approaches to resolve them. As the literature reviewed by Marek and Antle (2008) documents, there is strong evidence for nurse management of medications among community-dwelling elders. Their review described how such nurse medication management enables: (1) medication reconciliation to identify redundant medications and discrepancies between prescribed medications and medications actually taken; (2) improved patient education about the purpose of medications and side effects; and (3) identification and resolution of barriers to medication adherence due to functional or cognitive limitations. The medication management practices used by the care coordinators in the four programs are consistent with the evidence base described in the literature.

Facilitator of communication

The program care coordinators served as facilitators of communication among providers and between patients and their providers. A growing body of research documents the importance of effective communication between multiple providers for better patient outcomes; this holds true in routine primary care but is of special importance when patients transition between care settings (Coleman & Berenson 2004; Stille *et al.* 2005). Previous research has shown that advanced practice nurses (APNs) working with frail, older adults can play an integral role in facilitating communication between providers as well as helping physicians to understand patients' global needs and to adapt their care management strategies accordingly (McCauley *et al.* 2006). Furthermore, APNs have been shown to be an effective link among fragmented systems of care for the most vulnerable populations, including individuals with both serious mental illness and HIV (Kutney *et al.* 2006). Little has been documented about the ability of nurses who are not prepared at the advanced practice level to achieve the same success. The findings from these four programs suggest that experienced registered nurses can also serve as an effective link between multiple health care providers. This finding is important, given the scarcity and higher cost of APNs.

Comprehensive approach to managing care transitions

Medicare spending for roughly half of all beneficiaries identified in 1997 as having multiple chronic conditions was nearly 60% higher over the subsequent four years than for the typical beneficiary (CBO 2005). These high Medicare expenditures are driven primarily by hospital admissions and readmissions (Medicare Payment Advisory Commission 2008). Hospitalization may be a "teachable moment" that motivates patients to improve adherence to recommended self-care more than would a routine education session. However, a hospital admission often results in changes to a patient's medication regimen, such as the addition of new drugs and discontinuation of old ones, and patients may not fully understand all of the changes. Further, despite no longer needing acute inpatient care, patients may not be completely stable at discharge and may need to perform even more intensive self-monitoring and self-care than usual. Finally, health and health-related services need to be coordinated following discharge to avoid excessive testing, fragmented care, and costly rehospitalization.

Coleman and colleagues' (2006) transition management program consisting of medication review and reconciliation and education of patients and caregivers in self-management skills delivered by nurse practitioners has been shown to substantially reduce hospital readmissions among high-risk elderly patients after hospital discharge. In addition, Naylor and colleagues (2004) reported that an intervention consisting of discharge planning, patient education, coordinating care across settings, and direct clinical care conducted by nurse practitioners led to large reductions in hospital readmissions among elderly patients hospitalized for heart failure. Although none of the four programs fully adopted the Coleman or Naylor models, their responses to hospitalizations contained many elements of these models. One notable difference is that the interventions in the studies by Coleman and Naylor were delivered by advanced practice nurses.

Opportunities for face-to-face physician contact

Care coordinators had to distinguish themselves to physicians from the multitude of insurance company staff, pharmaceutical salespersons, and others vying for physicians' attention. Thus, it was essential that the care coordinators had opportunities to have face-to-face contact with physicians formally or informally so that they could make themselves known to physicians. The four programs fostered opportunities for care coordinators to have face-to-face contact with physicians, for example, by having care coordinators accompanying patients to appointments with physicians, or in Mercy's case, co-locating care coordinators with primary care physicians. Research shows that nursing care management without collaboration from primary care physicians does not yield positive patient and cost outcomes (Leibel *et al.* 2007). While it appears that care coordinator-physician face-to-face contacts may contribute to developing collaborative relationships and improving communications, the most effective mechanism for promoting collaboration is still not completely understood. Further, contrary to some expectations, payments to physicians for such contacts were not associated with success in reducing hospitalizations.

Case study

Mr. Johnson is a 76-year-old male who was referred to case management services after a hospitalization for an acute myocardial infarction and stent placement. His medical history includes obesity, hypertension, hyperlipidemia, osteoarthritis, and irritable bowel syndrome-constipation dominant. The care manager (CM) *completed a comprehensive assessment* during an initial home visit with Mr. Johnson and his daughter, Amy. In collaboration with Mr. Johnson and Amy, the care manager determined Mr. Johnson's goals: (1) managing daily activities without his wife who recently died unexpectedly; and (2) taking medication as prescribed. Because his wife was his caregiver and made sure he took his medications as prescribed, Mr. Johnson was unaware of his medication regimen. He also had difficulty bathing his lower extremities, performing household tasks such as vacuuming, mopping, obtaining groceries, and he has never prepared meals. He also had given up driving and his wife always drove him where he needed to go.

The CM *called the physician's office to verify Mr. Johnson's current list of medications* which included: Plavix 75 mg daily, aspirin 81 mg daily, simvastatin 40mg at bedtime, lisinopril 40 mg daily, and hydrochlorothiazide 25 mg daily. Mr. Johnson also reported he took two additional 500 mg aspirin at bedtime for pain, milk of magnesia 30 cc as needed, Ginkgo for memory, and a multivitamin daily. During the conversation, the physician requested that Mr. Johnson stop the Ginkgo and substitute acetaminophen for the aspirin at bedtime. The *CM requested refills* of the Plavix, simvastatin, lisinopril, and hydrochlorothiazide to be called to the pharmacy. Prior to ending the phone call a follow-up appointment was made for Mr. Johnson the next week.

In prioritizing his care, the CM, Mr. Johnson, and Amy decided that it was necessary to develop an immediate plan for medication management. The CM *reviewed all of Mr. Johnson's medications with him* including how and when they were to be taken, what the expected therapeutic effects were, potential side effects, what to do if he missed a dose or took an extra one. Until a medication box could be purchased they obtained envelopes to store and organize the medication by time of administration so the Mr. Johnson would know when he was to take them. Amy *would take him to the pharmacy to pick up the medication and a medication box*. While at the pharmacy they were to *make arrangements for medication to be mailed* to Mr. Johnson upon the request of him or Amy. A *medication list was completed*, a copy would be provided to Mr. Johnson and one to his physician's office.

To help manage his activities of daily living *arrangements were made with the local grocery store to have groceries delivered every 2 weeks* and he would learn to cook. For household chores Mr. Johnson and Amy were provided information regarding a local homemaker agency and together they would *arrange for someone to assist him every 1 to 2 weeks for 4 hours for household cleaning and laundry*. While at the pharmacy Amy and Mr. Johnson would *pick up a shower chair* so he could bath his lower extremities.

Mr. Johnson did well for several weeks until he fell at home and was taken to the local ED. The ED providers determined that Mr. Johnson's fall was due to being septic from a urinary tract infection; his blood sugar was over 550. He was admitted for a course of IV antibiotics and treatment of his elevated blood sugar. The CM *provided the hospital with a list of Mr. Johnson's current home medications*. The hospital discharge planner, Mr. Johnson, and the CM decided that Mr. Johnson would return home after discharge.

The CM *visited Mr. Johnson the day after he returned home. When reviewing his medication*, he had a new medication listed, glucophage 1000 mg daily and Plavix was not listed on his discharge instruction sheet. The CM *contacted the physician's office and obtained an order to restart the Plavix* and *made an appointment for Mr. Johnson* that week. The CM also *obtained an order from the physician's office to enroll Mr. Johnson in Diabetes Management classes*. The CM *assisted Mr. Johnson to complete a new medication sheet adding the new medication*, glucophage. The CM would *provide a new copy of the medication sheet to Mr. Johnson's physician*.

Prior to completion of the home visit the CM *assessed Mr. Johnson's knowledge of and ability at performing blood sugar checks* and recording them. The CM found that he knew he was supposed to do these activities but was not sure he wanted to. The CM concluded he was in the preparation phase of behavior change. He was aware of the need to perform the tasks but not sure he could stick himself to draw blood. The CM *explained the importance of self blood-sugar monitoring* and what the results meant to Mr. Johnson. She *assisted him in performing the blood sugar check* with precise instructions as to how to prick his finger. Mr. Johnson agreed to try and perform the activity the next morning and call the CMs office and report the test results and they would *discuss further what the results meant*.

Conclusion

The reductions in hospitalizations for patients at high-risk suggest that pursuing care coordination programs similar to those operated by HQP, Hospice of the Valley, Mercy, and Washington University makes sense, if the programs can operate at a cost that is equal to or less than the savings generated. As noted above, several interventions that have improved patient outcomes use APNs. APNs demand a higher salary than RNs without masters-level preparation, which has cost implications for program operation. The four programs described in this chapter reduced hospitalizations using experienced RNs. Although further research should examine the comparative effectiveness of APNs versus experienced RNs, these findings show that using RNs as care coordinators can improve outcomes for high-risk Medicare beneficiaries.

In sum, regardless of whether care coordination is implemented as part of a medical home, accountable health care organization, or DM/care coordination program, lessons learned from the evaluation of the MCCD suggest that certain features are necessary to reduce hospitalizations. The potential impact of care coordinator caseload on effective implementation must be considered to ensure regular opportunities for face-to-face contact with patients and their providers.

Notes

1. Effective coordinated care interventions are defined as those that result in better self-care and adherence to recommended treatments while reducing health care costs.
2. To determine whether care coordination improves the quality of care and reduces Medicare expenditures, the Balanced Budget Act of 1997 mandated that the Secretary of Health and Human Services implement and evaluate care coordination programs in the Medicare fee-for-service setting. In early 2001, CMS authorized 15 demonstration programs for the MCCD to operate for four years; 11 of the 15 programs later requested, and were granted, two year extensions and continued to operate into 2008. Of these 11 programs, those sponsored by Mercy Medical Center (Mercy) and Health Quality Partners (HQP) were most successful in reducing hospital use or Medicare costs and were granted another two year extension by CMS. Mathematica conducted site visits to both programs in late 2008 to gather more detailed information about their interventions. Subsequent analysis showed that two other programs, Hospice of the Valley and Washington University, reduced hospializations for high-risk subgroups. In early 2009, Mathematica requested that the nine programs extended only through 2008 update standardized descriptions prepared for the original evaluation; seven programs did so. Detailed findings from the evaluation have been published elsewhere (Peikes *et al.* 2008; Schore *et al.* 2009; Peikes *et al.* 2010).
3. High-risk patients are defined as enrollees which chronic obstructive pulmonary disease (COPD), congestive heart failure (CHF), or coronary artery disease (CAD) and at least one hospitalization in the prior year or any of 12 chronic conditions and two or more hospitalizations in the prior two years (Schraeder *et al.* 2009; Peikes *et al.* 2010).
4. CMS paid each of the 15 programs a negotiated monthly fee for each beneficiary in the treatment group. The evaluation showed that when these care coordination fees were included, none of the 15 programs generated net savings to Medicare over the original four-year evaluation period (through 2006), nine programs definitely increased net costs, three probably increased costs, and three appeared to be cost neutral.
5. Mathematica is the independent evaluator of the Medicare Chronic Care Practice Research Network (MCCPRN), which was established in 2008 to investigate "real world" research questions and to improve the value, enhance the quality, and/or lower the cost of the Medicare program across sites experienced in providing care management services. Nine of the original 15 MCCD sites participate in the MCCPRN.
6. The program was initially jointly developed through partnership with Washington University and a DM vendor. The program used local care coordinators employed by Washington University who contacted patients by telephone and in person and used California-based care managers employed by the vendor who contacted patients only by telephone. The partnership dissolved in 2006. Program impacts were observed only after termination of the partnership.
7. Mercy staff reported that caseloads increased to 100 patients per care coordinator at the end of the two year extension.
8. Mercy's access was by virtue of the program being part of the Mercy Health Network, which also owns the hospital. HQPs access to Doylestown hospital system was by virtue of an arrangement whereby the hospital employed the care coordinators and

leased them back to the program. HQP tried to make similar arrangements with other area hospitals, but privacy concerns and other considerations were major barriers. Washington University obtained access as a result of developing an ongoing collaborative relationship with the main hospital in the Barnes-Jewish-Christian (BJC) network.

9. At the end of 2008, roughly 25% of HQPs patients had been categorized as "high risk with geriatric frailty" and just under 66% as "high risk without geriatric frailty."

10. As noted earlier, HQPs program had a chart abstractor to assist the care coordinators but had to eliminate the position in August 2007 due to cost constraints.

11. Data on care coordinator monitoring frequency and location, collected systematically by the programs for the evaluation, are for patients who enrolled during the first year of the demonstration (April 2002 through March 2003) and cover each patient's first year after enrollment. Thus, these data do not reflect changes in in-person contacts as programs matured.

12. This model posits that individuals move through five distinct stages (or levels of readiness) for behavior change and that relapse or regression to an earlier level is a common part of the process (Prochaska & DiClemente 1983).

13. Motivational interviewing is a patient-centered counseling style based on empathy, identifying discrepancies between patient goals and current behaviors, assuming that the patient is responsible for the decision to change, accepting resistance to change rather than confronting it, and supporting patient self-efficacy and optimism for change (Emmons & Rollnick 2001).

14. HQPs focus on improving patient health behavior stemmed, in part, from research suggesting behavior change (such as weight loss, increased physical activity, and smoking cessation) is more important than health care in reducing morbidity and mortality (Schroeder 2007).

15. At the end of 2008, just under 66% of all HQP patients had participated in at least one of its 10 group education programs; participation ranged from 44% among patients in the program's highest risk group to 84% among those in its lowest risk group.

16. Although Washington U did not initially perform in-person contacts, they did so once their relationship with the DM vendor dissolved in 2006.

17. Opportunities for some face-to-face contact with physicians ere important for care coordinators to distinguish themselves from other clinicians; however, these opportunities do not suggest that care coordinators always had strong collaborative working relationships with physicians. In addition, the frequency to which care coordinators took advantage of these opportunities is not known.

References

Bandura, A. (1977) Self-efficacy: toward a unifying theory of behavioral change. *Psychological Review*, 84, 191–215.

Bodenheimer, T., Lorig, K., Holman, H., *et al.* (2002) Patient self-management of chronic disease in primary care. *Journal of the American Medical Association*, 288, 2469–2475.

Bodenheimer, T., & Berry-Millett, R. (2009) *Care Management of Patients with Complex Health Care Needs*. Research Synthesis Report No. 19, The Robert Wood Johnson Foundation, Princeton, NJ.

Bott, D., Kapp, M., Johnson, L., *et al.* (2009) Disease management for chronically ill beneficiaries in traditional Medicare. *Health Affairs*, 8(1), 86–98.

Boyd, C.M., Shadmi, E., Conwell, M., *et al.* (2008) A pilot test of the effect of guided care on the quality of primary care experiences for multimorbid older adults. *Journal of General Internal Medicine*, 23, 536–542.

Brown, R. (2009) *The Promise of Care Coordination: Models that Decrease Hospitalizations and Improve Outcomes for Medicare Beneficiaries with Chronic Illness*. A report commissioned by the National Coalition on Care Coordination. Available at: http://www.socialworkleadership.org/nsw/Brown_Executive_Summary.pdf.

Coleman, E.A., Eilersten, T.B., Kramer, A.M., *et al.* (2001) Reducing emergency visits in older adults with chronic illness: a randomized controlled trial of group visits. *Effective Clinical Practice*, 4(2), 49–57.

Coleman, E.A., & Berenson, R.A. (2004) Lost in transition: challenges and opportunities for improving the quality of transitional care. *Archives of Internal Medicine*, 141, 533–536.

Coleman, E.A., Mahoney, E., & Parry, C. (2005a) Assessing the quality of preparation for posthospital care from the patient's perspective – the care transitions measure. *Medical Care*, 43, 246–255.

Coleman, E.A., Smith, J.D., Raha, D., *et al.* (2005b) Posthospital medication discrepancies: prevalence and contributing factors. *Archives of Internal Medicine*, 165, 1842–1847.

Coleman, E.A., Parry, C., Chalmers, S., *et al.* (2006) The care transitions intervention: results of a randomized clinical trial. *Archives of Internal Medicine*, 166, 1822–1828.

Congressional Budget Office. (2004) *An Analysis of the Literature on Disease Management Programs*. Congressional Budget Office, Washington, DC.

Congressional Budget Office. (2005) *High-Cost Medicare Beneficiaries*. Congressional Budget Office, Washington, DC.

Counsell, S.R., Callahan, C.M., Clark, D.O., *et al.* (2007) Geriatric care management for low-income seniors: a randomized controlled trial. *Journal of the American Medical Association*, 298, 2623–2633.

Counsell, S.R., Callahan, C.M., Tu, W., *et al.* (2009) Cost analysis of the geriatric resources for assessment and care of elders care management intervention. *Journal of the American Geriatrics Society*, 57, 1420–1426.

DeBusk, R.F., Houston Miller, N., Parker, K.M., *et al.* (2004) Care management for low-risk patients with heart failure: a randomized, controlled trial. *Annals of Internal Medicine*, 141, 606–613.

Dorr, D.A., Wilcox, A.B., Brunker, C.P., *et al.* (2008) The effect of technology-supported, multidisease care management on the mortality and hospitalization of seniors. *Journal of the American Geriatrics Society*, 56, 2195–2202.

Emmons, K.M., & Rollnick, S. (2001) Motivational interviewing in health care settings: opportunities and limitations. *American Journal of Preventive Medicine*, 20(1), 68–74.

Ewing, J.A. (1984) Detecting alcoholism: the CAGE questionnaire. *Journal of the American Medical Association*, 252, 1905–1907.

Folstein, M.F., Folstein, S.E., & McHugh, P.R. (1975) Mini-mental state: a practical method for grading the cognitive state of patients for the clinician." *Journal of Psychiatric Research*, 12, 189–198.

Galbreath, A.D., Krasuski, R.A., Smith, B., *et al.* (2004) Long-term healthcare and cost outcomes of disease management in a large, randomized, community-based population with heart failure. *Circulation*, 110, 3518–3526.

Gravelle, H., Dusheiko, M., Sheaff, R., *et al.* (2007) Impact of case management (Evercare) on frail elderly patients: controlled before and after analysis of quantitative outcome data. *British Medical Journal*, 334(7583), 31–34.

Flacker, J., Park, W., & Sims, A. (2007) Hospital discharge information and older patients: do they get what they need? *Journal of Hospital Medicine*, 2, 291–296.

Heinik, J., Vainer-Benaiah, Z., Lahav, D., *et al.* (1997) Clock drawing test in elderly schizophrenia patients. *International Journal of Geriatric Psychiatry*, 12, 653–655.

Jacox, A., Carr, D.B, Payne, R., *et al.* (1994) *Management of Cancer Pain: Clinical Practice Guideline, No. 9.* AHCPR Publication No. 94-0592. Agency for Health Care Policy and Research, U.S. Department of Health and Human Services, Public Health Service, Rockville, MD.

Jencks, S.F., Huff, E.D., & Cuerdon, T. (2003) Change in the quality of care delivered to Medicare beneficiaries, 1998–1999 to 2000–2001. *Journal of the American Medical Association*, 289, 305–312.

Kutney, L.A., Hanrahan, N.P., Aiken, L.H., *et al.* (2006) Perceived facilitators and barriers to the implementation of an advanced practice nursing intervention for HIV regime adherence among the seriously mentally ill. *Journal of Psychiatric and Mental Health Nursing*, 13, 626–628.

Liebel, D.V., Friedman, B., Watson, N.M., *et al.* (2007) Review of nurse home visiting interventions for community dwelling older persons with existing disability. *Medical Care Research and Review*, 66, 119–146.

Lorig, K.R., Sobel, D.S., Stewart, A.L., *et al.* (1999) Evidence suggesting that a chronic disease self-management program can improve health status while reducing hospitalization: a randomized trial. *Medical Care*, 37(1), 5–14.

Mahoney, J.E. (2010) Why multifactorial fall-prevention interventions may not work. *Archives of Internal Medicine*, 170, 1117–1119.

Marek, K., & Antle, L. (2008) Medication management of the community-dwelling older adult. In *Patient Safety and Quality: An Evidence-Based Handbook for Nurses*, (ed. R.G. Hughes), pp. 499–536. Agency for Healthcare Research and Quality, Publication No. 08-0043, Rockville, MD. Available at: http://www.ahrq.gov/qual/nurseshdbk/.

Mattke, S., Seid, M., & Ma, S. (2007) Evidence for the effect of disease management: is $1 billion a year a good investment? *American Journal of Managed Care*, 2007, 670–676.

McCauley, K.M., Bixby, B.M., & Naylor, M.D. (2006) Advanced practice nurse strategies to improve outcomes and reduce cost in elders with heart failure. *Disease Management*, 9, 302–310.

Medicare Payment Advisory Commission. (2008) *A Databook: Healthcare Spending and the Medicare Program.* Medicare Payment Advisory Commission, Washington, DC.

Morse, J.M., Prowse, M.D., Morrow, N., *et al.* (1985) A retrospective analysis of patient falls. *Canadian Journal of Public Health*, 76, 116–118.

Naylor, M.D. (2003) Transitional care of older adults. *Annual Review of Nursing Research*, 20, 127–147.

Naylor, M.D., Brooten, D.A., Campbell, R.L., *et al.* (2004) Transitional care of older adults hospitalized with heart failure: A randomized, controlled trial. *Journal of the American Geriatrics Society*, 52, 675–684.

Nutrition Screening Initiative. (1991) *Report of Nutrition Screening I: Toward a Common View.* Nutrition Screening Initiative, Washington, DC.

Peikes, D., Brown, R., Chen, A., *et al.* (2008) *Third Report to Congress on the Evaluation of the Medicare Coordinated Care Demonstration.* Mathematica Policy Research, Princeton, NJ.

Peikes, D., Chen, A., Schore, J., *et al.* (2009) Effects of care coordination on hospitalization, quality of care, and health care expenditures among Medicare beneficiaries: 15 randomized trials. *Journal of the American Medical Association*, 301, 603–618.

Peikes, D., Peterson, G., Schore, J., *et al.* (2010) *Effects of care coordination on hospitalization, quality of care, and health care expenditures among Medicare beneficiaries: 11 randomized trials.* Unpublished Manuscript, Mathematica Policy Research, Princeton, NJ.

Pham, H.H., Schrag, D., O'Malley, A.S., *et al.* (2007) Care patterns in Medicare and their implications for pay for performance. *New England Journal of Medicine*, 356, 1130–1139.

Pfeiffer, E. (1975) A short portable mental status questionnaire for the assessment of organic brain deficit in elderly patients. *Journal of American Geriatrics Society*, 23, 433–441.

Prochaska, J.O., & DiClemente, C.C. (1983) Stages and processes of self-change of smoking toward an integrative model of change. *Journal of Counseling and Clinical Psychology*, 51, 390–395.

Schore, J., Peikes, D., Peterson, G., *et al.* (2009) *Fourth and Final Report to Congress on the Evaluation of the Medicare Coordinated Care Demonstration.* Draft Report, Mathematica Policy Research, Princeton, NJ.

Schraeder, C., Shelton, P., Brown, R., *et al.* (2009) *Report to MedPAC. Appendix D: MCCD Best Practice Sites: Interventions, Similarities and Differences.* Available at: http://www.mccprn.com/Documents/Network_Documents/MCCPRN.ReporttoMedPAC.March2009/pdf.

Schroeder, S. (2007) Can we do better – improving the health of American people. *New England Journal of Medicine*, 357, 1221–1228.

Smith, B., Forkner, E., Zaslow, B., *et al.* (2005) Disease management produces limited quality-of-life improvements in patients with congestive heart failure: evidence from a randomized trial in community-dwelling patients. *American Journal of Managed Care*, 11, 701–713.

Sochalski, J., Jaarsma, T., Krumjholz, H., *et al.* (2009) What works in chronic care management: the case of heart failure. *Health Affairs*, 28(1), 179–189.

Stille, C.J., Jerant, A., Bell, D., *et al.* (2005) Coordinating care across diseases, settings, and clinicians: a key role for the generalist in practice. *Annals of Internal Medicine*, 142, 700–708.

Sylvia, M.L., Groswold, M., Dunbar, L., *et al.* (2008) Guided care: cost and utilization outcomes in a pilot study. *Disease Management*, 11(1), 29–36.

Ware, J.E., & Sherbourne, C.D. (1992). The MOS 36-item short-form health survey (SF-36). *Medical Care*, 30, 473–483.

Wheeler, J.R. (2003) Can a disease self-management program reduce health care costs? *Medical Care*, 41, 706–715.

Yesavage, J.A., Brink, T.L., Rose, T.L., *et al.* (1983) Development and validation of a geriatric depression screening scale: a preliminary report. *Journal of Psychiatric Research*, 17(1), 37–49.

Section 2

Transitional care models

Chapter 13

The care transitions intervention

Susan Rosenbek and Eric A. Coleman

Introduction

The Care Transitions Intervention[SM] (CTI) is a patient-centered intervention designed to improve quality and contain costs for patients with complex care needs as they transition across settings. During an episode of illness, patients may receive care in multiple settings, often resulting in fragmented and poorly executed transitions. Because patients and their caregivers are often the only common thread moving across settings, together they comprise an appropriate target for an intervention designed to improve the quality of transitional care.

During the four-week intervention, patients with complex care needs receive specialized tools and learn self-management skills for ensuring their needs will be met when their conditions require that they receive care across multiple settings. Patients who have received this intervention experienced improved self-management knowledge and skills – primarily in the areas of medication management and condition/disease management – and greater confidence about what was required of them during the transition and beyond. Increased knowledge and confidence in self-care skills translated into an enhanced ability for patients (and family caregivers) to ensure that a greater proportion of their needs were being met during this vulnerable time.

Background

The intervention research was conducted in collaboration with a large, non-profit, capitated delivery system in Colorado. When the study began, the 30-day hospital readmission rate for the targeted population was approximately 15%. The delivery system contracted with one hospital, several skilled nursing facilities, and one home health agency. While in the hospital, patients received care from hospitalists. After discharge from the hospital, patients were seen by a different team of health professionals in each post-hospitalization care setting.

Comprehensive Care Coordination for Chronically Ill Adults, First Edition. Edited by Cheryl Schraeder and Paul Shelton.
© 2011 John Wiley & Sons, Inc. Published 2011 by John Wiley & Sons, Inc.

Outcomes

Data from a randomized controlled trial of 750 subjects suggest that coaches are highly effective in reducing hospital readmissions and costs, even in a heavily penetrated Medicare Advantage market in which the reduction of hospital use has been an explicit focus for many years. Key findings from the study include the following:

- Reduced readmission rates: Intervention patients had 20% to 40% lower overall hospital readmission rates (that is, readmissions for any reason) than did control subjects at 30, 90, and 180 days post-discharge. The differences, adjusted for age, sex, education, race/ethnicity, chronic disease score, and other factors, were statistically significant at 30 and 90 days. Intervention patients were approximately 50% less likely to be rehospitalized at 30, 90, and 180 days for the same condition that caused the initial hospitalization.
- Cost Savings: Although a formal cost-effectiveness analysis was not conducted, the hospital-cost data suggest an annual cost savings of just under $300,000 (savings represent the difference in hospital costs at 180 days post-discharge between the intervention group and the control group, which includes the subtraction of the cost of the intervention). These estimates may be conservative since the health care delivery system that participated in this trial had already made great progress in reducing hospital readmissions compared to the national average of 15% to 25%. Therefore, there would be greater potential for reduction in hospital utilization and costs in the average delivery system (Coleman *et al.* 2006).

Rationale

There were several key steps in the planning and development process of the CTI. The first step was a patient and caregiver survey. Patients and caregivers were surveyed on factors that are necessary and important to them during a care transition. Listening to patients' experiences through focus groups revealed that they often did not feel prepared for the care they needed in subsequent settings. Being prepared included not only knowing what was to occur next, but also understanding their roles in the process. They also reported receiving conflicting advice on how to manage their conditions, not knowing who to contact with questions, and having to complete tasks that health care providers had left undone. This information was used to establish the conceptual domains on which the intervention was based.

The second step was development of patient-influenced conceptual domains. Conceptual domains were developed to assist the patient with medication self-management, use of a patient health record that is owned and maintained by the patient or caregiver to share information with other members of their care team, follow-up with the primary care or specialty care physician within a specified time, and a list of indicators that, if seen, could indicate a worsening condition, as well as a plan for how to respond to them. These domains became the Four Pillars of the intervention.

Intervention

Goal

The goal of the CTI is to improve care transitions by providing patients with the tools and support to learn self-management skills that will ensure their needs are met during the transition from hospital to home. The Transitions Coach is key to encouraging the patient and family caregiver to assume a more active role in their care. Training Coaches do not fix problems and they do not provide skilled care. Rather, they model and facilitate new behaviors and communication skills for patients and families to feel confident that they can successfully respond to common problems that arise during care transitions. Thus, in the role of patient empowerment facilitator, the Transitions Coach provides information and guidance to the patient and/or family for an effective care transition, improved self-management skills, and enhanced patient-practitioner communication (Coleman 2008).

Targeting

In the original research, patients were eligible for the CTI for the following 11 diseases: stroke, congestive heart failure (HF), coronary artery disease, cardiac arrhythmias, chronic obstructive pulmonary disease, diabetes mellitus, spinal stenosis, hip fracture, peripheral vascular disease, deep venous thrombosis, and pulmonary embolism (PNE). In the dissemination phase, many of our partners have developed their own risk identification approaches to determine which patients to target. In some cases, this is a risk algorithm for readmission drawn from administrative data. Other partners respect that their 30-day Medicare readmission rates for HF, myocardial infarction (MI), and PNE are publicly reported so they begin there. Moreover, some partners allow for a hospitalist or primary care nurse to override the targeting approach when they feel the patient's situation warrants inclusion. Each adopting organization determines its exclusion criteria, as well as which patients to target. Since this is a self-management model, exclusion criteria can include dementia with no caregiver, or primary psychiatric diagnosis with psychotic elements and active drug or alcohol use.

Structure of the intervention

The CTI is based on Four Pillars. One, medication self-management – the patient is knowledgeable about his/her medications and has a medication management system. Two, use of a patient-centered record – the patient understands and utilizes the Personal Health Record (PHR) to facilitate communication and ensure continuity of the care plan across providers and settings. The PHR is managed by the patient of the informal caregiver. Three, primary care and specialist follow-up – the patient schedules and completes a follow-up visit with their primary care or specialist physician and is prepared to be an active participant in these interactions. Four, knowledge of red flags – the patient is knowledgeable of indicators that his/her condition is worsening and demonstrates knowledge of how to respond.

Key elements of the intervention

Transitions coach

Advanced practice nurses, registered nurses, social workers, occupational therapists, and other professionals have all served in the role of Transitions Coaches. Patients and their families work with a Transitions Coach for the first 30 days after leaving the hospital (Parry *et al.* 2003). The Transitions Coach focuses on providing continuity of care across settings by facilitating the transfer of information across the various sites that care for the patient. This is accomplished through supporting the patient in developing and maintaining a Personal Health Record; helping the patient and family members to understand when and how to obtain timely follow-up care (both primary and specialty care); coaching patients to ask the right questions to the right health care providers to get their needs met across the various follow-up settings; helping patients and their families to play a more active role in managing their conditions and to develop self-care skills, including self-management and increased awareness of symptoms, and recognizing "red flags" and warning signs that trigger the need for care, along with instructions on how to respond to them.

Personal health record

The Personal Health Record (PHR) is maintained by the patient. It is a paper tool that consists of key information needed to facilitate continuity of the care plan across settings. The patient brings the record to each appointment. The PHR includes the patient's health conditions (in their own words); medications and allergies; advance care directives; warning symptoms or signs that correspond to the patient's chronic illness(es); and space to record their and their caregiver's questions and concerns in preparation for the next physician encounter (Parry *et al.* 2003).

Sequence of the intervention

Hospital visit

The Transitions Coach first meets with the patient/family in the hospital to establish rapport, introduce the PHR, and discuss the home visit.

Home visit

The home visit ideally takes place within 48 to 72 hours of discharge. Key coaching activities during this visit include:

• Actively engaging patients in medication reconciliation (from before and after the hospitalization, including over-the-counter medications and medications prescribed to someone else that are being taken by the patient) and developing a clear, easily understood medication regime. The Transitions Coach models the behavior for how to address common medication discrepancies that occur during transitions, such as duplicative or missing medications.

- Using role playing and other techniques to educate patients and family members on communicating care needs effectively during subsequent encounters with health care professionals.
- Reviewing a list of any "red flags" that indicate a worsening condition, and strategies for how to respond to these red flags, should they manifest.

Follow-up phone calls

The Transitions Coach calls the patient three times during the intervention. Calls focus on reviewing the patient's progress toward established goals, discussing any encounters with health care professionals, reinforcing the importance of maintaining and sharing the PHR, and supporting the patient's self-management role. Each patient's follow-up phone call is tailored to the needs of that patient and the events that have transpired since the last contact. The follow-up calls also provide an opportunity to revisit the key coaching areas and patient action items identified in the home visit. (Additional details of the four pillars of CTI activities are provided in Table 13.1).

Staffing

Transitions Coaches can be nurses, social workers, occupational therapists or other professionals who have the experience and competence in helping patients advocate and care for themselves. As a conservative estimate, each Transitions Coach can provide care for 24 to 28 recently discharged patients at a time, or approximately 300 per year. The caseload is determined more by the geographic spread of patient's residences rather than the skills of the Transitions Coach.

Skills needed

Thoughtful selection of the Transitions Coach is essential to the success of the intervention. A good Transitions Coach will have a demonstrated patient-centered focus and excellent communication skills. The person should be an experienced, empowered health professional comfortable with home visits and open to learning the role. Because this is a new role for most health professionals, training by the Care Transitions Program is essential. In training, new coaches learn to identify the difference between their prior "doer/educator" roles and the new coaching role of skill transfer (Coleman 2007).

Sample costs

At the time of the research in 2003, total annual costs to support one advanced practice nurse were $74,310. The primary expense was salary and benefits ($70,980), cell phone and pager ($650), mileage reimbursement ($2,500) and photocopying of the PHRs and other supplies ($180). As noted earlier, the potential savings appear to exceed these costs by a significant amount.

Table 13.1 Care Transitions Intervention Activities by Pillar and Stage of Intervention 2

| Stage of Intervention | Four Pillars | | | |
	Medication Self-Management	Patient-Centered Record	Follow-Up	Red Flags
Goal	• Patient is knowledgeable about medications and has a medication management system.	• Patient understands and utilizes a Personal Health Record (PHR) to facilitate communication and ensure continuity of care plan across providers and settings. The patient manages the PHR.	• Patient schedules and completes follow-Up visit with Primary Care Provider/Specialist and is empowered to be an active participant in these interactions.	• Patient is knowledgeable about indications that condition is worsening and how to respond.
Hospital Visit	• Discuss importance of knowing medications and having a system in place to ensure adherence to the regimen.	• Explain PHR.	• Recommend Primary Care Provider follow-up visit.	• Discuss symptoms and drug reactions.
Home Visit	• Reconcile pre- and post-hospitalization medication lists. • Identify and correct any discrepancies.	• Review and update PHR. • Review discharge summary. • Encourage patient to update and share the PHR with Primary Care Provider and/or Specialist at follow-up visits.	• Emphasize importance of the follow-up visit and need to provide Primary Care Provider with recent hospitalization information. • Practice and role-play questions for Primary Care Provider.	• Discuss symptoms and side effects of medications.
Follow-Up Calls	• Answer any remaining medication questions.	• Remind patient to share PHR with Primary Care Provider/Specialist. • Discuss outcome of visit with Primary Care Provider or Specialist.	• Provide advocacy in getting appointment, if necessary.	• Reinforce when/if Primary Care Provider should be called.

Case studies

The CTI has been successfully implemented in both rural and urban areas. Payers include Medicare, Medicaid, and private health plans. Patients coached represent great diversity with respect to education level, health literacy, primary language, race/ethnicity, and presence of a family caregiver. Health care organizations implementing the CTI include, but are not limited to health plans, accountable care organizations, Area Agencies on Aging, home health agencies, hospitals, independent practice associations, quality improvement organizations, and state agencies. Following are two case studies we will use to demonstrate how the CTI model works. They are a combination of our experience and do not represent specific individuals.

Case study #1

Miss R is a 76-year-old teacher who lives alone in an urban high rise apartment. She has a niece who lives in the city, about 10 miles away. Miss R has a history of HF. She is a 20-year breast cancer survivor, is hypertensive, and will soon be discharged from the hospital following an acute MI.

Hospital visit

The nurse on the cardiac unit noted that Miss R meets the screening criteria for the CTI. She notified the Transitions Coach of Miss R's admission. Several days later, the nurse called the Transitions Coach with Miss R's tentative discharge date.

The Coach met with Miss R and explained the intervention. Miss R was exhausted but intrigued. There was a pile of teaching sheets accumulating on her bedside stand, but she had been too tired to read them. The resident physician mentioned that she'd be starting a new medication that morning. He left before she could ask any questions. Miss R welcomed the support of the Coach and agreed to the CTI. The Coach gave Miss R her bright green PHR with the Coach's name and phone number on it. They reviewed the PHR together. The Coach pointed out the Discharge Checklist and encouraged her to talk with her inpatient care team about these topics, including questions about her new medication. Miss R mentioned that her doctor told her she would be discharged home on Tuesday. They agreed the Coach would come and see her in her home on Thursday at 11:00 AM.

Home visit

After calling to confirm a good time to meet, the Transitions Coach arrived at Miss R's apartment. As they moved toward the kitchen table, the Coach asked Miss R to gather all of her medications (prescribed and OTC) and any paperwork she got from the hospital. Sitting down to talk, the Coach explained that this would be a different kind of visit from the others Miss R has had, such as those from the Visiting Nurse. The focus of their time together was to help Miss R be better prepared to take care of her health conditions so she would not have to go back to the hospital. Miss R and the Coach would work together to review the medications, prepare her for her next doctor's visit, and help her to better understand her health conditions.

Miss R located her PHR and handed it to the Coach. The Coach reminded Miss R the PHR belongs to her and handed it back. The Coach asked Miss R to identify one goal she would like to achieve as they work together for the next 30 days. Miss R was stumped. The Coach inquired if there was an activity she enjoyed doing before she went into the hospital. Miss R said she would love to get back to meeting her friends for coffee in the apartment building coffee shop on Wednesday mornings. Miss R wrote down that goal in her PHR. Now she had something positive to work toward. Together they discussed small steps Miss R could take to achieve this goal. Miss R listed these steps under her goal in her PHR. Miss R was uncertain how much walking she should do. She wrote this question in her PHR to discuss with her doctor.

Miss R and her Coach began the medication review. The Coach asked Miss R to show her what medication she takes and how she takes it. As they reviewed each bottle, Miss R recorded in her PHR each medication as she was actually taking it. If there was a discrepancy between the bottle instructions and what she was taking, they stopped and Miss R wrote down a question in her PHR for her care team (doctor, nurse, or pharmacist) about how to resolve this difference. Miss R also wrote down all the non-prescription medications, supplements, and herbs she was taking. Once she completed the list, the Coach and Miss R compared that list with the medications listed on her discharge instructions. They discovered a medication Miss R's cardiologist started her on in the hospital. She had a prescription for the medication but had not gotten it filled. Miss R usually walks to her pharmacy two blocks away, but does not yet have the stamina to get there. They discussed possible solutions, such as Miss R asking her niece to the medication filled, or Miss R calling the pharmacy to see if they deliver. Miss R decided to try the pharmacy delivery option first and made a note in her PHR to remind her to make the call. Miss R and the Coach also discovered that the discharge instructions had a different dose of her blood pressure medication than she was taking. Miss R made a note in her PHR to discuss this with her primary care doctor.

Miss R's Coach asked her if she had an appointment with her primary care doctor. Miss R said no; she thought the hospital would be making the appointment for her. Miss R dislikes calling her PCP's office for an appointment because the clerk usually says she cannot be seen for months. The Coach shared statements that will be more likely to get her an appointment sooner. "I was just in the hospital for a heart attack." "My medications were changed and I have questions I need to discuss with the doctor." "I need to be seen next week." Miss R and the Coach practiced. The Coach also suggested Miss R ask for the office nurse when she calls. Miss R was still nervous about making the call, so they planned to have Miss R make the call before her Coach left for the day.

Miss R noticed the section of the PHR labeled Medical History and Red Flags. The Coach asked Miss R to list her health conditions in her own words in her PHR. Miss R listed breast cancer, bunions, high blood pressure, and heart attack. The Coach asked her to describe how she was feeling before she went into the hospital. Miss R said she thought at the time she had a stomach problem and was a little short of breath. Miss R wanted to better understand what she should watch for and know when to call the doctor. The Coach agreed this was an important question for the doctor and Miss R added this to her list of questions for her follow-up visit.

At the end of the visit, the Coach reminded Miss R that this would be the only time they would meet face-to-face. The Coach said she would call Miss R Friday after her office visit to see how it went: whether she got her questions answered and how she progressed toward her goal. They reviewed the questions Miss R had written down to discuss with her doctor. She promised to take her PHR to the visit and to update it with any changes to her medications. The Coach reminded Miss R her name and number could be found on the front of her PHR and that Miss R could call with any questions or concerns.

Follow-up phone call

The Coach called Miss R at noon on Friday and asked how she was doing. Miss R said she was walking a bit more each day and was feeling stronger. She talked with the doctor at her office visit about increasing her activity. He said walking would be good. He thought her goal of getting back to seeing her friends was great. The Coach asked if she got her other questions answered about what signs to watch for indicating her condition could be getting worse. Miss R said yes, and she now has an action plan about what to do if that occurs. Miss R let the coach know she took her PHR to the visit and it helped her remember to ask about the dosage change for her high blood pressure medication. The Coach asked her to read her PHR to make sure the medication list was current. Miss R also shared that she had called the pharmacy and they agreed to deliver her pills. The Coach celebrated Miss R's follow through and asked if she had any other questions. They agreed the Coach would call her in a week to see how her walking was progressing and how close she was to getting back to see her friends in the coffee shop. The Coach reminded Miss R that she could call her if she thought of questions or concerns before their next scheduled call.

Case study #2

Mr. T is an 82-year-old tribal elder from northern Wisconsin. He lives with his son and his family, who are fishing guides. Mr. T was also a guide until his health began to decline. He has a history of diabetes, HF, and a total hip replacement. He was recently hospitalized for shortness of breath related to his HF.

Hospital visit

The Transitions Coach, Tom, was notified of Mr. T's admission by the discharge planner at the local hospital. In addition to identifying patients who are eligible for the Care Transitions program, the discharge planner has agreed to introduce the CTI to eligible patients. When she told Mr. T his Coach's name, he realized he knew Tom from a community organization in town whose services he used in the past. Tom is someone he can trust. Mr. T is worried about the changes in his medications and how he and his family will manage once he is discharged back home.

Tom stopped in to see Mr. T in his hospital room and chatted with him about the day center Mr. T used to visit. Tom explained the CTI and showed Mr. T the PHR. Mr. T shared that he was unsure of what he was supposed to do once he got home. There were changes in his medication and his diet. Tom showed Mr. T the Discharge Checklist in the PHR and encouraged him to ask his hospital team to sit down and discuss these items. Mr. T was glad to hear that Tom would visit him at home. They decided on a day and time. Mr. T said his daughter-in-law had been helping with his medications and planned to ask her to be there for Tom's visit. Tom requested that Mr. T have all of his medications and hospital-related paperwork gathered for them to review at the home visit.

Home visit

When Tom arrived for his home visit with Mr. T and Sally, his daughter-in-law, they settled at the kitchen table where all of Mr. T's pill bottles and papers were in a big bowl. Tom explained that this visit and their interactions for the next 30 days would be different from the service coordination he provided before. Together they will work to help Mr. T be better prepared to take care of his health conditions so he does not have to go back to the hospital. They would review Mr. T's medications, prepare Mr. T and Sally for his next doctor's visit, and help him to better understand his health conditions. Sally told Tom she had been giving Mr. T his medications and taking him to his office visits. She said she was told Mr. T should be weighing himself every day, but Mr. T thinks it's a waste of time. Tom acknowledged this as an important topic they will address.

First, Tom asked Mr. T if he could share an activity he would like to get back to – something fun he has not been able to do lately. Mr. T looked out the window at the river. Although he could no longer handle the canoe, he would like to fish from the dock. His legs have been too swollen and his breathing too labored to fish since the season opened. Tom encouraged Mr. T to write his goal in his PHR.

Getting back to the daily weight issue, Tom asked Mr. T to talk about how he was feeling before going into the hospital. Mr. T said his feet got increasingly swollen and his breathing got to the point he could only sleep sitting up in his recliner. It was terrifying and Mr. T said he really did not want this to happen again. Tom asked Mr. T to tell him what he understood about his health condition. Mr. T said a nurse talked with him about his HF in the hospital and said that weighing himself every day could give him an important clue about when he was getting into trouble. Tom reminded Mr. T of his goal to go fishing. Mr. T agreed to try the daily weighing. If keeping better track of his health can get him fishing it's worth it.

Tom, Sally, and Mr. T began the medication review. Mr. T said "Sally takes care of all my pills, talk to her." Sally confirmed she been giving him his pills for the past year. Tom asked Sally to show him what medications Mr. T was taking and how he took them. As they reviewed each bottle, Sally listed each medication in the PHR and how Mr. T was taking them. If there was a discrepancy between the bottle instructions and what Mr. T was taking, they stopped and Sally wrote down a question in the PHR for Mr. T's care team about how to resolve this difference. Sally also wrote down all the non-prescription medications, supplements, and herbs Mr. T was taking. Once Sally completed the medication list in the PHR, they compared that list with the medications listed in Mr.

T's discharge instructions. Sally discovered discrepancies in the dosage of Mr. T's water pill. Tom suggested Sally add that to the questions for the doctor in the PHR.

Mr. T said he likes his doctor, but has so little time with him at the office visits. Tom shared that doctors are busy, but not too busy to answer patient questions. Taking his PHR to the office visit would actually save the doctor time. Mr. T could share his list of medications and have his top three questions listed there too. Tom asked Mr. T if he would feel comfortable when he and Sally went to see his doctor, saying right at the beginning of the visit, "I have three questions I need to ask you before I leave today." Mr. T said he felt comfortable saying this and asking the questions. Tom asked if they had a follow-up visit scheduled with Mr. T's primary care doctor. Sally and Mr. T said no. They were planning on calling some time this week. Now that they had discovered the discrepancies in his medications, they would call that afternoon and ask for an appointment that week.

Tom asked if they had any questions. Sally said the discharge instructions listed a low salt diet. She was not sure how to go about this. Mr. T wanted to be part of that discussion because he does not want his food to be bland. Sally and Mr. T added a question to the PHR for the doctor regarding how to learn more about the diet.

Tom asked Mr. T and Sally to review the questions they have down in the PHR for the doctor. Tom told them he would call tomorrow to make sure they were able to get the doctor's appointment. He encouraged Sally and Mr. T to call him if they had any questions or concerns.

Follow-up phone call

Tom called the next day. Mr. T said they were able to talk to the office nurse. She not only made an appointment for next Friday, she arranged for Sally and Mr. T to see a dietician. Tom asked Mr. T if he had had a chance to weigh himself. Mr. T said yes and told Tom he was writing each day's weight on the wall calendar. That day, he went out on the dock and tomorrow he planned to walk half way to the dock! Tom celebrated Mr. T's success and said he would call next week to see how the doctor's appointment went.

Lessons learned

Planning for adoption of the care transitions intervention

If planning to adopt the CTI, explore the web site in depth (www.caretransitions.org) and contact the Care Transitions Program to guide you through the adoption and training process. Engage the support of senior and clinical leadership. Find a champion for this program – someone who is willing to make an investment in patient care. It is also important that this person think beyond the immediate quarter and instead focus on long-term goals.

Create and maintain positive relationships with community-based organizations. Interaction with various health care organizations in the community is a must for this model, so a positive relationship helps to smooth the transition for the patient. Open communication and a less "siloed" community help to reduce barriers to care for patients.

Training and practice

Transitions Coaches must complete an interactive face-to-face training with the Care Transitions Program Team. This training is essential to ensure model fidelity. Successful adoption of the CTI requires a distinct role change for new coaches. Many health care professionals feel they have been coaching throughout their careers. However, they have been educated and rewarded for doing things for patients. The Transitions Coach focuses on skill transfer and modeling of behaviors. The Coach does not perform assessment of skilled services. It takes practice and focused feedback to make the change from "doer" to Coach.

After initial training, Transitions Coaches need time to practice with colleagues and receive focused feedback. Shadowing each other's home visits and then debriefing has also been very effective.

Model fidelity

To achieve the best outcomes, adopt the model as designed. We have found the home visit is essential for true patient engagement and skill transfer. The focus of the intervention and movement through the four pillars must flow directly from the patient's goal, not the Coach's. This is a cultural change for many organizations.

Model execution

It is important to have a set of clearly defined goals and outcome measures which are aligned with the strategic plan for the organization. Criteria for patient targeting and exclusion should be specific and agreed upon by all stakeholders. Include information technology leadership early in the planning process to make sure that data needs (status report parameters and outcomes measurement) are given priority.

Establish an engaged, consistent, and committed stakeholder group. This must include the hospital. The stakeholder group creates the well-defined workflows from the time of admission to the end of the intervention. All stakeholders must agree on the workflows and the timelines. Plan ongoing meetings to discuss results and modifications needed in the workflows. Include both stakeholders and coaches in these meetings. This provides a safe place to problem-solve operation issues and to celebrate successes.

Support to sustain the model

Planning must continue beyond the launch of the program. Early on, identify a contingency plan for staff turnover in the Transitions Coach role and define criteria for program expansion. This plan should include the recruitment and training of additional Transitions Coaches. Continually refine the business case in response to the changing health care environment and plan for how you will communicate your success, both inside and outside your organization.

Summary

The CTI is an evidence-based four week program where patients with complex care needs and family caregivers receive specific tools and work with a Transitions Coach to learn self-management skills that will ensure their needs are met during the transition from hospital or skilled nursing facility to home. This is a low-cost, low-intensity, scalable intervention comprised of a hospital visit, home visit, and three phone calls. Patients who received this program were significantly less likely to be readmitted to the hospital, and the benefits were sustained for five months after the end of the one month intervention. Thus, rather than simply managing post-hospital care in a reactive manner, imparting self-management skills pays dividends long after the program ends.

References

Coleman, E.A., Parry, C., Chalmers, S., *et al.* (2006) The care transitions intervention: results of a randomized controlled trial. *Archives of Internal Medicine*, 166, 1822–1828.

Coleman, E.A. (2007) *The Care Transitions Intervention: Improving Transitions Across Sites of Care Users Manual*. Division of Healthcare Policy and Research, University of Colorado, School of Medicine, Denver, CO. Retrieved at http://www.caretransitions.org.

Coleman, E.A. (2008) Transition coaches reduce readmissions for Medicare patients with complex postdischarge needs. Agency for Healthcare Research and Quality Innovations Exchange, Rockville, MD. Retrieved from http://www.innovations.ahrq.gov/content.aspx?id=1833.

Parry, C., Coleman, E., Smith, J., *et al.* (2003) The care transitions intervention: a patient-centered approach to ensuring effective transfers between sites of geriatric care. *Home Health Services Quarterly*, 22(3), 1–17.

Chapter 14

Enhanced Discharge Planning Program at Rush University Medical Center

Anthony J. Perry, Robyn L. Golden,
Madeleine Rooney, and Gayle E. Shier

Introduction

Rush University Medical Center's Enhanced Discharge Planning Program (EDPP) is a telephonic social-work-based transitions of care model that provides a psychosocial intervention and short-term care coordination for at risk older adults as they transition from hospital to home. The goals of EDPP are to promote patient safety and satisfaction; to improve the quality of life for older adults and caregivers; and to reduce unnecessary health care costs, particularly those related to preventable rehospitalizations and emergency department visits. To achieve this, EDPP social workers utilize a bio-psycho-social framework for assessing post-discharge adherence to the treatment plan including medication compliance, physician visits, strategies for coping with care demands, and other issues that impact health and quality of life.

In our current system, there is limited recognition of the non-medical factors that impact health outcomes, such as cultural beliefs, socioeconomic status, and social supports. Patients are being discharged faster with minimal preparation into post-discharge structures that are siloed and inefficient. This results in duplication, gaps in service, and frustration. Older adults in particular are known to be more vulnerable to poor transitions because of multiple chronic conditions, physical and cognitive limitations, social isolation, and financial stressors. EDPP takes a holistic approach to helping these patients with the belief that change and efficiency are possible through collaboration between providers around common goals and interests keeping the patient as the central focus. EDPP social workers work on establishing these partnerships and communicating post-discharge information back into the medical record for use by the inpatient team if future care is required.

The model's use of master's-prepared social workers to coordinate care ensures equal importance is placed on the psychosocial and environmental factors that impact health outcomes when older adults transition home. Professionally, social workers are well suited for this role as they are trained to view individuals in the context of their environment, possess extensive knowledge of community resources, and have expertise in care coordination and navigating complex systems. EDPP social workers create a bridge between

Comprehensive Care Coordination for Chronically Ill Adults, First Edition. Edited by Cheryl Schraeder and Paul Shelton.
© 2011 John Wiley & Sons, Inc. Published 2011 by John Wiley & Sons, Inc.

the hospital and community by making sure patients understand and are able to comply with the medical plan of care, by facilitating communication between providers, and by connecting patients to vital community resources.

The EDPP intervention has been templated for evaluation, replication, and dissemination by a team of EDPP social workers, medical staff, and researchers at Rush University Medical Center. The development of the model has gone through three phases: 1) problem analysis and concept development, 2) program pilot and refinement, and 3) a randomized control trial of the intervention with the goal of building evidence to inform future policy and practice. It is currently being utilized within the medical center as a way to measure discharge effectiveness and as a strategy to improve patient safety and quality outcomes.

Background

Rush University Medical Center in Chicago is a not-for-profit academic medical center encompassing a 676-bed hospital for adults and children and the Johnston R. Bowman Health Center. The Johnston R. Bowman Health Center provides acute inpatient rehabilitation and day rehabilitation services for older adults and adults with disabilities and has apartments for moderate to low-income seniors. It also houses the Anne Byron Waud Patient and Family Resource Center which provides services to older adults and caregivers including a helpline for information and referral and in-person assistance with securing community resources, counseling, health education, support groups, and computer training.

The resource center and EDPP are specific services under the Older Adult Programs department (OAP) created at Rush to wrap around and integrate with the clinical, educational, and applied research services provided by the medical center to the community. Rush maintains a strong commitment to the community through linkages such as the Rush Community Services Initiatives Program, an umbrella for student-led outreach programs to address the social and health care needs of residents in the community and Rush Generations for older adults and caregivers. Rush Generations is an 8,000 member senior affinity and health promotion program which incorporates disease management, evidence-based caregiver support programs, and educational services.

The mission of Rush University Medical Center is to provide the best care for our patients and to be recognized as the medical center of choice in the Chicago area. The hospital is home to one of the first medical colleges in the Midwest and has one of the nation's top-ranked nursing colleges, as well as graduate programs in allied health, health systems management, and biomedical research. The hospital offers highly selective residency and fellowship programs in medicine, surgery, and other subspecialties. This unique combination of research and patient care has earned Rush recognition in 11 of 16 specialty areas the *U.S. News and World Report*'s 2010 "America's Best Hospitals" issue.

Rationale

The Enhanced Discharge Planning Program was established in 2007 as a collaboration between Older Adult Programs and the Department of Case Management at Rush. The program was created in response to a need identified by hospital staff to address shorter lengths of stay and concern about the complicated needs of older adults or caregivers who were identified as being at risk for complications post-discharge. Inpatient discharge planners recognized time demands made it difficult for them to contact patients after hospitalization to follow-up on issues of concern. Social workers in Older Adult Programs were identified as viable partners who had the knowledge base and skills to deal with the needs of this special population.

The program was initiated on three inpatient medical/surgical units and one inpatient rehabilitation unit, each with a significant number of patients over the age of 60 and with inpatient discharge planners who were willing to be included in this innovative approach to care. The discharge planners for these units subjectively assessed risk and referred patients either by telephone or through the electronic system already in use for referrals to outside providers. No formal risk criteria were defined or utilized during the pilot period and referral reasons and rates varied widely across inpatient discharge planners. During the pilot period for this program (March 2007 to June 2009), inpatient discharge planners referred 1,186 patients to EDPP social workers for follow-up. The most common reasons for referral were concerns about complex care, questions about the status of referred services, problems coping with new treatments and illnesses, and caregiver stress.

Upon receipt of referrals, the EDPP social worker reviewed notes documented by the inpatient discharge planner about the discharge needs and medical plan of care. Initially, patients and caregivers were contacted by telephone within 72 hours of discharge to complete a bio-psycho-social assessment of the post-discharge situation and to intervene around identified issues. The goals of the intervention were to stabilize the situation, ensure follow-up with medical providers, establish appropriate health care and community based services, and to provide emotional and technical support to the patient and caregiver.

EDPP social workers completed 4,152 calls with patients, caregivers, physicians, home health agencies, and other relevant parties during the two-year pilot period (Altfeld *et al.* 2009). Each case required an average of 3.5 calls over 4.6 days to resolve post-discharge problems. The most common areas requiring intervention were: follow-up needed on referred services (78%), difficulty adjusting to a new illness or treatment (28%), the need for emotional support for caregivers (20%), and issues regarding increased patient frailty and dependence on others (19%).

Data were collected manually to identify gaps in services, systems issues, and referral trends which were used to template the intervention and to structure a randomized control trial (RCT) which began in June 2009. Goals of the RCT were to measure EDPP's impact on 30-day readmissions, emergency department visits, adherence to the discharge plan, effect on patient satisfaction, self-management and caregiver burden, and the extent to which EDPP affected communication between patients and their physicians. Formalized referral criteria were selected through the process of a literature review, an analysis of the pilot data, and interviews with the inpatient discharge planners who had participated in the pilot. A research advisory team of professionals within the medical center helped refine the risk criteria and research protocols.

The goals of EDPP are achieved in part by two parallel approaches that create the intervention. One approach is through enhancing coordination among care providers across disciplines and settings. In the typical transition environment, it is common for care providers to practice in silos, impeding the transfer of information and knowledge across disciplines. EDPP enhances transitions by acting as a conduit for information across settings while encouraging communication among disciplines. This ensures coordination and enables the patient to successfully transition from hospital to home.

The second approach is through the template psychosocial evaluation and subsequent focused intervention. During the RCT planning phase, steps were made to determine a standard intervention protocol for commonly encountered post-discharge issues. This ensured continuity across clinicians and allows for improved analysis of the intervention. It also creates the basis for program replication.

Intervention

Overview

The Enhanced Discharge Planning Program (EDPP) operates with three guiding tasks to reach the goal of preventing avoidable adverse events post-discharge:

1. Ensure patients understand the discharge plan of care and receive recommended services while screening for unidentified medical or social needs.
2. Connect patients to outpatient health services (such as home health care, dialysis, radiology, laboratory services, or specialty care) with particular emphasis on the first physician follow-up appointment.
3. Support caregivers to reduce stress and burden.

EDPP social workers engage in the intervention process within 48 hours after discharge. This process has four distinct components which will be explained in detail: referral, pre-assessment, assessment, and intervention.

Referral

Referral criteria include demographic, medical, and psychosocial factors that have been shown to influence patient risk for readmission. Referred patients must meet an algorithm of risk criteria developed to identify individuals who are at a high enough risk to require post-discharge follow-up but at a low enough risk to benefit from such services. Eligible patients are identified on all adult inpatient units in a daily report generated through an automated analysis of the documentation completed by nurses and inpatient discharge planners in the hospital electronic medical record. The integration of referrals into normal work patterns was identified as a priority in order to capture all patients appropriate for EDPP services regardless of inpatient providers' workloads or weekend versus weekday discharges. To be eligible for inclusion in the RCT, patients had to meet one baseline risk criteria and have at least one additional risk factor present (Table 14.1).

At baseline, patients needed to be age 65 or older, have seven or more prescribed medications, and be returning home under their own care or with home health services. Additional risk factors for inclusion in the RCT were identified in transitional care literature as reasons patients experience adverse events post-discharge. These include: living

Table 14.1   EDPP Eligibility Criteria

EDPP Eligibility Criterion
Must meet all the following criteria: Aged 65+ Discharged to Community Polypharmacy of 7+ medications
Must meet one additional criterion: Lives alone Is without a source of emotional support Is without a support system for care Discharged with a service referral High risk for falls Inpatient hospitalization in past 12 months Identified in-depth psychosocial need High-risk medication prescribed

alone, frequent hospital admissions, an unstable or nonexistent support system, and high falls risk. Others were taken from a section in the medical record completed by the inpatient discharge planners for identification of in-depth psychosocial needs. They are defined as any non-medical factor that may present significant barriers for the patient or caregiver in having a successful post-discharge outcome (Table 14.2). The most common reasons for referral during the RCT were prior admissions, living alone, high risk for falls, and one or more in-depth psychosocial needs identified.

Pre-assessment

Once a referral is received, EDPP social workers perform a pre-assessment of the patient's discharge plan of care. This pre-assessment allows the EDPP social worker to gather medical and psychosocial information relevant to the inpatient stay and to identify

Table 14.2   In-Depth Psychosocial Needs

Difficulty adjusting to or coping with an illness or diagnosis Safety issues in the home Complex care needs Mental health concerns Issues with the teaching or learning of new treatments or regimens Suspected compliance issues with the treatment regimen Rehabilitation needs post-discharge Issues relating to the patients' support system Patient or family concerns, particularly related to caregiving Risk of harm in the post-discharge environment Financial constraints Substance and/or alcohol abuse End of life issues Legal issues Noncompliance Palliative care needs Patient or family conflict

potential barriers to a successful transition. The EDPP worker will consider the following to formulate questions in the pre-assessment: admission reasons, treatments provided, changes in functional status, coping or mental health issues for the patient or caregiver, capacity for self-management, support system at home, financial or insurance barriers to care, presence of a primary care physician, and presence of complex care. The following questions are used to guide the pre-assessment:

- What was the reason for admission? Was it elective or an emergency?
- What is the follow-up plan of care? What is the plan for:
  - Home health services
  - Medical follow-up appointments
  - Blood work
  - Durable Medical Equipment
  - Pain management
  - Wound Care
  - Medications
- What was the outcome of the hospital stay? Is the patient awaiting any results? Were there any complications, new diagnoses, or new treatments during the hospital stay?
- What psychosocial factors are already known about the patient's situation?
- Who is the patient's emergency contact? Is one present?
- Which potential community and/or diagnosis-related resources could aid this patient?

With this information, the EDPP social worker creates a picture of what happened during the inpatient hospital stay and what may be happening at home as a result. The pre-assessment also identifies what is not known about the patient's home environment that may impact health and well-being. At the end of the pre-assessment, the EDPP social worker generates a list of questions addressing potential problem areas and unclear issues to direct the next step of the process, which is assessment.

Assessment

The goals of the assessment phase of the intervention are to verify understanding and ability to comply with follow-up recommendations and to ensure patients are receiving appropriate health and community-based services. The EDPP social worker seeks answers to the following questions.

Follow-up medical care

- Do patients have a copy of the discharge instructions?
- Have patients filled their prescriptions? Do they have any questions about their medications?
- Have home health services started? Did the nurse reconcile the patients' medications? Did other services start (physical therapy, occupational therapy, social work, speech therapy)? Do patients know their schedules and understand the services they are receiving?
- Are patients aware of their follow-up appointments? Do they anticipate any barriers in getting to them?

- Do patients have a primary care physician? Does that doctor know they were hospitalized? Do they know the process to transfer their medical records to an outside physician?
- Do patients know whom to contact should they need information about their medical care?
- Do they have any other concerns or issues relating to medical care?

Support

- Do patients have a family member or friend that can help?
- Do patients belong to a faith community or social group that can help?
- How confident are patients that they can rely on these people if assistance is needed?
- Do patients need additional community services? Which needs are not currently being met?
- How are patients coping? With whom can they talk to about their emotional issues?
- How is the caregiver? Do they need support or resources?
- What other psychosocial factors need counseling and/or resources?

With the advent of diagnostic related groups (DRGs) and other changes in insurance reimbursement, patients are leaving hospitals in shorter periods of time often with complex care needs. Many patients and caregivers are unable to anticipate issues while in the hospital or do not disclose information for a number of reasons: limited time to talk about issues of concern, they don't think the issues are important, or sometimes emotional issues like shame and guilt prevent disclosure of important information. For this reason, many new issues come to light after the patient returns home to assume self-management of care without the support of hospital staff. Even the best discharge planning cannot account for all possible scenarios.

EDPP is able to identify post-discharge problems and provides intervention promptly to stabilize the situation. Patients self-report an increased willingness to be honest and share openly with EDPP social workers about their home situation and care needs, things they may not share with their medical providers. Once these issues are disclosed, EDPP social workers are able to address the psychosocial and environmental factors that impact health outcomes while creating linkages to sources for medical intervention.

Intervention

Issues identified during the initial assessment are addressed during the EDPP intervention phase. During this phase, patients and caregivers are encouraged to take an active role in care with the support of the EDPP social worker. EDPP social workers engage in the process of collaboration with health care and community-based providers to resolve immediate discharge issues and to establish a plan of care for management of ongoing needs. New issues are often identified while others are resolved. For this reason, the duration of the intervention varies from one day to a month or longer depending upon the patient's situation, the responsiveness of the outpatient providers, and the availability of resources to meet patient needs.

At the conclusion of the intervention phase, each patient and caregiver are provided with contact information for the EDPP worker or the Anne Byron Waud Patient and Family Resource Center should future issues arise. Information about the post-discharge intervention is documented in the hospital system for review if patients require future care.

Findings

A randomized controlled trial with 746 participants examined the impact of the EDPP intervention: 360 participants received the full EDPP intervention upon discharge while 384 participants received the usual care a patient can expect upon discharge. The typical intervention was completed in 8 days with an average of 5 calls required to resolve the issues identified during the initial EDPP post-discharge assessment. The EDPP social workers identified issues in 83% of intervention group participants. For 74% of these individuals, the problems did not emerge until after hospital discharge. Common problem areas largely centered on patient self-management, coping, education, and service needs. Common interventions involved educating, providing emotional support, and facilitating communication.

Surveys completed during the first intervention phone call and again 30 days post-discharge revealed that patients receiving the EDPP intervention reported:

- Increased understanding of the purpose for taking their prescribed medications.
- Decreased stress managing their health care needs.
- Decreased caregiver stress managing patients' health needs.

When compared to the usual care groups' survey responses at 30 days post-discharge, participants receiving the EDPP intervention reported:

- Greater understanding of their responsibilities for managing their health.
- Greater communication with physicians within 30 days of hospitalization.
- Greater scheduling of follow-up medical appointments.
- Greater attendance at follow-up medical appointments.
- Decreased mortality rates.

Analysis of the EDPP model reveals that the social-work-based intervention may be having a positive impact on mortality rates within the first 30 days post-index discharge.

There should not be a paragraph indentation here. It is the second sentence of the paragraph. Intervention group participants in the RCT had a mortality rate of 2.2% compared to 5.3% in the usual care group.

Case study #1

Referral

The patient is an older adult, recently paralyzed from gunshot wounds, referred to EDPP for high-risk prescribed medications, and a questionable support system to sustain his care.

Pre-assessment

In the pre-assessment review of the medical chart, the EDPP social worker identified several areas that needed to be considered in the patient's continuity of care. The patient did not have insurance, but he qualified for Rush's Charity Care program. The patient did not have a community primary care physician (PCP). The patient was discharged with a referral to the Illinois Community Cares Program (CCP), a state administered program, funded by a Medicaid waiver, intended to support older adults and disabled persons to maintain independence in their homes and communities versus a more costly alternative of moving into a skilled nursing facility. CCP services assist with household tasks, including cleaning, shopping, laundry, and meals and some personal care tasks (www.IDOAhomecare.org). Based on literature and EDPP experience with older adult and disability issues, the EDPP social worker premised that the patient's caregivers might need additional support and that the patient might experience depressive symptoms as a critical component of pain.

In summary, the EDPP social worker identified the following areas as important factors involved in the assessment of and intervention in the patient's care coordination: Rush Charity Care insurance limitations in accessing Rush and non-Rush provider systems; the need for a PCP in coordination and management of patient care; CCP referral for community services; caregiver stress; pain management with high risk medications; and possible depression or mental health concerns.

Assessment

The EDPP social worker communicated with the patient's primary caregiver, a 26-year-old relative with four children under her care. She related that the patient was having a difficult time in communicating with his providers. The patient's caregiver expressed that their immediate concern was that the brace the patient received during the recent hospitalization at Rush was causing him acute pain. The conversation also identified the following issues: the patient could not afford the prescribed pain medication and Rush Charity Care insurance does not cover medications. The patient's caregiver indicated that she had obtained a generic medication, but she was not sure if it had an equivalent potency compared to the name brand. In order for the patient to resume outpatient rehabilitation (OP Rehab) services in the community, the patient needed a doctor's order, yet the patient's caregiver did not know how to obtain an order. The patient did not have a PCP that he and his caregiver could collaborate with in getting health and medication issues resolved.

In discussing the difficulty the patient was having in communicating with his providers, the caregiver described that the patient exhibited agitation, lack of interest, change in sleep patterns, and reduced appetite – all of which are depressive symptoms. In addition, the patient and caregiver were confused about the plan for care, and this confusion was exacerbated by the patient not having insurance to access non-Rush provider systems.

The patient's caregiver indicated that she did not understand how to follow through on the CCP referral for in-home support services. The caregiver reported feeling overwhelmed in providing care to the patient and her children and shared that she coped by "taking one day at a time."

In summary, the major areas to consider in the intervention are: resolution of pain caused by the brace; addressing financial constraints to obtain medications; obtaining a doctor order required to resume OP Rehab services; addressing depressive symptoms, health literacy, and confusion around coordination of patient plan of care; obtaining CCP referrals and other community service options; and diffusing caregiver stress.

Intervention

The EDPP social worker collaborated with providers and the patient's caregiver in approximately 15 calls placed over five days.

Resolution of pain caused by brace   The EDPP social worker identified the brace manufacturer (known from other cases) and contacted the provider's office on the Rush campus (most convenient to patient). The office representative agreed to see the patient on a walk-in basis.

Financial constraints to obtaining medications   The EDPP social worker collaborated with a social worker who works with older adults at the local county health clinic on a plan for the patient to see a PCP at the clinic and thereby obtain prescriptions, at no charge, through the clinic.

Obtain doctor order required to resume OP Rehab services

The EDPP social worker confirmed with the OP Rehab provider that a doctor order was necessary for the patient to resume services. The EDPP social worker then requested that the Rush hospitalist complete a fax order and verified receipt of the order by the OP Rehab provider. The EDPP social worker assured a Rush hospitalist that a goal of the care plan was to connect the patient to a PCP who could monitor the patient's care.

Depressive symptoms, health literacy and confusion around plan of care

The EDPP social worker collaborated with OP Rehab therapists in regard to patient difficulty with communication, depressive symptoms, and the caregiver's confusion around coordinating the patient care plan. The therapists offered that the patient's rehab team included a psychological counseling resource and encouraged ongoing collaboration among the care providers to reinforce a cohesive structure for health literacy, patient advocacy and patient self-determination. The therapist suggested that collaboration among the care providers to reinforce health literacy and patient responsibilities would benefit patient care. The EDPP social worker facilitated communication between the patient, caregiver and providers.

CCP referral and other community service options   The EDPP social worker followed up with the CCP program to determine the status of the referral and facilitated new referral when original was not located in CCP system. The social worker provided the caregiver with information to access community older adult and disability resources.

Caregiver stress

The EDPP social worker and patient caregiver discussed caregiver stressors and acknowledged the universality of the impact on caregivers as described in caregiver literature. The caregiver expressed an interest in attending a caregiver support group to share and learn skills and strategies for effective caregiving. The EDPP social worker educated the caregiver about a program, Powerful Tools for Caregivers, that is provided at the Rush Older Adult resource center.

Case study #2

Referral

The patient is a 78-year-old woman admitted to the hospital for complications after a hip replacement. She was referred to EDPP due to a prior hospitalization in the past 12 months and a high risk for falls.

Pre-assessment

In the pre-assessment review of the medical chart, the EDPP social worker identified a medical follow-up appointment scheduled. The patient was discharged with wound care and pain management needs, as well as limited mobility. Home physical therapy and nursing services were ordered before discharge. Potential areas for focused intervention included: ability to attend scheduled follow-up appointments; wound care and pain management; changes in mobility; and home health services.

Assessment

During the assessment with the patient, the EDPP social worker learned that the patient was experiencing declines in cognitive and physical functioning and was in severe pain, as she had run out of pain medications. Her daughter, who usually assists with medications, was out of town for the weekend, and the patient had forgotten to refill them.

The patient shared her medical history and experiences with non-traditional medicine. She noted how her life changed after her accupressurist of 30 years died. She felt her accupressurist has kept her pain to a minimum. After her accupressurist died, she sought assistance from traditional medicine which included a hip replacement. The patient states she lost her ability to walk since this procedure and the subsequent seven surgeries. Two years ago, the patient fell, fracturing her neck. She has experienced short term memory loss since the fall.

The patient felt her support system was generally available, and she expressed appreciation for assistance provided by her daughter and spouse. However, she felt they did not understand or believe the severity of her pain and its impact on her functioning. Her husband was still working and according to the home health staff, minimally involved in her care. Additionally, the patient expressed frustration at her daughter's and spouse's lack of understanding or empathy for the cognitive changes she was experiencing. According to the patient, her family members' expectations of what she should be able to do were unrealistic given her new limitations. The patient reported being home alone most of the day, which was a challenge due to her mobility issues, high risk for falls, and memory loss.

The EDPP social worker assessed the presence of depressive symptoms due to the patient's functional decline, loss of independence, chronic health problems, pain, and family conflicts. She expressed frustration with "being old and sick" and felt like a burden to her family. The patient expressed feeling overwhelmed by her current care needs and had difficulty organizing her care plan. This was compounded by her family's frustration around her healing process, as they perceived her as "not trying hard enough."

In later conversations, additional barriers relating to incontinence was identified. Due to her changes in mobility, the patient was unable to go to the bathroom successfully in public restrooms that did not have grab bars. Her shame led to loss of dignity and feelings of greater social isolation. Issues for intervention included: coping with pain and obtaining medications; depression and coping; conflict with support system; caregiver stress; functional and cognitive decline; and incontinence.

Intervention

Coping with pain and obtaining medications

The EDPP social worker communicated with the home health nurse and physical therapist about the patient's pain and safety issues. They communicated their awareness of the severity of her pain and cognitive issues that may have contributed to the medications going unfilled. With the help of the home health nurse, the social worker ensured that the family was able to monitor administration of medications and refills as needed. She also spoke with the home health nurse and surgeon for a better understanding of pain expectations for use in conversations with this patient.

Depression and coping

The EDPP social worker allowed the patient to share her feelings around her many physical and cognitive losses and changes and validated the patient's experience. The EDPP social worker contacted the home health agency about adding a master's-level social worker to the home health service plan and spoke with that social worker about this patient's depression, including a potential need for medications. The EDPP social worker referred the patient to a community-based mental health counseling service, a friendly visiting program, and alternative medicine resources within the community.

Conflict with support system

The EDPP social worker allowed the patient to share her feelings regarding her support system and sought input from the home health nurse around the family's dynamics. The EDPP social worker then facilitated a phone conference with both the patient and caregiver, mediating the communication. Based upon the conference, the EDPP social worker recommended increasing the hours of a private duty caregiver to provide care in the hours the caregiver could not to relieve both patient and caregiver stress (patient was financially ineligible for in-home services through The Department of Aging). The

EDPP social worker encouraged the caregiver's and patient's willingness to accept help and provided support around the loss of independence.

Caregiver stress

The EDPP social worker spoke to the daughter individually, allowing her to share her emotions and receive support around the challenges she faced in her role as a caregiver. The EDPP social worker provided education to the daughter about memory loss and discussed the meaning of the patient's changed role and functioning.

Functional and cognitive decline

The EDPP social worker assessed the patient's ability to address her own care due to her cognitive changes. She educated the family about realistic expectations and the need for increased supervision during the day. The EDPP social worker provided resources for additional therapy such as neuropsychological testing and, as such, coordinated with the home health social worker around the need to increase private duty caregiver assistance. She provided emotional support to the patient around the loss of dignity, increased shame, and increased dependence.

Incontinence

The EDPP social worker talked to the home health nurse (who would follow-up) about incontinence issues, including resources shared with the patient to assist with toileting in public restrooms. Her daughter was made aware of these resources as well.

Lessons learned

Effective transitional care requires collaboration of many entities from different disciplines, settings, and educational backgrounds. As with any model, it is necessary to keep stakeholders involved and invested in the success of the program. This can be done by keeping lines of communication open and promoting honesty and accountability among care providers. Patients respond positively to the collaboration of providers and are better able to take responsibility for their self-care when there is a structure around them to support this endeavor.

Successful study of clinical and coordination interventions requires focused attention on the substance of the intervention as well as a willingness to thoughtfully characterize and categorize the intervention to allow for appropriate study of the program.

Summary

The Enhanced Discharge Planning Program (EDPP) is a program providing telephonic short-term social work care coordination for patients discharged from Rush University

Medical Center after an inpatient hospital stay. It is tailored to provide assistance to older adults at risk for an adverse event once home from the hospital. The program's goal is to prevent avoidable adverse events post-discharge by: (1) ensuring patients understand the discharge plan of care and receive recommended services while screening for unidentified medical or social needs; (2) connecting patients to outpatient health services with particular emphasis on the first physician follow-up appointment; and supporting caregivers to reduce stress and burden. Outcomes from a RCT of the model suggest that many transitional care issues do not arise until patients return home and begin to engage in self-management roles. For this reason, it is important to provide a bridge between the hospital and home that addresses the medical and non-medical factors contributing to health and well-being post-discharge. EDPP links "silos" of care, bridging the great divide between social and medical models.

References and suggested reading

Altfeld, S., Golden, R., McFolling, S., *et al.* (2009) An innovative model for transitional care: enhanced discharge planning program. *Collaborative Case Management*, 7(2), 7–9.

American Hospital Association. (2009) *Hospitals in the Pursuit of Excellence Case Study: Social Workers Enhance Post-Discharge Care for Seniors.* American Hospital Association, Chicago, IL. Available at: http://www.hpoe.org/case-studies/4340001768.

Brown, R. (2009) *The Promise of Care Coordination: Models that Decrease Hospitalizations and Improve Outcomes for Medicare Beneficiaries with Chronic Illness.* Mathematica Policy Research, Princeton, N.J. Available at: http://www.socialworkleadership.org/snw/Brown_Executive_Summary.pdf.

Section 3

Integrated models

Chapter 15

Summa Health System and Area Agency on Aging Geriatric Evaluation Project

Kyle R. Allen, Joseph L. Ruby, Susan Hazelett,
Carolyn Holder, Sandee Ferguson, and Phyllis Yoders

Introduction

Historically, the clinical course for older patients with chronic illnesses was a steady decline in health punctuated by frequent symptom exacerbations requiring acute hospitalizations, with each hospitalization accelerating the rate of decline. More recently there has been a growing trend for hospitalized patients to be cared for by a Hospitalist, as well as any number of specialists, leading to fragmentation of care. Communication among medical providers is not routine and the patient's primary care physician (PCP) is rarely aware of the discharge plan or, often, that the patient was admitted to the hospital at all.

The medical model has dominated patient care and little, if any, consideration is given either to the prevention of functional decline during or after an acute hospitalization or to the psychosocial issues that might impede the medical plan of care. Traditionally, little effort was put forth for discharge planning, which typically involved a written set of instructions given to the patient as he/she walked out the door. Patients were discharged to home or to another care setting with no post-discharge follow-up. Patients returned to their homes often to find that they did not understand the plan of care or medication changes, they faced new functional deficits, and they had no knowledge of the resources available to help them overcome the psychosocial barriers that impeded optimal health. PCPs faced a health care system, financed mainly through Medicare and private pay, which encouraged disease treatment over prevention, limited time for office visits, little formal training in geriatrics, and little knowledge of the community resources available to their patients. Even further siloed were community-based long term care providers who had no way to communicate with hospital discharge planners, outpatient geriatrics staff, health plan or health maintenance organization case managers and the PCP, so no single provider had a complete picture of the patient's overall status, and no one was responsible for making sure all aspects of the discharge plan of care were implemented. As a result, these complex patients frequently suffered potentially avoidable illness exacerbations which brought them back to the hospital, more debilitated each time, to undergo the same chain of events.

Comprehensive Care Coordination for Chronically Ill Adults, First Edition. Edited by Cheryl Schraeder and Paul Shelton.
© 2011 John Wiley & Sons, Inc. Published 2011 by John Wiley & Sons, Inc.

In the early 1970s a number of demonstration projects were undertaken to try to establish effective ways to deliver chronic illness care in the community setting. In the early 1980s the Omnibus Budget Reconciliation Act was passed which allowed states to deliver home and community-based services to Medicaid recipients. In the 1990s the Social Health Maintenance Organization (S/HMO) demonstrations and the Program for All Inclusive Care for the Elderly (PACE) were initiated (Harrington & Newcomer 1985; Branch *et al.* 1995) which provided better links between acute and long-term care services. With today's focus on health care costs and accountable care organizations, models of care that effectively integrate acute and long-term care are needed.

This chapter describes the development of a unique collaboration between a health care system and a community-based long-term care provider whose goal was to mend known gaps in care by integrating the social and biomedical models of care and coordinating funding streams.

The beginning: a new model of acute care for chronically ill older adults

In the mid 1990s, the Division of Geriatric Medicine at Summa Health System (SHS) in Akron, Ohio, was participating in a randomized trial testing the effectiveness of a model of care known as the Acute Care for Elders (ACE; Palmer *et al.* 1994). SHS is an integrated, not-for-profit health care delivery system that provides a coordinated continuum of services to its patients. It includes its own health insurance plan, skilled home care, hospice, a foundation, an independent and employed medical staff, and several joint ventures. It is the major teaching hospital for Northeastern Ohio Universities Colleges of Medicine and Pharmacy. In 1995, Summa was just two hospitals, Akron City and St. Thomas, with 963 beds; now Summa is composed of six community teaching hospitals with more than 2,000 beds. SummaCare Health Plan currently has over 150,000 covered lives, including a Medicare Advantage plan of 23,000.

The ACE concept tested at Summa was a model of hospital care delivery aimed at improving the functional status and clinical outcomes for hospitalized older adults. Many of the concepts used in the ACE Model are adaptations of the principles of Wagner's model for chronic illness care (Wagner *et al.* 1996a). This model makes heavy use of interdisciplinary teams and has been shown to be effective in ensuring comprehensive care of patients with chronic diseases in numerous studies (Stuck *et al.* 1993; Stewart *et al.* 1999; Wagner *et al.* 1996b; Hansen *et al.* 1995). The results of the ACE trial showed improved care processes, as well as patient and provider satisfaction, without increasing costs. ACE patients also showed fewer declines in functional status and fewer nursing home admissions at discharge and at one year post-discharge.

The success of the ACE model in the acute care setting prompted the investigators to extend it to other inpatient units, outpatient clinics, and long-term care entities. Summa's geriatric care delivery model was one of "consult and support" to collaboratively manage and assist PCPs in caring for their chronically ill elderly patients.

Expansion of the ACE model of care

Despite the comprehensive nature of these programs within the health care setting, the impact they were having on post acute outcomes was not optimal. What was missing was a patient connection in the outpatient setting, which is emphasized by Wagner's model.

As an integrated delivery system, Summa needed to expand its reach to elderly patients across the continuum of care, so Summa created the Center for Senior Health (CSH) at around the same time the ACE research trial was taking place. The CSH is an outpatient consultative service that supports the PCP through interdisciplinary comprehensive geriatric assessment, high risk assessment, a geriatrics resource center, a clinical teaching center, in-patient geriatric consultation, and post-inpatient consultation follow-up. CSH blends the medical and social models, attempting to treat the whole patient by addressing acute and chronic medical needs, psychosocial needs, and holding family conferences.

A major limitation of the CSH was that it did not have access to patients in their homes nor could it provide long-term case management. CSH began to rely heavily on community-based, long-term care agencies to access in-home assessment information, as the home is the setting where most chronic illness care occurs. Thus, it made sense to formally integrate with the local Area Agency on Aging (AAA) since they already provided the case management for Ohio's Medicaid waiver community-based long-term care program called PASSPORT.

Summa's community-based care partner: the area agency on aging

Ohio's AAA 10B Inc., is an independent, private, nonprofit corporation that serves more than 20,000 elderly consumers in northeast Ohio. The AAA is designated by the Ohio Department of Aging to develop a network of services to assist older adults and their families. Its mission is to provide older adults and their caregivers with long-term care choices, consumer protection, and education, so they can achieve the highest quality of life. In addition to its community care coordination programs and its elder rights division, the AAA administers the state's Medicaid waiver program, PASSPORT, which is a social model of care delivery that addresses the functional, social, psychological, and behavioral needs of low-income, chronically ill older adults whose functional status qualifies them for nursing home placement. A primary goal of PASSPORT is to delay or prevent nursing home placement.

Around 1995 the AAA found itself managing a growing number of consumers with functional decline, geriatric syndromes, and multiple chronic illnesses. As much as 10% of their total client population fell into this high-risk category. The AAA leadership recognized that there was a great need to be integrated with the acute medical sector because of the limitations they were seeing on their ability to reduce permanent nursing home admissions, manage polypharmacy, geriatric syndromes and chronic diseases, interface with PCPs, and the limitations of only "brokeraging" social services versus a more comprehensive approach to improving overall outcomes for their consumers.

At the time the AAA leadership was planning a paradigm shift from service provision to care management. Nevertheless, the AAA still operated under a social model. When a consumer became acutely ill and required hospitalization there was no formal communication process among PASSPORT care managers and health care providers. Without access to input from medical professionals to manage chronic illnesses in the home, too many consumers were prematurely institutionalized. Indeed, every year almost 50% of PASSPORT consumers were transferred to a nursing facility and another third died.

Rationale for integration

Current health care reform posits that a solution to improving quality of care and financial outcomes, particularly for patients with chronic diseases, is a redesign in payment and quality monitoring which will drive integration of services and providers, and thus enhance clinical and financial outcomes. However, clinical, financial, and inter-institutional integration rarely exists, and, without strong incentives, is fairly elusive in the U.S. health care sector.

The AAA and Summa's Senior/Post-Acute Care service-line identified a lack of continuity of care related to communication problems and fragmentation of care for the complex population that each was serving. The silos of Medicare and Medicaid funding enabled this fragmentation, creating two infrastructures (Medicare for medical issues and Medicaid for social issues) and no incentive for these to become integrated. Each was faced with having to provide more services to a growing population with increasingly complex needs and limited resources. It was recognized that in the medical model, acute medical needs were of paramount importance, and psychosocial and functional issues were least likely to be addressed, and in the social model the opposite was true. What was needed was a model that "spanned the boundaries" between the two (that is, a bio-psycho-social model).

While recognizing and wanting to build off of the strengths of the programs they had established, geriatric medicine leaders from Summa and the AAA also recognized the challenges and deficits they faced in providing continuity of care, and began meeting to discuss how they could build a new model of care. This new model needed to integrate multidisciplinary geriatric services in an acute hospital and community-based care to eliminate duplication or gaps in services, and improve outcomes of care for their mutual consumers/patients. They also realized that everyone involved shared a common goal for their consumers, and that these goals could be better met through streamlined communication across the continuum from the medical to the community setting.

The SAGE project

Thus, Summa and the AAA 10B, Inc., embarked upon the SAGE project (Summa Health System/Area Agency on Aging, 10B/Geriatric Evaluation Project). SAGE provided the organizational structure to develop the resources and processes to effectively integrate geriatric medical services and community-based long-term care services. There were no development or planning grants, integrated funding mechanisms or contractual relationships to work from – just a collaborative effort and strong leadership on behalf of both organizations to meet common goals and coordinate funding streams. The goal of SAGE

was to provide a coordinated care delivery model to improve linkage to community resources and reduce fragmentation of care to improve the health, functional status, and
prevent institutionalization of older adults at risk for nursing home placement. The SAGE
project furthered the goals of both organizations and provided a "value added" benefit.

The CSH/AAA task force

The first step in the SAGE project was to form what was called the CSH/AAA Task
Force. This was begun in 1995. It provided a forum to promote communication, provide
feedback, and create initiatives to bridge the acute and community aging network. Task
force members included: a Summa geriatrician, an ACE and CSH social worker, an
ACE Clinical Nurse Specialist, the AAA Screening and Assessment Director and Care
Management Supervisor, and a PASSPORT care manager and social worker. This task
force eventually expanded to include representatives from Summa's Home Care, a non-
Summa owned and skilled nursing facility with a short-stay geriatrics rehabilitation unit,
Summa's Internal Medicine and Family Practice Centers, and SummaCare's Medicare
Managed Care program.

The task force met monthly for two years, then changed to quarterly meetings. Its
objectives were to:

1. Develop initial screening, communication and referral protocols to identify at-risk older
   adults on PASSPORT waiver who required integrated care management services.
2. Establish mechanisms for sharing information and resources.
3. Identify gaps and potential duplication in service delivery.
4. Outsource an AAA case manager at the CSH as part of the interdisciplinary planning
   process.
5. Educate staff of both institutions on scope of skills and services.
6. Collect information on referrals, outcomes, and statistical data.
7. Identify and address barriers to implementation of protocols.

During this first phase, a centralized contact person was identified at each institution
to streamline communications. The task force developed forms for CSH referrals to the
AAA, for AAA referrals to the CSH, and for acute care referrals to the AAA. Follow-up
protocols were developed for AAA patients who were admitted to Summa's ACE and
geriatric rehabilitation unit to inform the AAA care manager about their patient's status.
Follow-up protocols were also developed with Summa's Internal Medicine Center, Home
Care and Family Practice Center with the same purpose – to improve continuity of care
with PASSPORT.

Hospital and skilled nursing facility providers identified that they could often identify patients/consumers who could benefit from community-based long-term care but
who were often discharged before any referrals were made, which often contributed to
readmission and emergency department (ED) visits. Patients were often discharged with
skilled home care services and not referred to PASSPORT until after 30 to 60 days post
discharge, causing a lag in services until Medicaid was approved. A program was needed
to bridge the gap between the acute medical and community-based aging network to
expedite services without duplication and optimize the success of the transition to home.

Thus, in 2000, an in-hospital AAA nurse (RN) care manager assessor program was piloted by the SAGE task force. Initially the SAGE group piloted the idea of bringing an "outsider" like the AAA RN assessor into the acute care hospital, integrated with the hospital discharge planning teams. The ACE Unit had a well developed interdisciplinary team to trial this RN assessor program. After a brief overview of ACE processes, the RN assessors attended daily interdisciplinary team rounds where they learned roles of ACE Unit staff and hospital processes. The RN assessors then worked closely with the ACE team, including the social work and discharge planning nursing staff, to screen for patients who could benefit from community-based services, including PASSPORT. Additionally, legal and compliance departments were consulted to assure that proper processes were in place to be compliant with the Health Insurance Portability and Accountability Act (HIPAA) rules and regulations.

This project targeted dually eligible (Medicare and Medicaid) patients who were at high risk for institutionalization while they were in the acute-care hospital setting, and offered them an assessment, care planning and referral to community resources. The RN assessor program was a new model for the AAA because traditionally the AAA RN assessors do these assessments/enrollments in the home of the consumer and must travel from house to house. Screening tools were developed to identify areas of need and to provide specific interventions to achieve desired clinical outcomes without duplication or gaps in services. After a successful pilot on the ACE Unit, leadership from the SAGE task force met with nursing leadership at SHS to expand this program to both Akron City and St. Thomas Hospitals using two AAA RN assessors.

The final AAA RN assessor program

Under the system-wide AAA RN assessor program, when an appropriate patient is admitted to the hospital, the admitting nurse notifies the AAA using the referral protocols that were developed by the task force. The AAA assessor assesses the patient prior to hospital discharge to begin a PASSPORT eligibility assessment, working collaboratively with hospital social workers and discharge planners in communicating their findings and outcomes of their assessment, and acting as a liaison to the hospital staff regarding aging network and AAA services. Individuals who are willing and eligible are enrolled into the PASSPORT program, or if not eligible, back to the AAA screening and assessment division for linkage to other community resources. Also, when an established PASSPORT consumer is admitted to SHS, the PASSPORT care manager is notified by CHS staff so that they can share the PASSPORT care plan with the hospital. At discharge, hospital staff shares the discharge plan with the PASSPORT care manager.

Compliance with these communication protocols was monitored and feedback was provided to the hospital and task force. In addition, the AAA care manager uses a screening tool developed by the task force to identify community dwelling high-risk elderly and refers these consumers to Summa's outpatient Center for Senior Health (CSH) upon release from the hospital or after they are discharged from a short stay at a skilled nursing home. At the CSH an Advanced Practice Nurse, social worker, and Geriatrician perform a comprehensive geriatric assessment. The results of that assessment are presented at an interdisciplinary team conference that includes the AAA care manager. At this conference the team generates a plan of care which is then shared with the patient, family, and their PCP. After the plan is agreed upon by all, the AAA assumes the main management of the patient, in collaboration with the PCP and periodic geriatrics follow-up. If the patient is readmitted to the hospital, the admitting nurse notifies the AAA and the process begins again.

Outcomes from SAGE

The RN assessor program facilitated improved capacity management for complex patients in the acute hospital. It improved AAA care managers' communication with PCPs and hospital staff to reduce repeat hospitalizations, ED visits, and nursing home placements. The extra support from the case manager improved outcomes for complex patients who previously were often readmitted and very costly, and decreased discharges from PASSPORT to nursing homes.

During the AAA assessor pilot program referrals to PASSPORT care managers from the hospital doubled (184 to 415) and enrollments into PASSPORT also doubled (32 to 64). After the model went system-wide, PASSPORT referrals increased by 94% and enrollment increased by 725%.

SAGE impacted four main groups: consumers, the health care delivery system, staff, and the community. Consumers saw improvement in function, reduced hospitalizations and increased patient and caregiver satisfaction with care. The health care delivery system saw improved communication among all caregivers, integration of the medical and social models of care, coordination of two funding streams, the establishment of direct organizational linkages, opportunities to develop research studies for extramural funding, decreased disenrollment from PASSPORT, decreased fragmentation of care, and decreased costs. Staff and PCPs reported savings in staff time by streamlining communications and tasks, as well as positive feedback regarding patient outcomes, their ability to better serve patients, a better understanding of each discipline's internal operations, and a better understanding of the "big picture" of health care delivery, funding streams and access to expert resources. Finally, the community (taxpayers, legislators) saw individuals maintained at home at a cost of no more than 60% of the Medicaid cost of nursing home care, and the informal integration of two funding sources (Medicare and Medicaid) to maximize benefits to consumers without duplication or cost shifting, contributing to a reduction in costs.

Barriers

A number of barriers had to be overcome in order for the SAGE project to succeed. The most important was leadership, requiring the involvement of visionary leaders who understood both the medical and social sectors. These "boundary spanners" are individuals who have connections in both sectors so they know who to contact for specific issues. They have credibility in both sectors which helps new members establish trust. Boundary spanners are good facilitators because they can see the collaboration from multiple perspectives simultaneously, and they know the language of both sectors. Finally, they know the needs of both sectors, enabling them to help shape an end product that is more responsive to the needs of everyone involved.

These individuals can be any professional with training in both sectors. For SAGE we found that a physician was the best choice to spearhead the collaboration because of their experience with geriatrics, community-based long term care, administration, research, and academia. The executive director of the AAA also served as a boundary spanner by demonstrating vision and leadership and wanting to move the organization from a social services brokerage provider to an organization that could be more integrated with the health care system.

The next barrier was constructing an effective multidisciplinary working group. Most problems involving collaborations revolve around the relationships of the parties involved. Regardless of the group, two major factors are critical to success: commitment and communication. Collaborations bring together a broad range of individual organizations, some of whom may be competitors, which can result in tensions when participants have different languages and values. In our case, the task force members were initially fearful of losing control over their day to day routine, their professional or institutional operations, the direction of the collaborative, or their own "trade secrets." It must be made clear that participants do not have to agree about everything to work together successfully. The group needs to build a common language and support group for decision making, making sure to keep all members informed about what is going on, enabling members to learn about each other's concerns, values, and work, and enabling them to air disagreements. It is important that participants feel free to talk about what they think is not working. Furthermore, the parties involved must perceive a compelling need to work together and be willing to do so (buy-in). In our case, each participant had a different problem needing to be addressed by the collaboration and realized that only by working together could they achieve the benefits neither could achieve alone, so long as the benefits of one participant were not achieved at the expense of another. Eventually, participants began to see the benefits of collaboration and began to rely on each other's resources and skills.

Time is another barrier for most health professionals. Hospitals cannot afford to allow doctors to participate unless the project has a direct impact on increased revenues, cost savings, and/or quality. Thus, the argument must be made to each entity that the collaboration will positively impact the bottom line by, for example, creating savings in staff time due to streamlined communications and tasks, or increased referrals, or decreased readmissions/ED visits. As health care reform is enacted it will be of paramount importance that more strategic partnerships are forged because with the "value based purchasing" focus of the health care reform legislation these partnerships will be vital for improving accountability, quality, and cost effectiveness.

Generalizability

The SAGE project can be easily adapted to any organization. It requires no additional funding or formal contractual agreements – merely a commitment from each institution to provide in-kind staffing. It brings together a broad range of individuals and organizations, many of whom do not have a history of working together. A partnership like SAGE can align these historically separate entities for future collaborative projects.

Outgrowths of the SAGE partnership

1. The RN Assessor program was replicated in five other local community hospitals (which were not Summa owned or affiliated).
2. Legislators in the state and in the Ohio Department of Aging have been encouraging other AAAs to replicate a similar model in their region.
3. Health policy has been impacted as result of the SAGE partnership, and with testimony and advocacy, has persuaded Ohio legislators to expand PASSPORT services to other at-risk individuals.
4. A high-risk case management program, which screened individuals at the time of PASSPORT enrollment, was developed by the AAA in conjunction with the U.S. Administration on Aging, the Ohio Department of Aging, and SummaCare. The project was funded by the Administration on Aging's Integrated Care Management Grants. The project focused on health promotion and illness prevention with the goal of decreasing disenrollment to a nursing facility and increasing patient/family satisfaction. Most of the individuals in the high risk program had multiple chronic medical and social service needs, and were at risk of hospitalization, nursing home placement, or death due to declining functional and health status. This high risk program was thought to promote cost-effective care by maximizing coordination/collaboration, minimizing fragmentation, and facilitating consumers' navigation of the care system.
5. Successful grant application from the Administration on Aging to integrate AAA case management with the SummaCare health plan Medicare Managed Care division to maximize Medicare and Medicaid benefit coverage. This grant brought about better working relationships between the AAA PASSPORT case managers and the SummaCare Care Coordination case managers by facilitating their ability to share care plans through electronic case management software programs.
6. During phase two of the Administration on Aging's Integrated Care Management Grants, Summa and the AAA developed the Care Management Interdisciplinary Team (CMIT), which brings geriatric medicine and an interdisciplinary team directly to the PASSPORT case managers via regular meetings at the AAA itself to more effectively change its culture. CMIT is attended by a geriatrician and pharmacist from the health system, as well as hospice social worker, and is facilitated by an AAA supervisor advanced practice nurse. The PASSPORT case managers bring difficult and high risk cases to this weekly team for discussion, review, and problem solving. Recommendations are made to the PCP using "academic detailing" and rationale for changes in treatment plans (such as medication dosages or elimination of high-risk drugs) with suggested alternatives. The PASSPORT case manager also amends their care plan for interventions that do not require a physician order.
7. Formal research proposals have resulted in two major randomized controlled trials and other small projects. These projects have received extramural support from the Agency for Healthcare Research and Quality, the National Palliative Care Research Center, and other local foundations.

Conclusion

Today, our health care agencies and institutions agree that continuing on separate tracks is no longer in the best interest of medicine, managed care, or community-based long-term care, and certainly not in the best interest of the consumers we share. In the years ahead, with the projected significant growth in the older population and with the pressures to contain budgetary expenditures, the development of new health care delivery models designed to respond to the complex needs of this population, such as the SAGE project, will become a necessity.

A new era is emerging in health care reform after the "quality era" and several decades of attempts at integration of hospital and physician practices that is called the "accountable care era." Though the social HMO (SHMO), Program of All Inclusive Care (PACE), and the Special Needs Plans for Medicare and Medicaid have had some success, the SAGE model provides a broader, more scalable and more integrated model. This program could be enhanced with funding for documentation and analysis of outcomes.

References

Branch, L.G., Coulam, R.F., & Zimmerman, Y.A. (1995) The PACE evaluation: initial findings. *The Gerontologist*, 35, 349–359.

Hansen, F., Poulsen, H., & Sorensen, K. (1995) A model of regular geriatric follow-up by home visits to selected patients discharged from a geriatric ward: a randomized controlled trial. *Ageing Clinical and Experimental Research*, 7, 202–206.

Harrington, C., & Newcomer, R.J. (1985) Social/health maintenance organizations: new policy options for the aged, blind, and disabled. *Journal of Public Health Policy*, 6, 204–222.

Palmer, R., Landefeld, C., Kresevic, D., *et al.* (1994) A medical unit for the acute care of the elderly. *Journal of the American Geriatrics Society*, 42, 545–552.

Stuck, A.E., Siu, A.L., Wieland, G.D., *et al.* (1993) Comprehensive geriatric assessment: a meta-analysis of controlled trials. *Lancet*, 342, 1032–1036.

Stewart, S., Vandenbroeck, A., Pearson, S., *et al.* (1999) Prolonged beneficial effects of a home-based intervention on unplanned readmissions and mortality among patients with congestive heart failure. *Archives of Internal Medicine*, 159, 257–261.

Wagner, E.H., Austin, B.T., Von Korff, M. (1996a) Organizing care for patients with chronic illness. *Milbank Quarterly*, 74, 511–544.

Wagner, E., Austin, B., & Von Korff, M. (1996b) Improving outcomes in chronic illness. *Managed Care*, 4(2), 12–25.

Chapter 16

Program of All-Inclusive Care for the Elderly (PACE)

Brenda Sulick and Christine van Reenen

Introduction

This chapter focuses on the Program of All-Inclusive Care for the Elderly (PACE), a fully integrated, provider-sponsored model of care designed to meet the specific health care needs of Medicare and/or Medicaid beneficiaries with both chronic medical conditions, and functional and/or cognitive impairments. It describes key features of the PACE model and highlights innovations at three PACE organizations that intended to address specific needs within their communities.

As Baby Boomers age, demand for and use of long-term services and supports (LTSS) will grow dramatically. LTSS include a range of supportive services needed by people who have limitations in their ability to care for themselves because of a physical, cognitive, or mental disability or condition (O'Shaughnessy 2010). According to the U.S. Administration on Aging (2009), the number of Americans aged 65 and over is expected to increase from 35 million in 2000 to 40 million in 2010 (a 15% increase) and then to 55 million in 2020 (a 36% increase for that decade.) The number of Americans aged 85 and over – those most likely in need of services – is projected to increase from 5.5 million in 2007, to 5.8 million in 2010, and then to 6.6 million in 2020 (a 15% increase for that decade).

Rapid growth in the numbers of older Americans will put pressure on states' Medicaid programs and other sources of funding for long-term care. In 2008, the amount spent on long-term services and supports was $191.1 billion, of which Medicaid accounted for $119 billion, or 62.3% of the total. Out-of-pocket costs contributed $43.5 billion (22.7%). Private sources, including long-term care insurance and spending for nursing home and other home health services, were 11.7% ($22.3 billion). Other public sources, including all other public spending for nursing homes, home health services, continuing care retirement communities, assisted living facilities, and on-site nursing care facilities, were 3.3% ($6.2 billion; O'Shaughnessy 2010).

As states consider how to respond to a growing need for LTSS and its associated costs, one approach is to put greater emphasis on home and community-based versus institutional care (Henry J. Kaiser Family Foundation 2010). States' efforts to "rebalance" their

Comprehensive Care Coordination for Chronically Ill Adults, First Edition. Edited by Cheryl Schraeder and Paul Shelton.
© 2011 John Wiley & Sons, Inc. Published 2011 by John Wiley & Sons, Inc.

long-term care systems are already well underway. From 1997 to 2008, the percentage of Medicaid long-term care dollars spent on institutional care declined from 76% to 57%, with home and community-based services (HCBS) spending increasing from 24% of 43% of states' long-term care spending (O'Shaughnessy 2010). States' efforts to rebalance their long-term care systems from institutional to LTSS reflect the need to manage growth in long-term care expenditures, but also reflect older adults' preference to remain in their homes as an alternative to institutional care (American Association of Retired Persons 2010). If current trends continue, the importance of effective home and community-based programs, including PACE, in addressing the needs of older Americans will increase.

The PACE model

The Program of All-Inclusive Care for the Elderly (PACE) is a recognized leader in the delivery of comprehensive, integrated care to adults with chronic illness, and functional and/or cognitive impairments. For more than 25 years, PACE organizations have integrated Medicare and Medicaid covered services into a single, comprehensive benefit package for a frail, nursing home qualified, largely dual-eligible population. PACE was one of the first home and community-based models designed to maximize program participants' function and independence as an alternative to permanent nursing home placement.

The first PACE program, On Lok, which means "peaceful happy abode" in Cantonese, was established in San Francisco in 1973. On Lok's success led to Congressional support for additional demonstration projects to test the PACE model, and, in 1997, PACE became a permanent Medicare provider and Medicaid state plan option. Currently, there are 75 operational PACE organizations, and approximately 40 additional health care organizations in various stages of PACE-site development. Nationwide, PACE organizations currently serve approximately 22,000 participants in 29 states. The number of PACE organizations has significantly increased in the past five years. This is due, in part, to grant funding for 15 providers to develop PACE organizations serving older adults in rural areas, and a growing recognition among new sponsors that PACE is an economically viable model of integrated and coordinated care.

PACE organizations enroll an exclusively high-cost Medicare beneficiary population. To qualify for the PACE program, a person must be 55 years of age or older, live in a PACE service area, and be certified by the state to need nursing home-level care. The typical PACE participant is very similar to the average nursing home resident. On average, the person is 80 years old, has 7.9 medical conditions, and is limited in approximately three activities of daily living. Approximately half of PACE participants have been diagnosed with some form of dementia. Although all PACE participants are assessed as clinically eligible for nursing home level of care by their states, on any given day, about 90% of PACE participants reside in their homes (National PACE Association 2010).

PACE is a unique health care delivery model with detailed regulatory requirements related to patient assessment, care management, the role of the comprehensive PACE interdisciplinary team, staffing, and participant input. PACE organizations are health care providers and not large insurers like most Medicare Advantage plans.

As both direct care providers and payers for care, PACE organizations create comprehensive, fully integrated health care delivery systems. PACE fully integrates the delivery of all Medicare and Medicaid covered benefits into a single benefit package, including medical care, and community-based and institutional long-term care at the individual beneficiary level. Interdisciplinary teams made up of physicians, nurse practitioners, nurses, social workers, physical, occupational, and recreational therapists, pharmacists, dietitians, personal care, and transportation providers, and others, regularly assess participants' needs and develop comprehensive care plans specific to each individual. PACE programs are fully accountable for the overall quality of care provided by all providers, both employed and contracted, across all settings, and over time.

PACE organizations directly employ a broad range of health care providers, including physicians, nurses, therapists, health care aides and others, and must comply with extensive requirements related to the composition of the PACE interdisciplinary team and its role in assessment and care planning.

A full range of individualized health care services are provided to PACE participants without benefit limitations, co-pays, or deductible requirements, including all Medicare and Medicaid covered services, as well as those additional services determined medically necessary but not covered by Medicare or Medicaid. PACE organizations cannot shift the responsibility for providing care or incurring costs to other providers or payers. Further, PACE is prohibited by law from responding to payment reductions by altering program benefits or imposing deductibles and co-payments.

Research on various aspects of the PACE model indicate the benefits of its integrated, interdisciplinary approach to caring for frail older adults. Hirth's and colleagues' (2009) literature analysis found that PACE programs had "greater adult day health care use, lower skilled home health visits, fewer hospitalizations, fewer nursing home admissions, higher contact with primary care, longer survival rates, an increased number of days in the community, better health, better quality of life, greater satisfaction with overall care arrangements, and better functional status" (p. 158). They also noted that the PACE participants who improved the most were the ones with the most severe conditions when entering the program.

Despite the recognized value of the PACE model, several barriers have limited the program's growth. One challenge is the amount of time and start-up capital required for developing a PACE organization. On average, it takes approximately 18 to 24 months to plan for and initiate PACE. Establishing a new PACE program requires providers to develop comprehensive care delivery systems encompassing all medical care and long-term services and supports required by the PACE participant population, all of whom meet their states' criteria for nursing home level of care.

A second challenge is the lack of awareness and understanding of the program. For many states, PACE is a new concept of care delivery and it takes time for them to consider how PACE best fits into its existing institutional and community-based long-term care system. A third challenge is that some potential PACE participants choose not to enroll because they do not want to switch from their current physician to a PACE primary care physician or participate in the activities held at the PACE Center. PACE organizations are addressing these concerns, particularly in rural communities, by contracting with community primary physicians to supplement their PACE team.[1]

Best practice elements of the PACE model

The entire PACE model can be considered "best practice" because of its effectiveness in providing high-quality integrated care to a vulnerable population of older adults (Substance Abuse and Mental Health Services Administration 2007). All PACE programs are required to meet extensive regulatory requirements that are intended to assure coordination and integration of care across the full continuum of medical and long-term care services they provide. Important elements include comprehensiveness of services provided; an interdisciplinary team approach to needs assessment, care planning and care delivery; bundling of payment with the objective of aligning payer, provider, and patient incentives; and the use of high-quality standards. The following briefly explains these components.

Services

PACE participants receive a comprehensive package of services and benefits, including all Medicare and Medicaid covered benefits, from the PACE organization. For participants, there is never a co-pay or deductible. Unlike many other health care and long-term care models, PACE organizations provide medical care *and* social support, including preventive, acute, and long-term care services. Services provided by PACE include: 1) PACE Center Services: physicians (community-based primary care physicians are also available in some locations), nurse practitioners, nurses, social workers, physical therapy, occupational therapy, speech therapy, recreational therapy, nutrition counseling, personal care, chore services, transportation, meals, and escort services; 2) in-home services: home health care, personal care, homemaker/chore services, and meals; 3) specialist services: medical specialists, audiology, dentistry, optometry, and podiatry; and 4) inpatient services: hospital, nursing home, and inpatient specialists (Greenwood 2001). In addition, PACE participants receive other services determined necessary by the interdisciplinary team to improve and maintain their health status.

Interdisciplinary team

Each participant works with an interdisciplinary team that is responsible for initial and periodic assessments, care planning, and coordination of 24-hour delivery of care. The interdisciplinary team is required to include the following members: primary care physician, registered nurse, social worker, physical therapist, occupational therapist, recreational therapist or activities coordinator, dietitian, PACE center manager, home care coordinator, personal care attendants, and drivers.

The team process is "patient-centered," and participants, family members, and other caregivers are encouraged to actively participate in the care-planning process. Additional members of the team may be included (for example, nurse practitioners, pharmacists, and others) in response to participants' individual needs.

Assessment

Each participant receives an initial comprehensive assessment, plus reassessments on a semiannual and annual basis, with specific outcomes to be achieved identified. Additional reassessments are conducted in response to significant changes in participants' health status, or at the request of participants and/or their caregivers. PACE participants' assessments are robust, comprehensive, and include measures of physical and cognitive function and ability; medication use; participant and caregiver preferences for care; socialization and availability of family support; current health status and treatment needs; nutritional status; home environment, home access; participant behavior; psychosocial status; medical and dental status; and participant language. The assessment in each area is consolidated into a single care plan.

Comprehensive written care plan

Each PACE participant receives a comprehensive written plan of care that meets their needs for all care settings 24 hours a day, every day of the year. Care plans are developed by the PACE interdisciplinary team, the participant, and the participant's family and other caregivers, and are continuously updated to respond to participants' changing needs. The plan is used by PACE organizations to assess participant health care needs, manage participant care, and collaborate with providers, participants, and caregivers (Centers for Medicare & Medicaid Services [CMS] 2010).

PACE center

The PACE Center is the hub for delivery of PACE services. It is the location where participants go to socialize and receive services provided by their PACE interdisciplinary team. Additionally, it provides a central location for the interdisciplinary team to meet. The PACE Center must provide space for delivery of primary care, social services, restorative therapies (including physical and occupational therapies), personal care and supportive services, nutritional counseling, recreational therapy, and meals.

Capitated payment

PACE organizations receive monthly Medicare and Medicaid capitation payments for each participant. The majority of PACE participants (over 90%) are dually eligible (receive benefits from both Medicare and Medicaid). Medicare eligible participants who are not eligible for Medicaid pay monthly premiums equal to the Medicaid capitation amount, but no deductibles or co-insurance apply.

PACE providers assume full financial risk for participants' care without limits on amount, duration, or scope of services. PACE organizations receive monthly payments for all Medicare and Medicaid covered benefits, as well as additional services necessary to maintain participants' health and well-being. These funds are pooled so services are provided without regard to payer source. Because PACE payments are fixed, the incentives are strong to eliminate duplicative or unnecessary services, prevent avoidable hospitalizations, intervene in response to changes in participants' health status, and provide timely preventive and primary care services to develop community-based alternatives to institutional care. Regular oversight and monitoring by CMS and the state assures the quality of care provided by PACE organizations.

Quality assessment and performance improvement

Each PACE organization is required to have a quality assessment and performance improvement (QAPI) program in place that evaluates the services it offers. A written QAPI plan is developed and outlines how the PACE organization proposes to meet minimum levels of performance set by CMS and the State. The plan is reviewed annually by the PACE organization's governing body and must identify objective measures that demonstrate improved performance in various areas. These include: 1) utilization of PACE services, 2) caregiver and participant satisfaction, 3) outcome measures derived from data collected during assessments, 4) effectiveness and safety of staff-provided and contracted services, and 5) nonclinical areas, such as grievances and appeals, transportation services, meals, life safety, and environmental issues. Outcome measures must be based on current clinical practice guidelines and professional standards applicable to the care of PACE participants.

In brief, several elements of the PACE model may be considered as "best practice" because they are effective in caring for a population of vulnerable older adults with multiple chronic conditions, and may be replicated by other health care or care coordination models. Additionally, PACE organizations continue to develop innovative ways to meet the needs of their participants and communities.

Examples of best practice: urban and rural PACE organizations

While PACE regulatory requirements specify standard expectations of all PACE organizations, the model allows for flexibility and the development of new and innovative practices. The following are examples of innovative practices developed by PACE organizations in urban and rural settings. Additional information about these best practices can be obtained by contacting the organizations directly or the National PACE Association.

Best practice in an urban setting: co-location of a PACE organization with federally assisted housing, Community LIFE

Co-location, in this context, refers to providing access to PACE services to eligible individuals in senior housing facilities, such as federally assisted or public housing.[2] This arrangement enables them to "age-in-place" (that is, live in their homes for as long as possible) and makes it safe for them to do so.

One PACE organization that has been successful with co-location is Community LIFE, located in Pittsburgh, Pennsylvania. Community LIFE is co-sponsored by Presbyterian Senior Care, the University of Pittsburgh Medical Center (UPMC) Health System, and the Jewish Association on Aging. Community LIFE has PACE centers in East Liberty, Homestead, McKeesport, and Tarentum, PA. Combined, the four Community LIFE centers serve approximately 370 PACE participants.

Community LIFE partnered with its local public housing authority in Allegheny County in 2002, to build a PACE center on the Homestead property, a 240-unit apartment building owned by the county. The Homestead Apartments are a mixed housing development for persons 62 years of age and older. With a HOPE VI grant from the U.S. Department of Housing and Urban Development, the Homestead apartment building had access to funding for revitalization of distressed properties. Using this funding, a 14,000 square foot Community LIFE center was built within the Homestead apartment complex to offer comprehensive services to both Homestead residents and individuals in the surrounding community who are eligible and wish to enroll in PACE. Currently, approximately 10% of Homestead residents participate in the Community LIFE program.

This co-location project has benefited multiple stakeholders. PACE participants in the Community LIFE Homestead program receive health care services in a convenient and familiar setting, enabling them to remain in their homes for as long as possible rather than move into institutional care. The broader community benefits because Community LIFE Homestead sponsors events for not only their participants, but the entire community, such as holding an "Ask the Doctor Day," administering flu shots, and providing a mobile farmers market. Community LIFE benefits from co-location because it leases its center at reasonable rates from the housing authority, serves a number of PACE participants with their home-health needs efficiently through the economy of scale afforded by serving several participants in the adjacent housing, and receives visibility and access to future participants. The Allegheny Housing Authority benefits by being able to provide some of its most frail residents with quality health care. Additionally, providing services on a campus will likely reduce eventual vacancies and turnover that could result with the aging of its residents.

Best practice in a rural setting: the use of community physicians, Senior Community Care

An innovative practice used by some PACE organizations is contracting with community-based primary care physicians (PCPs). Senior Community Care (SCC), a service of the Volunteers of America, is a PACE program located in Western Colorado that has been successful in using community PCPs in their rural program. SCC serves all of Delta County and two-thirds of Montrose County, and had 186 participants in their program as of October 2010.

PACE organizations generally use a staff model, in which the primary physicians are employed by the program. In contrast, SCC contracts with community physicians in Delta and Montrose counties to provide medical care to their PACE-eligible participants. Community physicians' responsibilities include working closely with the entire SCC team to coordinate all participant services, providing 24-hour care as part of a physicians' call group, and acting as the attending physician when a participant requires hospitalization or care in a skilled nursing facility. In addition to the community physicians, SCC has a medical director that oversees all medical care and manages a caseload of about 20% of program participants. The community physicians provide the primary care for the remaining 80% of participants.

SCC was a recipient of the Rural PACE Pilot Grant Program, established by Congress under the Deficit Reduction Act of 2005, and administered by CMS. The practice of including community-based PCPs was built into the program when it was established in 2008, in order to provide prospective participants with an option to continue receiving their services from community-based PCPs. Some of their potential participants may have been unwilling to give up their relationship with their doctors, who, in some cases, had provided care to generations of their families.

Community PCPs have become an integral part of SCC's interdisciplinary team. They call into the team meetings to discuss a participant's intake, initial assessment, care plan, monthly updates, as well as participate in quality improvement activities. The SCC medical director and nurse practitioner also attend all team meetings. If a medical concern arises, the medical director and nurse practitioner provide medical care until the community physician is contacted. Physicians are reimbursed for phone conference calls, team meetings, and office visits. The SCC program also provides ongoing training to community physicians through personal meetings, conferences, and regular communication with its clinical staff.

The use of community physicians has proven to be highly beneficial for SCC. The participants benefit by being able to keep their current physicians with whom they are comfortable. The SCC program benefits by contracting with community physicians and eliminating a potential barrier to program enrollment (that is, requiring participants to change doctors). Finally, the community physicians like the program because they value the care coordination component, and are able to maintain their relationships with long-term patients and continue caring for them as they age and require more services. For organizations interested in exploring the possibility of contracting with community physicians for their program, SCC recommends having a clear understanding of the needs of your market and clientele, physician motivation, and the local systems of practice.

Building on the experience of an urban site to expand into a rural community, LIFE Geisinger

The LIFE Geisinger program, located in Danville, Pennsylvania, is considered a model of best practice because of its success in developing and implementing both a rural and an urban PACE program. LIFE Geisinger is part of the Geisinger Health System, a physician-led system that provides health care services, education, and research to 38 counties in Pennsylvania. Building on the experience they gained from its first site located in an urban area, LIFE Geisinger was able to expand to a second site located in a rural area. Additionally, managing PACE programs in difference environments allows LIFE Geisinger to make comparisons between the programs and share best practice that may be useful to other organizations. The following briefly describes the programs and best practices, along with lessons learned.

In 2006, LIFE Geisinger opened its urban PACE program in Scranton, Pennsylvania, serving Lackawanna and portions of Luzerne counties. The urban facility was developed in collaboration with a religious order of Sisters, with Geisinger taking on the financial risk for the new facility, and the religious order providing for 100% of the participants when it opened. As of October 2010, the urban program had 88 participants.

In 2008, LIFE Geisinger's rural program was established in Northumberland County to serve four rural counties. This program was funded, in part, through a federal grant to expand the PACE model into rural areas. This program is co-located on property owned by a local housing authority, which is an old neighborhood school that includes independent apartments and a community-college outreach program for nurses wishing to obtain Registered Nursing licensure. LIFE Geisinger was interested in the school because it had a large vacant gymnasium suitable for the center with a small addition. The local housing authority partnered with Geisinger and financed $1.3 million in leasehold improvement costs to renovate the space to accommodate a PACE center. LIFE Geisinger currently leases the space at fair market prices, including the cost to cover the $1.3 million over a 10-year term. As of October 2010, LIFE Geisinger's rural site had 71 participants enrolled in the program.

Best practice/lessons learned

LIFE Geisinger applied the experience and lessons gained from operating an urban PACE program to their second program established in a rural community. Best practices that were applied from LIFE Geisinger's urban program to its rural program include assessing community need and support for a new program, identifying successful partners, and designing a facility that fits well with the community.

The first practice is assessing the community's needs to determine if there was sufficient demand for the program and interest in supporting a new PACE organization. This includes the availability of referral networks that will help build the program and contract opportunities that will allow the organization to meet the PACE participants' needs.

With the rural site, there were initially some challenges with program enrollment because the PACE model was unfamiliar in the community, and people thought it sounded "too good to be true." A lack of trust also stemmed from the community's past experience with a Medicare+Choice program that had withdrawn its plan from several counties. This made the community cautious about taking a risk on another new program. However, once individuals began to understand and trust the LIFE Geisinger program, the number of participants steadily increased. Within 14 months of operation, the LIFE Geisinger's rural facility had a positive cash flow and was able to start returning the start-up investment made by their parent institution.

The second practice is to identify and work with successful partners that believe in the PACE philosophy. Both LIFE Geisinger's urban and rural partners supported the PACE model and were vested in the program's future success. Based on its experience, LIFE Geisinger recommends clarifying the partner's role and desired level of involvement in the project in advance to avoid any misunderstandings. This is especially important if new construction is involved and the PACE program accepts the majority of the financial risk.

A final practice is to design a facility that not only meets the needs of the PACE organization, but also fits in with the community in order to gain acceptance. Regardless of whether a new building is being constructed or renovations are being made on an existing property, organizations should determine whether the size of the facility will meet the required regulations for offering PACE services, and whether the facility's design and appearance is compatible with the local environment. The urban facility was a newly constructed structure with a contemporary design while the rural site involved renovations to a former school that was already a part of the community's landscape.

LIFE Geisinger's programs benefit all parties involved. The Sisters were able to participate in the development of a program that provides high-quality health care to frail, older adults. LIFE Geisinger was able to expand the PACE model in a rural community. Finally, the housing authority was able to renovate and rent a vacant property to a responsible partner that would help meet the health care needs of older adults in the community.

Summary

For over 25 years, the PACE model has successfully provided high quality and effective care to a targeted segment of the older adult population, those 55 and older who are nursing-home eligible. Because of the PACE program, many vulnerable individuals have been able to remain in their homes longer and avoid costly and unnecessary institutionalization. As the Baby Boom population continues to age over the next few decades, demand will grow for home and community-based programs like PACE. To help meet this need, PACE organizations are exploring and developing new opportunities to expand to other populations that would benefit from the PACE care model such as veterans, younger populations with disabilities, and middle-income older adults.

Acknowledgments

The authors appreciate the assistance they received from several persons in the preparation of this chapter. These include Richard A. DiTommaso, Executive Director, Pittsburgh Care Partnership/Community LIFE; Amy Minnich, Executive Director, LIFE Geisinger; Wayne Olsen, Senior Vice President, Volunteers of America; and Shawn Bloom, President/CEO, National PACE Association.

Notes

1. In order to engage community-based primary care physicians as PACE interdisciplinary team members, PACE organizations must obtain waivers of PACE regulatory requirements with the approval of both their state administering agencies and CMS. PACE organizations' experience to-date points to the importance of identifying community-based physicians who understand and support the overall mission and objectives of PACE and commit to their role as interdisciplinary team members, which involves

active participation in interdisciplinary team meetings, care planning, and quality improvement activities in addition to providing primary care services.
2. Federally assisted rental housing includes public housing and Section 202 housing. Public housing, which is publicly funded and administered, provides housing to eligible low-income families, the elderly, and persons with disabilities. Section 202 provides rental housing for low-income adults age 62 or older.

References

American Association of Retired Persons Public Policy Institute. (2010) *Fact Sheet on Health Care Reform Improves Access to Medicaid Home and Community-Based Services.* American Association of Retired Persons, Washington, DC. Retrieved http://www.assets.aarp.org/rgcenter/ppi/ltc/fs192-hcbs.pdf.

Centers for Medicare & Medicaid Services. (2010) *Care Planning Guidance for PACE Organizations.* Centers for Medicare & Medicaid Services, Baltimore, MD.

Greenwood, R. (2001) *Center for Medicare Education Issue Brief: The PACE Model.* American Association for Homes and Services for the Aging, Washington, DC.

Henry J. Kaiser Family Foundation. (2010) *Medicaid and Long-Term Care Services and Supports.* Kaiser Commission on Medicaid and the Uninsured. Washington, DC. Retrieved from http://kff.org/medicaid/upload/2186-07.pdf.

Hirth, V., Baskins, J., & Dever-Bumba, M. (2009) Program of All-Inclusive Care (PACE): past, present, and future. *Journal of the American Medical Directors Association*, 10, 155–160.

National PACE Association. (2010) *Who Does PACE Serve?* National PACE Association, Alexandria, VA. Retrieved from http://www.npaonline.org/website/article.asp?id=50.

O'Shaughnessy, Carol. (2010) *National Spending for Long-Term Services and Supports (LTSS).* The George Washington University National Health Policy Forum, Washington, DC. Retrieved from http://www.nhpf.org/library/the-basics/Basics_LongTermServicesSupports_04-30-10.pdf.

Substance Abuse and Mental Health Services Administration. (2007) *National Registry of Evidence-based Programs and Practices.* U.S. Department of Health and Human Services, Washington, DC. Retrieved from http://www.nrepp.samhsa.gov/ViewIntervention.aspx?id=162.

U.S. Administration on Aging. (2009) *A Profile of Older Americans: 2009.* U.S. Department of Health and Human Services, Washington, DC. Retrieved from http://www.aoa.gov/AoARoot/Aging_Statistics/Profile/2009/4.aspx.

Section 4

Medicaid models

Chapter 17

Introduction to Medicaid care management

Allison Hamblin and Stephen A. Somers

Introduction

Many of those served by Medicaid are relatively healthy, with only routine health care needs and nominal annual health-related costs. Yet, a small subset of the program's beneficiaries includes many of the country's highest-need, highest-cost patients. This includes adults and children with physical and behavioral health disabilities, those with long-term care needs, as well as low-income frail elders. Roughly 5% of Medicaid beneficiaries account for close to 60% of total program expenditures,[1] with annual outlays estimated at approximately $190 billion.[2] Reducing even a fraction of spending for this high-cost population by improving care management can provide meaningful savings for states.

Implementing care management strategies is a key way for states to improve care delivery and address the high health costs of Medicaid's most complex need beneficiaries. Focusing on high-need, high-cost populations takes on even more importance with the Patient Protection and Affordable Care Act of 2010 expanding Medicaid coverage to around 25% of all Americans. This comes at a time when Medicaid agencies are facing strapped, over-extended budgets, and legislatures are looking to stem rising health costs. States will need to more effectively use existing resources to provide services for an expanded population, including the potential of many new beneficiaries with complex needs. Indeed, based on a recent review of existing state programs for low-income childless adults, the expansion population is likely to include a significant number of individuals with multiple chronic conditions, high levels of service use, and higher annual costs than generally healthy beneficiaries (Somers *et al*. 2010). It is likely that many of these new beneficiaries will be candidates for intense care management.

This chapter provides a glimpse at some of the innovative programs being implemented in states across the country that use care management approaches to address the complex physical, behavioral, and psychosocial needs of Medicaid's highest-risk populations. This first introductory section sheds light on the program's high-risk beneficiary subsets and outlines core elements essential for effective care management approaches.

Comprehensive Care Coordination for Chronically Ill Adults, First Edition. Edited by Cheryl Schraeder and Paul Shelton.
© 2011 John Wiley & Sons, Inc. Published 2011 by John Wiley & Sons, Inc.

Table 17.1   Mental Illness Among Medicaid's Highest-Cost Population

Prevalent Disease Pairs	Frequency Among Highest-Cost 5% of Medicaid Beneficiaries
Psychiatric illness and cardiovascular disease	40.4%
Psychiatric illness and central nervous system disorders	39.8%
Psychiatric illness and pulmonary disorders	28.6%

Source: Kronick *et al.* (2009)

Who are Medicaid's highest-need, highest-cost beneficiaries?

Understanding the unique care needs and requirements of Medicaid's highest-cost subsets is the first step toward developing appropriate care management interventions. The program's highest-need subset has multiple chronic physical health problems and typically faces a variety of socioeconomic barriers (such as unstable housing, lack of transportation, and so on) that impede access to care. Mental illness and substance abuse are also endemic among the program's highest-need, highest-cost beneficiaries. More than 50% of Medicaid beneficiaries with disabilities are diagnosed with mental illness (Kronick *et al.* 2009). This pervasiveness is particularly high among the program's most expensive 5% of patients, with mental illness present in three of the top five most prevalent pairs of diseases for this high cost subset (Table 17.1).

Mental illness is closely linked to poor health outcomes and the presence of mental illness can exacerbate problems related to chronic physical conditions. For example, a recent analysis demonstrated that health care spending is substantially higher for Medicaid beneficiaries with chronic physical conditions who also have a mental illness. Among those with common chronic physical conditions (for example, asthma, diabetes, hypertension, coronary heart disease), the presence of a co-occurring mental illness is linked with health care costs that are 60% to 75% higher than those without a mental illness.

Yet despite the high prevalence, as well as the human and financial costs of mental illness, the majority of Medicaid beneficiaries with mental illness are in fragmented systems of care. Behavioral health services are typically provided separately from physical health care with little to no coordination between the two delivery systems. As a result, patients typically receive care from a confusing array of disparate providers that are frequently unaware of the individual patients' overall needs as well as the treatments and prescriptions they are receiving from other providers.

The programs outlined in this chapter showcase innovative care management approaches that integrate the full array of physical health, behavioral health, and psychosocial services. These best practices can serve a starting point to guide program design and evaluation for other states and health plans.

Core elements of care management

Most of Medicaid's highest-cost, highest-need beneficiaries receive care through fragmented and uncoordinated fee-for-service delivery systems. In this context, care

Table 17.2   Core Elements of Medicaid Care Management
Programs

1. Stratification and triage by risk/need.
2. Integration of services.
3. Designated "care home" and personalized care plan.
4. Consumer engagement strategies.
5. Provider engagement strategies.
6. Information exchange among all stakeholders.
7. Performance measurement and accountability.
8. Financial incentives aligned with quality care.

management programs can serve as a vital mechanism for helping individuals achieve better access to needed care, navigate their way through complex systems, and increase the self-management and self-advocacy skills necessary to function as informed and "activated" health care consumers. Within fee-for-service systems, states contract with care management organizations of various kinds to deliver these services (or in some cases build this capacity internally). In the case of managed care, states are increasingly requiring their health plan partners to offer targeted care management strategies to beneficiaries with complex needs.

Across the country, innovative states are implementing programs that provide "high touch" care management for targeted groups of beneficiaries. Best practices from around the country suggest the following core elements should be considered in the design of complex care management programs (see Table 17.2).

The following section briefly outlines each of these elements and provides specific state examples to illustrate how these strategies can be incorporated into care management approaches. The states highlighted in this section are participants in the *Rethinking Care Program,* a national initiative developed by the Center for Health Care Strategies (CHCS) to design and test better approaches to care for Medicaid's highest-need, highest-cost beneficiaries. Through support from Kaiser Permanente, four state pilot demonstrations – in Colorado, Pennsylvania, New York, and Washington – are testing and refining how to implement the following core program elements to best serve Medicaid's "high-opportunity" beneficiaries.

Stratify and triage beneficiaries by level of risk and need

Determining how to invest limited program resources to effectively meet the needs of Medicaid's highest-risk, highest-cost beneficiaries, is a conundrum faced by every state. Identifying the patients who are most likely to benefit from care management and designing programs tailored to meet their needs is an extremely valuable, but not necessarily clearly defined, endeavor. Stratification efforts typically use claims data to identify one or more of the following characteristics: high medical expenditures (historic or expected), high hospitalization or emergency department visit rates (historic or expected), and specific types or numbers of existing diagnoses.

Ideally, identification and stratification efforts should use additional data to supplement information available via health care claims, particularly in the case of new enrollees for whom limited claims history is available. Along these lines, upon enrollment, Medicaid programs should ideally have a mechanism in place to rapidly identify new beneficiaries who may have immediate physical health, behavioral health, or psychosocial needs. Promptly linking new patients with needed care management services can help reduce exacerbations of chronic conditions and avoid potential costs related to unnecessary emergency department visits or hospital stays. A variety of strategies can be used to identify the health needs of newly enrolled beneficiaries, including referrals from a provider or specialist, a beneficiary's own self-identification, or initial health screens.

An initial health screen can be used to quickly assess and identify high-risk beneficiaries with pressing health and care coordination needs. Such screens typically include questions that address both clinical and non-clinical issues to capture the full range of beneficiary needs. For the higher-risk subset, a state may choose to implement a more in-depth clinical assessment to more completely understand beneficiary needs, prioritize risk levels, and connect them to services that will best meet those needs. Both initial health screens and clinical assessments can be used on a periodic base to re-evaluate beneficiary level of need.

Another mechanism for states to assess the needs of beneficiaries on an ongoing basis is through predictive modeling. While predictive models are often used to forecast costs for rate-setting purposes, states can also use these tools to identify "high-opportunity" candidates for care management. Predictive models use data from various sources to estimate an individual's future potential health care costs and/or opportunity for care management. Adapting predictive models to address the Medicaid population's complex array of needs, including physical and behavioral health co-morbidities, as well as socioeconomic issues, is a critical consideration for states.

Washington State offers an example of an innovative use of predictive modeling. The state used internal resources to develop a customized predictive modeling tool to identify high-risk Medicaid populations for enrollment in care management programs. Based on the Chronic Disability Payment System (Kronick *et al.* 2000), Washington's tool uses a variety of information to target care management needs, including prescription drug use; preventive care opportunities; emergency room use; provider contact information; and mental health, substance abuse, and long-term care service use. The secure web-based tool is available for approved Washington State's Department of Social and Health Services staff, and is also available for use by contracted care managers as a source of timely information on enrollee care needs and service use.

Integration of services

As mentioned above, high-risk beneficiaries often have care needs spanning across and beyond traditional silos of the health care delivery system. These needs may include primary and specialty medical care, mental health care, substance abuse treatment, long-term care services, and community supports (for example, housing, transportation, energy, job training, and so on). Effective care management programs ensure the coordination of services across these domains, connecting providers and enabling the exchange of relevant information so that treatment for any one of the patient's needs recognizes the full range of those needs. Such coordination is essential to prevent a broad array of clinical mishaps, including adverse medication interactions, duplicative tests and/or treatments, and unrealistically complicated self-management regimens.

An example of integrated care management can be found in Pennsylvania, where the state has partnered with physical and behavioral health plans and providers in two pilots to better integrate physical and behavioral health care for adults with serious mental illness. In each pilot, a designated care manager is accountable for managing the range of physical and behavioral health needs of clients, and is supported in doing so through access to timely, integrated information on health needs, provider relationships, and service use across systems.

Establish a designated "care home" and personalized care plan

Establishing a consistent care home that is acknowledged by the consumer, provider, and care management organization provides a central hub to coordinate all physical, behavioral, and psychosocial needs. The care home is often a primary care provider practice or community health setting, but for beneficiaries with severe mental illness, the care home is just as likely to be a mental health provider in the community. Regardless of the setting, the care home should be supported by a team-based approach to care management that provides access to clinical, psychiatric, chemical dependency, social work, and pharmacy expertise. Within this care team, each beneficiary should have a dedicated "go-to person" serving as the primary care manager. Providing one go-to person is valuable for both the beneficiary in terms of familiarity and consistency and the primary care provider. Depending on the needs of the beneficiary, the go-to person may vary (for example, it may be a nurse, a care manager, or a social worker).

A personalized care plan that is accessible and approved by all the members of the multidisciplinary care team serves as the ongoing framework to guide care management decisions. The care plan is an individualized plan of care that maps out the beneficiary's physical, behavioral, and psychosocial needs, primary care and specialty providers, home environment, transportation needs, and so on. It documents an agreed-upon set of goals for the beneficiary and the care team. Care plans should be developed in concert with beneficiaries to help them set and prioritize attainable and compelling goals. In a Pennsylvania pilot program for adults with severe mental illness, an integrated web-based care plan automatically incorporates data from participating physical and behavioral health plans. Care managers can access and update information through an online interface.

Engage consumers at their levels to meet their needs effectively

Without meaningful consumer engagement even the best designed care management intervention is bound to fail. Effectively reaching consumers, understanding their needs and goals, and ensuring that care management efforts are aligned with those goals are essential to program success. Yet, engaging beneficiaries is perhaps one of the most difficult tasks of any Medicaid care management program designed to address complex physical and behavioral health issues.

Poor contact information, unstable housing, overwhelming socioeconomic challenges, and, in some cases, lack of trust, all intersect to make finding, enrolling, and engaging patients with chronic illnesses and mental health and substance use issues exceedingly difficult. That said, investments in creative and persistent approaches to locate and engage high-risk beneficiaries can yield positive results for care management programs.

In Washington State's Department of Social and Health Services, the Research & Data Analysis Division uses an innovative approach to finding beneficiaries that has substantially increased the state's engagement rate of a complex need, and in some cases, homeless population. Factors contributing to the success include a client-finding team that is dedicated to persistent outreach and sleuth-work; use of consumer incentives; and a highly personalized approach that focuses on messages that are compelling to consumers.[3]

Once consumers are enrolled in a care management program, consumer engagement continues to be an important element to program success. Taking the time to understand the consumer point of view can help care managers design programs that directly speak to beneficiary needs. Some states are employing motivational interviewing training and techniques to more effectively support beneficiaries setting and reaching goals for changing behavior. Motivational interviewing is "collaborative, person-centered form of guiding to elicit and strengthen motivation for change" (Miller & Rollnick 2009).

Engage providers as part of care team

Care management is most effective when it is closely integrated with care delivered by the patient's physicians and other treating providers. To this end, successful care management programs invest substantial effort in establishing and maintaining relationships with the provider community. Demonstrating the value of care management to providers can be key to engagement, and can be facilitated by seeking provider input in program development, accepting provider referrals into the program, and providing access to clinically valuable patient information (with patient consent, including, for example, pharmacy fills, diagnoses, and recent health care service utilization).

In some models, care managers are co-located at physician practice sites. For example, in Colorado and a number of other states, Medicaid health plans have placed care managers in high-volume community clinics to ensure close coordination between the care managers and the primary care physicians.

Establish information exchange among all stakeholders including consumers

The push for greater use of information technology in health care is rooted in the understanding that access to timely, relevant clinical information is key to identifying care needs, anticipating future health risks, and avoiding negative outcomes. As mentioned above, effective care coordination requires that relevant information be made available to all members of a care team as needed, including availability to consumers. This information may include basic data on diagnoses, lab results, service use including hospital admissions and emergency room visits, prescription medications and provider contact information. Ideally, it also includes alerts regarding potential gaps in care (such as annual screening exams for diabetics), potential adverse medication interactions, and real-time notifications of critical events such as hospitalizations to ensure coordinated discharge planning.

To note, while access to information technology, such as electronic health records, greatly facilitates the process of information exchange, much can be done in its absence. For example, in one of the Pennsylvania pilots mentioned above, integrated health profiles are developed and shared with all members of the care team in hard copy form pending the availability of an electronic solution.

Incorporate ongoing performance measurement and accountability

Promoting some measure of accountability, through shared risk, shared savings, or a combination thereof, is a critical element to influence a successful care management approach. By linking performance measures with financial incentives, states can align providers, including primary care, behavioral health, and other specialists, as well as care management organizations, to common goals. States should consider performance measures that go beyond standard HEDIS measures to recognize the complexities of the population. Prevention quality indicators, for example, are a set of measures that are used with hospital inpatient discharge data to identify beneficiaries with ambulatory care sensitive conditions.[4] These conditions are recognized as issues for which outpatient care can potentially prevent the need for hospitalization. Process measures can also be used to support the implementation of effective care delivery (for example, outreach and enrollment targets, completion of a patient-centered care plan, achievement of care plan goals, and so on). Once measures are established, processes must be put in place to ensure consistent and effective performance monitoring.

Establish financial incentives that align with high-quality, coordinated care

As with all aspects of health care delivery, payment mechanisms provide critical levers for driving desired processes and outcomes of care. "You get what you pay for" holds true in health care as in any other industry, and in the case of care management, states must consider how to most effectively align financial incentives with overall program goals. Incentives may need to be specifically designed to address any of the following goals, among others – maximizing enrollment, encouraging rapid assessment of health needs, reducing avoidable admissions and emergency room visits, coordinating care across systems, and transitioning patients out of care management as needs are stabilized. Alternative mechanisms for aligning incentives with these goals include: establishing different payment rates for different stages of patient engagement/enrollment; linking incentive payments (or withholds) to targeted thresholds of performance on a set of key measures; and developing gain-sharing arrangements that allow partners to share in the savings associated with reduced medical costs.

To align incentives for its physical-behavioral health integration pilots, Pennsylvania created a shared incentive pool that rewards the pilot partners for high performance on measures associated with effective integration. The performance measures can be influenced by both physical health and behavioral health care management partners, and both are jointly accountable for the measures. In the first year, the focus was on measures of cross-system collaboration and integrated care processes (such as member assessment, stratification, and jointly developed plan of care). In the second year, the measures evolve to capture intermediate outcomes, such as reduced use of emergency departments and reduced inpatient admissions.

Summary

Ensuring that patients receive the right care in the right setting at the right time is the underlying goal of care management. The innovative state programs profiled in this chapter are employing all or a majority of the elements outlined in this section to help Medicaid beneficiaries with complex needs achieve this critical goal. These elements can also be used as a framework to guide the evaluation and ongoing quality improvement of existing care management approaches. As states across the country prepare to absorb the new demands of the expansive population, employing such tools to advance effective care management models takes on even greater importance.

Notes

1. Kaiser Commission on Medicaid and the Uninsured and the Urban Institute estimate based on 2004 Medicaid Statistical Information System (MSIS) data.
2. CHCS estimate using the Urban Institute and Kaiser Commission on Medicaid and the Uninsured estimate based on the Centers for Medicare & Medicaid Services 64 reports, March 2009, and National Health Expenditure Projections 2009–2019.
3. Fore more information see resources from CHCS Webinar: *Strategies for Finding and Engaging Medicaid Beneficiaries for Complex Care Management*, October 5, 2010. Available at: http://www.chcs.org/publications3960/publications_show_htm?doc_id=1261169.
4. For more information see the Prevention Quality Indicators, Agency for Healthcare Research and Quality, March 2007. Available at: http//www.qualityindicators.ahrq.gov/.

References

Kronick, R., Gilmer, T., Dreyful, T., *et al.* (2000) Improving health based on payment for Medicaid beneficiaries: CDPS. *Health Care Financing Review*, 21(3), 29–64.

Kronick, R.G., Bella, M., & Gilmer, T.P. (2009) *The Faces of Medicaid III: Refining the Portrait of People with Multiple Chronic Conditions.* Center for Health Care Strategies, Inc., Hamilton, NJ.

Miller, W.R., & Rollnick, S. (2009) Ten things that motivational interviewing is not. *Behavioural and Cognitive Psychotherapy*, 37, 129–140.

Somers, S.A., Hamblin, A., Verdier, J.M., *et al.* (2010) *Covering Low-Income Childless Adults in Medicaid: Experiences from Selected States.* Center for Health Care Strategies, Inc., Hamilton, NJ.

Chapter 18

The Aetna Integrated Care Management model: a managed Medicaid paradigm

Robert M. Atkins and Mark E. Douglas

Introduction

With the U.S. economy struggling to recover, and as health reform implementation begins, the stage is now being set for how the new federal Patient Protection and Accountable Care Act (PPACA) will shape the future health care system. One change under PPACA that will dramatically impact state Medicaid programs is the new requirement to expand eligibility for individuals under the age of 65 with incomes up to 133% of the federal poverty level by 2014. An increased number of adults will have access to Medicaid during a time when states hampered by budget shortfalls are being forced to evaluate the financial viability of their current programs caring for what already is a very diverse, costly, and complicated population. Of the expanded population that will join the Medicaid ranks, 25% have at least one chronic disease, and nearly one in six rate their health as fair or poor (Guyer & Paradise 2010). This group of individuals typically has less access to primary care and the care received is often fragmented with little attention paid to prevention or wellness care. Further, many of these individuals experience behavioral health issues which can lead to decreased continuity of care and increased medical costs. The required Medicaid expansion will place additional pressure on states and other key stakeholders to rapidly find the most effective, evidence-based care strategies that contain costs and improve access and quality while providing services in an individualized manner.

The Aetna Integrated Care Management Model: a managed Medicaid perspective

Aetna has developed expertise providing advanced care management services while operating managed Medicaid programs throughout the United States. Over many years, Aetna has successfully implemented several innovative care management models that center on evidence-based outcomes using a multi-disciplinary, individualized approach. Much of the success experienced has been the result of developing care management strategies that address the complex needs of the aged, blind, and disabled (ABD) population, whose

Comprehensive Care Coordination for Chronically Ill Adults, First Edition. Edited by Cheryl Schraeder and Paul Shelton.
© 2011 John Wiley & Sons, Inc. Published 2011 by John Wiley & Sons, Inc.

care often drives increased costs and demands for health care services. In recent years, Aetna has intensified efforts to concentrate on appropriately targeting care to the broader Medicaid population while also identifying sub-populations and individuals who are most at-risk and will receive greater benefit from intensive care management services. The culmination of these efforts led to the development of the Integrated Care Management (ICM) model. The ICM model is a care paradigm that moves from a one-dimensional medical approach focused on managing limited clinical conditions or disease-related matters, to a multi-faceted model that redefines successful health outcomes with a member-centric aim. The ICM model evolved from a bio-psycho-social model of care based on five guiding principles:

- Shift from Disease to Individualized Focus – the care model shifts from a disease-oriented model to a true individual focus that recognizes each individual's physical, behavioral, and social risks that will affect their current and future health statuses.
- Appropriate Care Level and Intensity – each individual's care is facilitated in relation to a continuum of evidence-based services based on the timely delivery of interventions that reflect the proper intensity and complexity of each individual's specific care needs.
- Behavioral Engagement for Change – emphasis is placed on member engagement and activation strategies that are designed to motivate individuals to take ownership of their care leading to the eventual goals of autonomy, resiliency, and optimal self-management.
- Provider Collaboration – central to successfully maximizing health outcomes is creating trusting care relationships that promote collaboration with a member's primary care provider, community care team, and social support system combining core competencies in physical and behavioral health that support a comprehensive medical home.
- Promote a System of Care – the ICM model seeks to actively detect barriers and fragmentation of care to align all resources into an integrated system that is defined in the context of each member's individual needs and family and cultural community.

The ICM model is applied in the context of a Medicaid health plan providing services to assigned members. However, the principles can be adopted for use in a number of care settings. Further on, a more detailed discussion outlines the core components and operational considerations that define the foundation of the ICM model.

ICM model overview

The ICM model was designed to address an array of care needs for the Medicaid population. However, a key feature of the ICM model is the methodology and care process that emphasizes reaching and care managing those complex members at highest risk for poor health outcomes. The ICM model is posited on a conceptual framework that promotes aggressively managing the most complex, highest-risk population in order to make greater strides in controlling costs and improving the quality of care and quality of life members will experience. The model is based on a care paradigm that quickly identifies members most at-risk and engages them with intensive care management services. The model also maintains supportive care options for lower-risk members who will require targeted, episodic care management and population health services.

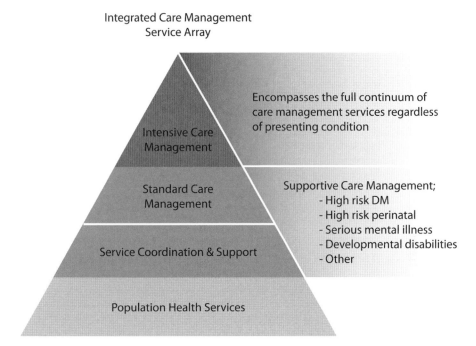

Figure 18.1   Care Management Pyramid

Targeting the right population with the right services

The ICM model is designed to provide specialized care management services to two larger groups of individuals that fall into complementary subdivisions of the Medicaid population: (1) complex, high-risk members; and (2) members that require various levels of episodic supportive care management services. A key feature of the ICM model is the strategic identification of a small subset of individuals with the most complex needs and fragmented care patterns for Intensive Care Management. Care management for these members is characterized by a longer-term relationship with a single clinical care manager who maintains a lower caseload solely dedicated to managing complex, high-risk members. Intensive Care Management services provided to complex, high-risk members, are frequent, high-touch (face-to-face), and sustained for long periods of time (typically several months) to ensure that members reach optimal stabilization and are moved into a lower risk stratification. Members in this group have most of their care management services coordinated by a clinical care manager, but as a member progresses toward stabilization and self-management, coordination needs can be met by non-clinical staff to ensure clinicians on the care team focus on clinical care management activities.

The Supportive Care Management category consists of individuals that have a single complex care issue or several less intensive care issues that will stabilize or resolve within a shorter period of time and require fairly straightforward problem-solving. Supportive Care Management services focus on standard, targeted interventions for specific health or

Table 18.1 Intensive Care Management Versus Supportive Care Management

		Supportive Care Management	Intensive Care Management
Member Needs	Risk of future utilization	Lower	Higher
	Bio-psycho-social complexity	Lower	Higher
	Required healthcare services	Low to moderate complexity	High complexity
	Effectiveness of current healthcare	Variable	Low
	Adequacy of social support	Variable	Low
Care Management (CM) Features	CM services	Condition-driven	Complexity-driven
	Typical duration	Episodic (days/weeks)	Extended (months)
	Frequency of contact	As needed: less frequent	As needed: more frequent
	Relationship	Consultative	Collaborative, coaching, continuity over time
	Case conceptualization	Simple and straightforward	Systematic and contextual
	Case load size	Large	Small
	Case load drivers	Demand for services	Case Manager capacity
Care Management Outcomes	Focus	Solving immediate, presented problem	Resolving pervasive, persistent problems
	Regression to mean	More likely	Less likely
	Goal	Return to baseline level of functioning	Change baseline level of functioning
	Value	Get to baseline faster, safer, more reliably	Sustained improvement without continuing high level of care management services

other care issues that may require varied intensity but services are typically more limited in scope and frequency. For example, an individual whose overall health is relatively stable except for an acute disease exacerbation (such as asthma) that may require a shorter term intervention. Individuals in this category might receive regular follow-up for a limited period, including education and regular assessments to ensure medication adherence and engagement with their primary care provider. The focus for members in this category is finding the safest and most appropriate and cost-effective resolution. Care and support for these individuals may require higher-level clinician involvement and oversight for limited periods, but the sustained, longer-term interactions can be primarily supported with non-clinical staff.

The key components of ICM that shape both Intensive Care Management and Supportive Care Management are described in more detail below. The primary driver for the ICM model revolves around the quick identification of high-risk members and their movement into Intensive Care Management.

ICM foundational care components

The Integrated Care Management model is designed around the following eight key components: Focusing on the Right Members; Right People, Right Skills; Individualized Relationship-Based Care; Bio-Psycho-Social Care Planning; Multi-disciplinary Case Rounds; Progression of Care; Outcomes Accountability; and Standardized Electronic Health Information Platform.

Focusing on the right members

ICM considers each member's complete needs as they relate to their current and future health. Success in correctly aligning needs with the proper level of care is achieved by employing evidence-based member identification and stratification. Aetna uses predictive modeling and self-report tools to fully integrate physical and behavioral health conditions along with psychosocial risks and protective factors to identify members who would benefit from care management and also to properly stratify members into intensive and supportive levels of service.

While all members might benefit from participation in care management, a subset of the Medicaid population can benefit most from targeted, intensive care management activities. Aetna has developed a proprietary system to identify those members who are at highest risk for having poor health outcomes and who are the best candidates for intensive care management. Aetna's proprietary predictive model is a specialized tool that harvests data from multiple sources, including claims data and medication profiles to predict utilization trends over a 12 month period. In addition to our standard predictive model, Aetna developed a companion risk-stratification model, the Consolidated Outreach and Risk Evaluation Analysis™ (CORE), that identifies those members who will most benefit from intensive care management services.

CORE is a powerful tool that groups members according to their risk of future health care utilization, as well as identifying members where the most impact can be made. CORE integrates the predictive model built primarily on cost of care with two other risk models that measure risk of inpatient and emergency department (ED) utilization. In addition, the tool identifies specific subsets of members that are at higher risk for ED utilization and inpatient admission. The CORE identifies the top 1% of individuals who have the highest cost, highest ED utilization, and highest inpatient utilization. This group also has the highest prevalence of mental illness and substance use disorders. The output of the monthly CORE analysis regularly informs each health plan about which of their members is at highest risk over the next 12 months and whom should receive Intensive Care Management.

In addition to the CORE, each member is outreached and provided a general intake utilizing Aetna's proprietary Health Risk Questionnaire (HRQ). The HRQ is designed to detect physical, behavioral, and psychosocial factors associated with significant health risks that can be influenced. The HRQ measures key indicators such as presence of a primary care practitioner or medical home, health literacy, medication adherence, alcohol or substance abuse, mental illness or cognitive impairment, housing stability, available support systems, mobility challenges, increased hospitalizations and health perception.

Once candidates are properly triaged, they are placed in the Intensive or Supportive Care Management track, or in Population Health. Each plan will also reconcile the identification of complex members with any contractually-obligated state mandates requiring care management. Members who are not identified as requiring Intensive Care Management through the above methods, but who are required to be care managed, are placed in Supportive Care Management until the screening can be completed.

Right people, right skills

Engaging complex members to achieve successful outcomes requires a qualified staff of clinical intensive care managers and non-clinicians that have the requisite knowledge, expertise, and skills. Under the ICM model, licensed independent clinicians, such as registered nurses and licensed clinical social workers, direct and lead the care plan and care coordination strategies for members. All staff on the ICM team receive education on specific principles and care strategies such as motivational interviewing and patient activation techniques, with special considerations for advanced disease and behavioral health care strategies.

Individuals in Intensive Care Management receive individualized care from a single intensive care manager that consists of primarily "high-touch," sustained interventions. As previously discussed, a goal of ICM is to have one clinical team member coordinate all care management activities for a high-risk, complex individual for as long as necessary for the member to progress to the Population Health level. Caseloads for ICM care managers are envisioned to be smaller with an average of 30 to 70 members, but may vary based on each plan's contractual requirement and expectations for outreach activities.

Additional staff support is provided by non-clinical staff who work in tandem with a clinical care manager to ensure all aspects of care coordination are covered. As members progress in their care and as a member becomes more proficient in self-management, the need for intensive clinical oversight will diminish. In this stabilization phase of care management, non-clinicians are in a better position to provide care coordination activities that will allow care managers to stay focused on practicing at the full scope of their license regarding important clinical matters.

Individualized relationship-based care

Member motivation and activation to change and manage their health can only come about through positive, supportive relationships. This requires a collaborative relationship between the member and their assigned care manager that continues throughout the duration of a member's care management. The ICM model is centered on the expertise of two individuals – the member and the care manager. In the ICM system, each complex, high-risk member is assigned an intensive care manager who serves as the point person for coordinating all aspects of the member's care management. While the intensive care manager is expected to have an on-going, highly interactive relationship with each assigned member, other members of the team may also assist with care management. For example, care management associates will assist with non-clinical activities, and other team members with additional subject matter expertise relevant to a particular member's needs will collaborate with the assigned care manager to assure the member's needs are met.

Additionally, the care management team supports the relationships of health care providers, human services providers, and community support systems important to the member's recovery and resiliency. Ensuring the member has access to the range of resources they need, and coordination among those resources, are essential steps. This includes working with family and other care givers, engaging the member with a primary care provider in a medical home, and connecting them with essential social and housing supports that match their preferences and needs.

Bio-psycho-social care planning

Care planning that aligns the member's highest priority issues with goals and interventions that make sense from the member's perspective is critical to successful care management. Given that complex, high-risk members have multiple physical and behavioral health and psychosocial challenges, addressing these issues with a concise clinical assessment that concentrates on the full range of a member's needs is the first step to understanding what is truly important to the member. The assessment process advances the dialogue to uncover areas of agreement that will set the foundation on how to address barriers that prevents the member's effective management of their own health.

The ICM care planning process begins with the Care Plan Interview (CPI). The CPI provides a systemic method for evaluating all current and relevant aspects of a member's care and support systems. The information obtained during the CPI gives rise to the care plan which is viewed as a dynamic "document" that is developed through reaching consensus with the member on goals and action items that are most significant for them. The care plan becomes a tool that is implemented under the guidance of a skilled care manager who is continually tracking and revising the plan to reflect goal attainment or when necessary, to re-align goals that reinforce changes in the member's individual needs, abilities, and desires. The care plan creates the central touch point from which the care manager can base coaching and mentoring strategies, as well as guiding the member toward self-reliance.

The care planning process, however, is not restricted to only the care manager and the member. The care plan is a centralized tool with shared access by all providers of care or services with a mutual commitment to positively impact the member. The care planning process identifies the member's strengths and critical barriers to drive a care plan that is actionable and effective. The care plan identifies all the critical people who are responsible for specific activities intended to help the member achieve their goals. Finally, the care plan enables the care manager and member to track and trend progress toward the member's goals by focusing on long-term outcomes to assure the benefits are sustained into the future.

Multi-disciplinary case rounds

In order to promote effective care management, each health plan engages in frequent multi-disciplinary case rounds that allow for the intensive examination of individual cases and discussion of evidence-based care management strategies. Multi-disciplinary case rounds offer the opportunity to leverage the collective strengths of the medical management team to produce the best possible outcomes for members. Regular case rounds serve many functions by encouraging a plan's clinical leadership to provide staff supervision, coaching and mentoring opportunities, and ensuring sound clinical judgment.

Other important aspects of case rounds include the following: each plan is encouraged to have, at minimum, bi-weekly case rounds; case rounds concentrate on care management strategies, recommendations, and strategic problem-solving; risk identification and risk mitigation are emphasized as part of a comprehensive review; collaboration with other health plans to exchange ideas and examine emerging best practices; and all care managers are expected to present cases on a regular basis highlighting successes, lessons learned, and challenges that require consultation.

Progression of care

Successful care management ensures that members are receiving the requisite level of care required to help them achieve optimal health and self-management. It is critical to match the intensity of care management services to the member's needs as the member moves through recovery toward self-management and autonomy. Throughout the care management process care managers must adapt the intensity of care management to the member's willingness and ability to effectively use that intensity of service. Achieving positive results will only take place when the members take greater accountability over their own health care needs, with the intensity of care management services they receive decreasing and responsibility shifting to each member, accordingly.

Complex, high-risk members should be viewed as moving through four "phases" of care management:

- *Working Relationship* – The member is engaged in an effective working relationship with a primary care manager.
- *Recovery* – The member shows a sustained decrease in their current, avoidable utilization and problematic symptoms, as well as sustained progression towards optimal quality of life and reduction/moderation of risk factors.
- *Resiliency* – The member decreases their risk of future utilization by decreasing current risk factors and enhancing current protective factors.
- *Autonomy* – The member takes responsibility for their own health and well-being, which includes managing their own health conditions effectively.

As part of the on-going relationship care managers are expected to continually evaluate their ICM members' progress, utilizing the care plan as the primary tool for accurately

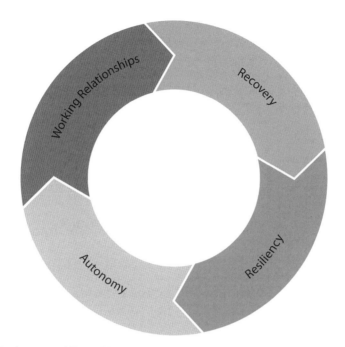

Figure 18.2 Autonomy Wheel Diagram

reflecting a member's position in the progression of care. Even though an individual's care will never progress in a completely predictable fashion, Integrated Care Management supports the member's motivation and activation to the point where they increasingly exhibit the ability to self-determine and choose the best course of action to positively engage in their health care.

Outcomes accountability

One hallmark of ICM is the commitment to create accountability at all levels of the organization and for the member. Instilling accountability for successful program outcomes will be directed by several key drivers which include consistent use of ICM principles; standardized reporting metrics to measure specific outcomes; ensuring the entire care management team understands and takes ownership of their respective roles; and performing regular auditing and monitoring of the program to ensure the plan is operating on-target with strategic objectives.

In addition, each plan is expected to support quality efforts to ensure alignment with the National Committee for Quality Assurance (NCQA) standards. While it may not be required that all plans acquire NCQA certification, each plan must operate with a quality improvement plan and be accountable for achieving and monitoring quality metrics, as devised at the organizational level and as mandated by each plan's state contractual obligations.

Standardized electronic health information platform

One overarching goal of ICM is to align the care team and all community providers with a member's care management data. This is accomplished in part by utilizing a unified, comprehensive electronic health information platform that can be accessed by providers and members through a secured portal. The platform links all member data, including demographics, evidence-based questionnaires, bio-psycho-social and condition-specific assessments, case formulations, care plans, detailed documentation of member interactions, claims data, and reporting. The electronic platform serves as a secure, communal portal for members and providers to readily exchange important care data to encourage cooperative care coordination and management.

Additional care strategies: surveillance, field-based assessments, and flow control

As previously discussed, the health care needs of individuals in the Medicaid population, especially those with persistent chronic illness, rarely follow a precise linear direction with respect to their health status (such as from acute illness episode, to recovery, to permanent stabilization). Often a member's health status will vacillate between additional acute episodes and intermittent periods of stabilization and destabilization. With the health status of the aged, blind, and disabled (ABD) population being driven by many dynamic factors that may alter the recovery and stabilization process, having the proper surveillance and control tools in place to find members at risk and match them with the appropriate intensity of care management services is critical.

Inpatient hospital notification and field-based assessment

As already noted, the ICM model is guided by the use of CORE™ to identify members most at risk who need intensive care management. Aetna has also developed several strategies involving inpatient hospital and ED notification as additional surveillance tools to identify members at risk for adverse outcomes. The ICM model recognizes that successful transitions in care require several stakeholders to work seamlessly together to prevent unnecessary readmissions and care fragmentation that can jeopardize a member's health and safety. Currently, many plans work closely with hospital providers and state officials to ensure collaborative discharge planning that addresses issues that may have contributed to the original admission, and to enhance communication that will ensure proper follow-up and continuity of care within the community.

Another powerful care management tool is community engagement of members. On-site assessments, or field-based care interventions conducted in the home or in any care setting, can have a powerful impact on continuity of care. While each Aetna plan has independent considerations for management of their individual populations, home assessments add value through a first-hand look at a member's personal environment. Information obtained from a home or care facility visit can yield important data about a member's strengths and barriers that will drive care planning and care coordination strategies.

Flow control

Further, the ICM model provides a flow control process which provides the ICM team the ability to match members with the right level of care management services in real time as new members are evaluated in relation to existing members progressing through care management. The flow control algorithm provides a well-defined but flexible process for incorporating a member into the right level of care. For example, a member may be new to the plan and it may not be initially clear whether the member needs Intensive Care Management or Supportive Care Management. The flow control process walks the team through a decision matrix that allows each member to be considered individually to ensure placement of the patient on the right track of care.

Application of the ICM process

In order to fully appreciate the ICM model, a hypothetical member history is provided below that depicts a general overview of the model. The care activities discussed below are only examples, and are not inclusive of all actions that might be used by the care management team.

Member history

Mr. Rose is a 54-year-old man with diabetes, hypertension, and congestive heart failure. Mr. Rose is Hispanic, lives alone, and is known to suffer from periods of depression and alcohol abuse. He smokes one pack of cigarettes per day. He has one daughter that visits periodically. He relies on neighbors in his apartment complex to assist at times. Mr. Rose is a self-professed "loner" but is personable. One month ago, Mr. Rose had three toes removed from his right foot and has been in the ED three times in the past two weeks with on-going wound management issues concerning his surgery site. His last primary care appointment was six months ago, which he missed. His most recent hemoglobin A1C was 9.0, his blood pressure was 148/98, and his urine tested positive for protein and glucose. Mr. Rose exhibits moderate symptoms of congestive heart failure marked by moderate fatigue with physical activity. The local hospital contacted the health plan to notify the care management team of his most recent ED visit. While Mr. Rose is a new member to the Medicaid plan, he was formerly on the plan six months ago and had previously been a member for over a year.

The ICM process

Intake and assessment

Initially, Mr. Rose will be outreached and provided a general intake utilizing the Health Risk Questionnaire (HRQ). Next, if adequate claims data exist, this information is run through the CORE analysis. For our purposes, Mr. Rose had previous claims data that identifies him as being among the most complex and high risk members of the plan but who could also benefit significantly from ICM. As a result, he will be assigned to an intensive care manager and placed in the highest level of ICM care.

Care management initiation

The intensive care manager assigned to Mr. Rose will take into consideration the HRQ results and will engage him in the Care Planning Interview (CPI). After analysis of the CPI and discussion with him about his care goals, if appropriate, the care manager will complete condition-specific assessments. For instance, specific tools may be used to assess his depression, diabetes, heart failure, personal safety, support systems, housing and food security, and alcohol and tobacco dependence. Based on these findings, available claims data, and Mr. Rose's own description and perception of his health status, results will be used to create a care plan, setting goals that are appropriate, achievable, culturally appropriate, and agreeable to Mr. Rose. Additionally, the care manager and Mr. Rose will coordinate care management activities with the primary care provider and other community parties, such as his daughter, neighbors or identified behavioral health providers. Mr. Rose, his primary care provider, and other appropriate providers will receive a copy of the care plan and have electronic access to monitor progress through the web portal. Mr. Rose's care will also be aligned with internal quality and outcomes measures, as well as any state contractual requirements.

At this stage, the care manager and Mr. Rose will begin care plan implementation activities. The care manager will use appropriate motivational interviewing and patient activation strategies to lay the groundwork for his engagement and accountability. In this case, a critical first medical step will be to ensure that the wound on Mr. Rose's foot is evaluated. Further, sending Mr. Rose to his primary care provider to re-engage with a medical home will also be a top priority. Following, an assessment of medication adherence and personal disease comprehension must be conducted. From there, the care manager will consider a series of educational activities and continuous assessments designed to address Mr. Rose's personal health management, behavioral health considerations, and that his community support systems are established and optimized.

Other considerations in Mr. Rose's care will be to outreach the hospital to discuss notification of any future admissions, to ensure care transitions are handled in a timely, effective, and collaborative manner. Further, an in-home assessment may also be warranted to evaluate personal safety issues and to observe Mr. Rose's self-care habits and abilities. Finally, a case conference with the primary care provider and plan's care team will be useful in aligning care strategies and in closely examining the collaborative goals and outcomes negotiated with Mr. Rose.

Outreach to Mr. Rose will be intensive in the beginning phases, perhaps several times a week telephonically for the first few months. During this time, a series of low and high-touch interventions will be used under the direction of the care manager in consultation with the medical management team and his primary care provider. Mr. Rose's care will also have a non-clinical care team member to assist with the coordination of non-clinical activities. Because Mr. Rose is in Intensive Care Management, continuity of the relationship with his care manager over time is a critical contributor to achieving sustainable long-term benefits. Mr. Rose will remain at the ICM level of service until his care needs stabilize and he can self-manage his health without the continued need for higher intensity care management oversight and services. When Mr. Rose reaches this stabilization point he will be discharged from intensive care management and continue to receive supportive care management health services.

Reference

Guyer, J., & Paradise, J. (2010) *Explaining Health Reform: Benefits and Cost-Sharing for Adult Medicaid Beneficiaries*. Henry J. Kaiser Family Foundation, Menlo Park, CA. Retrieved from http://www.kff.org/healthreform/8092.cfm.

Chapter 19

King County Care Partners: a community-based chronic care management system for Medicaid clients with co-occurring medical, mental, and substance abuse disorders

Daniel S. Lessler, Antoinette Krupski, and Meg Cristofalo

Introduction

King County Care Partners (KCCP) brings together organizations that serve medically vulnerable SSI-eligible Medicaid clients within King County, Washington, to improve clinical outcomes and decrease unnecessary utilization. They do this by providing community-based, registered nurse (RN)-led, multidisciplinary care management that empowers patients and enhances coordination, communication, and integration of services across safety-net providers. At-risk clients receive up to one year of intensive care management from a clinical team consisting of RNs and social workers. Care management includes an in-person comprehensive assessment, collaborative goal setting, chronic disease self-management coaching, joint physician visits of clients with care managers, frequent in-person and phone monitoring, connecting to community resources, and coordination of care across the medical and mental health systems.

Aging and Disability Services of Seattle-King County (ADS) is the contracting agency for KCCP; it is located in downtown Seattle and has a long history of providing care management services to homebound clients. ADS is particularly adept at connecting clients to community-based services and coordinating service delivery. ADS also has a history of collaborating in the development, evaluation, and dissemination of innovative and effective clinical practices that focus on the needs of its homebound clients. For example, ADS was a key participant in the Program to Encourage Active, Rewarding Lives for Seniors (PEARLS) intervention, which demonstrated the effectiveness of a home-based intervention for elderly patients with minor depression (Ciechanowski *et al.* 2004).

KCCP was created in response to a Request for Proposals (RFP) issued in July 2006, by the Health Recovery and Services Administration (HRSA) of the Washington State

Comprehensive Care Coordination for Chronically Ill Adults, First Edition. Edited by Cheryl Schraeder and Paul Shelton.
© 2011 John Wiley & Sons, Inc. Published 2011 by John Wiley & Sons, Inc.

Department of Social and Human Services (DSHS) which, at that time, administered the Medicaid program within Washington State. It has since been re-organized as the Medicaid Purchasing Administration (MPA). The RFP was developed based on insights gleaned from focus groups that Washington State DSHS conducted with safety-net primary care providers after initial attempts at disease management utilizing commercial vendors to provide telephonic disease-specific care management were unsuccessful. The RFP specifically sought proposals that would create a local chronic care management network within a defined geographic region for high risk, SSI-eligible Medicaid clients. A consortium of safety-net providers and human services organizations in King County successfully responded to the RFP, and KCCP was launched in March 2007. ADS contracts directly with MPA to provide care management services through KCCP.

The KCCP model

A key objective of KCCP is to enhance one-on-one community-based care management by developing a system of care that integrates the care management team with the safety net primary care practices that serve as medical homes for eligible Medicaid clients. The care model that makes such integration possible is illustrated in Figure 19.1.

To enable integration between the care management team and the safety-net primary care system, ADS sub-contracts with four large safety-net primary care clinic systems within King County, including Harborview Medical Center (the sole public hospital serving King County); Neighborcare Community Health Centers; Healthpoint Community Health Centers; and Sea Mar Community Health Centers. Each of the contracted clinic systems has between four and six primary care clinics, the latter three systems

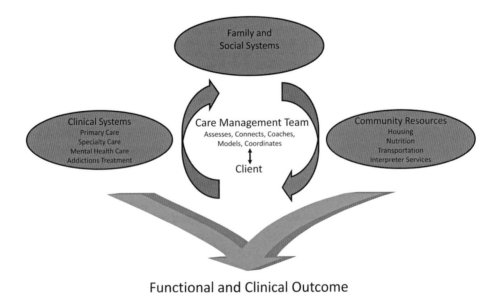

Figure 19.1   King County Partners Care Model: System Integration

Table 19.1   Demographic and Clinical Characteristics of KCCP's initial enrollees (*N* = 256)

Median age (years)	51
Female (%)	52
Non-white (%)	45
Median number of chronic conditions	5
Median number of prescribed medications	7
PHQ-9 score suggesting major depression (%)	48
Limited health literacy (%)	27
Pain in the last week that often or always interfered with things they needed to do (%)	49

are Federally Qualified Health Centers (FQHC). The contracted clinic systems care for large numbers of patients who have complex psychosocial needs (such as joblessness, homelessness, food insufficiency, low health literacy, and limited English proficiency), and co-occurring medical, mental health and substance abuse disorders. The extraordinary medical and psychosocial burden of these patients is reflected in aggregate results from assessments done on an initial group of program enrollees (See Table 19.1).

KCCP also provides a limited amount of financial support for each of the partnering clinic systems to hire one clinical care coordinator (CCC). The CCCs provide a link between the community-based ADS clinical team and the primary care medical homes within each of the partnering clinic systems. The CCCs assist with outreach to difficult-to-contact clients; assist the KCCP clinical team in communicating with primary care providers; assure that clinic-based services are coordinated and do not overlap with the services provided by the KCCP clinical team; champion the KCCP clinical team and program within their clinic systems; and assist in assuring a smooth hand-off back into the full care of the primary care medical home when clients transition from intensive care management.

In addition to the CCCs described above, there are three other key elements to KCCP systems integration: (1) information technology, (2) motivational interviewing (MI), and (3) participation in community forums. Each of these will be described below.

Information technology

KCCP has built a HIPAA-compliant, web-based clinical information system that enables sharing of patient-specific clinical information across the partnering organizations. This system allows documentation and tracking of client contacts, as well as reporting capability with respect to initial assessments and outcomes using validated clinical instruments (for example, PHQ-9). The KCCP clinical team has direct access to the Electronic Health Record (EHR) of one of the larger partnering organizations as well. The possibility of providing such EHR access across all partners is under active discussion.

Motivational Interviewing (MI)

KCCP's shared patient-centered approach to client interaction and care management is grounded in the spirit and method of MI (Rollnick *et al.* 2008). Individuals from all of

Table 19.2   Motivational Interviewing Training Components

- Initial two-day intensive MI workshop
- Monthly case conferences with MI coach
- Monthly one-to-one 30-minute mentoring sessions with MI coach
- Mid-year half-day workshop focused on using MI with the mentally ill
- Review and comment by MI coach on participants' taped interactions with actual clients

the partnering systems have jointly participated in extensive MI training – an activity designed to promote a consistent, client-centered experiences across clinical systems.

Participation in community forums

Members of the KCCP core clinical team participate in monthly meetings of community-based organizations whose services overlap with or may involve KCCP clients. These include the King County Healthcare for the Homeless program and Harborview Medical Center's High Utilizers Work Group.

The KCCP clinical team

The KCCP intensive care management clinical team is composed of three full-time RNs, two social workers (MSWs) with chemical dependency training, and a bachelor's level individual trained and experienced in chemical dependency counseling who serves as the "engagement specialist." These individuals have each received one year of intensive training and coaching in MI (See Table 19.2).

In addition, the clinical team participates in regular trainings that focus on behaviorally-oriented strategies for managing affective disorders commonly encountered in the chronically ill Medicaid population, such as depression and anxiety. The latter trainings are sponsored by a local, non-profit health plan as part of a state and locally-funded effort to improve access to mental health care for the poor and vulnerable populations seen in safety-net clinics. Thus, comprehensive ongoing training on relevant clinical skills, day-to-day clinical supervision by a nurse supervisor experienced in oversight of community-based clinical programs, and weekly case-conferences with the KCCP Medical Director, are essential underpinnings of KCCP's care management intervention.

Selection, engagement, and assessment of clients

High-risk patients eligible for intensive care management are drawn from a larger, target population of SSI-eligible Medicaid clients who reside within King County and have received care from one of the participating clinic systems within the prior 12 months. A predictive modeling computer program developed by DSHS is used to identify those clients within the target population who are at particularly high risk of future health care utilization. There are approximately 8,000 clients in the target population, of whom about 1,500 have been designated as high-risk based on predictive modeling. Because

KCCP is being evaluated using a randomized controlled trial (RCT) methodology that has not yet been completed, eligible clients are randomized either to receive the KCCP care management intervention, or to an abeyance group that will become eligible for the intervention after the RCT is completed.

A list of high-risk patients randomized to the intervention is provided to the ADS clinical team. A dedicated member of the clinical team (the engagement specialist) contacts those clients eligible for the intervention using a purposeful, informed approach that has yielded a greater than 50% engagement rate (defined as referred clients having completed an in-person comprehensive RN assessment; see West *et al.*, 2010). Key elements of the engagement approach include: (1) checking with the partnering clinic where the patient appears to be established for primary care to cross-reference and assure the most updated contact information;(2) scheduling work so that outbound calls can be made at different times of day including evenings and weekends; (3) utilizing the spirit and method of MI in interacting with patients; and (4) asking an individual from the clinic to contact the patient and encourage participation in KCCP if the patient is reluctant to speak with the engagement specialist.

After clients have agreed to enroll in KCCP care management, they are referred to an RN member of the clinical team who arranges for an initial in-person meeting and comprehensive assessment. Typically, this meeting occurs at the home of the client; when this is not possible, arrangements are made to meet the client at an alternative site (such as the physician's office). The initial assessment takes approximately 60 to 90 minutes, and includes administration of validated instruments to screen for common mental illness, substance abuse issues, and health literacy; assessment of chronic medical conditions, chronic pain, and functional status; review of medications; identification of psychosocial issues that may impact abilities to access care or follow through on care plans; and collaborative goal-setting that focuses on and takes account of the client's expressed needs, both medical and psychosocial.

Subsequent to the initial assessment, the RN arranges to join the client at one or more physician appointments, one of which must be with the client's primary care provider. Prior to the appointment, the RN coaches the patient regarding strategies that can improve the quality of communication between the client and the client's physician. Within the confines of the exam room, the RN may, with permission of the client, communicate important information that has been ascertained during the initial assessment and may be relevant to the patient's ongoing care. At this time, the goals established by the client with the help of the RN may be shared with the treating physician. The RN may also assist in assuring that clinical information is shared across providers (primary care, medical/surgical specialists, and mental health specialists) who are involved in the client's care.

Managing clients

Once clients are enrolled, assessed, and have had at least one joint appointment with their RN care manager and primary care physician, the RN may choose to engage one of the MSW team members in helping to connect the client to needed community resources, or provide assistance with the management of chemical dependency issues.

Table 19.3   Key Elements of the KCCP Care Model

- Engagement
- In-person assessment
- Goal-setting
- Coaching
- Self-advocacy
- Self-management (disease specific knowledge and skills)
- Health system access and navigation
- Modeling (joint visits to physicians)
- Ongoing support (frequent phone follow-up and monitoring)
- Coordination and communication
- Primary, specialty, and mental health care
- Referral and connection with community resources

Clients are provided with contact information (phone numbers) for their care management team (RN and/or MSW). The frequency of contact is at the discretion of the clinical care team and client. In general, more unstable or severely chronically ill patients receive more frequent contact, which may occur via phone or in-person. In-person contacts are typically arranged to coincide with physician visits. Physicians caring for patients enrolled in KCCP are also provided the care manager's contact information and encouraged to contact the care manager for assistance in caring for or concerns about the patient. Key elements of the KCCP care model are summarized in Table 19.3.

KCCP clinical staff has embraced the spirit and method of MI in their face-to-face interactions with clients. In case conferences with the KCCP Medical Director, the RNs and social workers have described in their own words the nature of these interactions. For example, one RN, in describing an interaction with a client, stated, "Affirm the client's perceptions and feelings, and suspicion melts away." This same RN indicated that she tells clients, "I'm not here to change you, or make you do anything you don't want to do" (Lessler 2010).

Collaboratively establishing client-centered goals is a priority for the care managers. The manner in which care managers approach goal setting – and, in particular, the content of their interactions with clients around a goal – is well captured in a key informant interview conducted as part of a qualitative analysis of the KCCP care management intervention. In the words of a member of the KCCP clinical team, "It helps us to know what their [the client's] agenda is. Our agenda might not be their agenda, and so when you're using MI and you're actively listening, a lot of times, without even talking, you can find out what's important to them, and so through that, I'm able to know where to go with them. I'm not going to spin my wheels working with them here because it's not important to them. They just said X, Y, and Z are important to them, so instead I'll put my energy there" (Cristofalo *et al.* 2010).

The application of MI principles and methods by the KCCP clinical team in their interactions with clients is well captured in the following vignette.

A.G. is a 38-year-old Native American man with generalized anxiety disorder and alcohol dependence, as well as several chronic medical conditions. At his initial meeting with the KCCP RN care manager, A.G. stated, "People have told me what to do; I don't want you telling me what to do." The RN responded to A.G., "I'm not going to tell you what to do; I'm going to walk beside you regardless of the path you take." At the third encounter between A.G. and the nurse, which happened to be in-person, A.G. stated, "I'm thinking about making a change, but I'm not ready today, and I'm not sure I will be ready in two days or two weeks." In subsequent meetings, both in-person and over the phone, the nurse describes reflections on the patient's ambivalence, affirmations for his thinking about change, and finally, more detailed problem-solving conversations. Ultimately, after six months in care management, A.G. enrolled in a 30-day inpatient chemical dependency treatment program (Lessler 2010).

Layered on top of the individual, patient-centered interactions that KCCP care managers have with clients, is a complex web of care coordination that includes advocacy and connection to community-based resources. The richness of this layer of care management is captured in the following summary of three months of care management provided by an RN care manager to her client:

> "Client one has significant cognitive deficits and substance abuse dependencies (narcotics and alcohol). Because of his cognitive deficits the client needed a tremendous amount of feedback and reminders regarding his goals, care, and appointments. He calls his RN care manager almost every day at times asking for reassurance and confirmation of appointments. On enrollment in KCCP, he did not have a primary care provider. Between March and mid-May 2009, the KCCP team helped the client establish primary care. During this time the RN care manager also attended a mental health appointment with the client and began the process of aiding the client in going to inpatient chemical dependency treatment by obtaining a letter of clearance for him. The RN care manager also got the client established with neurology rehabilitation specialty care, accompanying him to his first appointment, and coordinated care with a specialty clinic after the patient presented at an emergency room with an acute hand injury" (Krupski *et al.* 2009).

Evidence of program success

The overall success of the patient-centered model employed by KCCP is reflected in a recent phone survey of patients who were program participants (Krupski *et al.* 2010):

- 98% said they had a good, trusting relationship with their nurse or social worker.
- 92% said the health care goals they developed with their nurse included their most important health care needs.
- 91% said the program helped them feel they could take charge of their health.
- 90% were able to reach at least one of the health care goals they developed with their nurse.
- 82% said the program helped them get health care needs met that they could not have met on their own.

Likewise, in key informant interviews, physicians with enrolled patients indicated that the program was helpful to them in providing better care for their patients. For example, interviewed physicians perceived that the program increased the likelihood that patients would keep appointments with them; they commented that when nurses attended clinic appointments with patients they felt more informed about care that was being provided by other physicians involved in the patient's care (Cristofalo *et al.* 2010).

Overall, key elements of the success that KCCP has enjoyed to-date relate importantly to the program's core clinical team, and the clinic-based care coordinators having successfully embraced the spirit – non-judgmental, encouraging of client self-worth and following client authority – and methods of MI (Linden *et al.* 2010). Achieving this level of commitment to and demonstrated skill in using MI has required extensive training and ongoing support for developing and refining MI skills. Other factors that have contributed to KCCP's success include the face-to-face interaction of care managers with clients; the participation of care managers in physician visits; the monitoring and availability of care managers to clients (both in person and via telephone); and the ability of care managers to work with clients over a twelve-month time period, with more time allowed if needed.

Program challenges

The KCCP clinical team has also faced challenges. The clinical and psychosocial needs of clients in care management are often profound, and can be overwhelming for those involved in their care. Even with extensive training and institutional support, burn-out of care management team members is a considerable risk. KCCP has experienced RN turnover since its inception that has, at times, created program instability. In response to concerns about workload, KCCP has adjusted RN caseloads downward from approximately 100 clients per RN to 67 to 70 clients per RN/team.

KCCP has also been impacted by the challenges faced by its safety-net clinic partners. For example, the KCCP care management team has noted that primary care provider attrition within these clinics has sometimes interrupted continuity of care, making it difficult for patients to understand and follow through on care plans. More generally, the shortage of primary care providers has sometimes led to problems with timely access to care.

From a systems perspective, KCCP has attempted to knit together a community-based RN-led, multidisciplinary care management model with the safety-net clinics that provide medical homes for the vast majority of enrolled clients. Creating this system has been enabled by the fact that participating organizations share a mission of caring for underserved and vulnerable populations. In addition, the development of explicit contractual obligations, and the provision of financial resources to participating clinic systems has led to both commitment and accountability on the part of all partners.

Early in the development of KCCP, it became clear that, given the resources available, no one clinic system could adequately support an intensive care management model for its most severely medically and mentally ill, as well as socially and economically disadvantaged patients. KCCP centralizes intensive care management services for such clients within a single community-based agency (ADS) that is experienced in providing community-based care. This resource has now been leveraged across safety-net clinic systems in a manner that provides tight linkages between the clinic systems and the core service provider. It is especially important to note that ADS is not confined by the walls of a clinic; it is able to put a clinical team "on the ground" because it has a history of working with disabled and chronically ill clients who are homebound. Thus, it has at its disposal important infrastructure (for example, a motor pool for use by KCCP team members), knowledge, and experience that support putting a clinical team out in the community; clinic systems typically do not have this unusual blend of resources. In this way, KCCP has been able to provide intensive care management services that optimally leverage community resources, which are also integrally linked to the primary care medical homes of clients.

While celebrating a modicum of success, KCCP also faces considerable challenges. Previous research indicates that a key element of successful care management programs is the involvement and buy-in of treating physicians (Berenson & Howell 2009; Bodenheimer & Berry-Millett 2009). In this regard, a recent formative evaluation indicated that KCCP's ties to the physicians who worked within partnering clinics were not as strong as they could or should be. This evaluation also indicated that some of the physicians in clinic systems served by KCCP may not share KCCP's commitment to MI's approach for eliciting and strengthening motivation to change. Assuring more broad-based physician familiarity with and trust in KCCP's intensive care management program will require enhanced educational efforts by KCCP to clinic systems and physicians (Cristofalo *et al.* 2010).

Conclusions

Research indicates that successful care management programs include the following attributes: (1) patient selection, (2) in-person encounters including home visits, (3) specially trained care managers with low case loads, (4) multidisciplinary teams including physicians, (5) informal caregivers and family assisting the patient, and (6) use of coaching (Berenson & Howell 2009; Bodenheimer & Berry-Millett 2009). KCCP possesses, in varying degrees, the key attributes of a successful care management program for patients with complex health needs. It has the added strength of providing care management through a central, community-based organization that leverages an expensive and scarce resource across multiple safety-net clinic systems; it links care managers with the primary care medical homes and physicians of clients; and it connects clients and their families to community resources. Preliminary outcomes based on a formative evaluation of KCCP are encouraging; the extent to which KCCP is successful in affecting more definitive clinical (for example, mortality) and utilization (that is, costs) outcomes will be better understood when data from the ongoing RCT evaluating KCCP become available.

References

Berenson, R. & Howell, J. (2009) *Structuring, Financing and Paying for Effective Care Coordination*. The National Coalition of Care Coordination (N3C), Washington, DC.

Bodenheimer, T. & Berry-Millett, R. (2009) *Care Management of Patients with Complex Health Care Needs*. Research Synthesis Report Number 19. The Robert Wood Johnson Foundation, Princeton, NJ.

Ciechanowski, P., Wagner, E., Schmaling, K., *et al.* (2004) Community-integrated home-based depression treatment in older adults: a randomized controlled trial. *The Journal of the American Medical Association*, 291, 1569–1577.

Cristofalo, M., Krupski, T., Jenkins, L., *et al.* (2010) *Chronic Care Management Intervention: A Qualitative Analysis of Key Informant Account*. Center for Healthcare Improvement for Addictions, Mental Illness and Medically Vulnerable Populations, Seattle, WA.

Krupski, T., Cristofalo, M., Atkins, D., *et al.* (2009) *Qualitative Analyses of Client Contacts that Occurred During the First Three Months of the Rethinking Care Project*. Center for Healthcare Improvement for Addictions, Mental Illness and Medically Vulnerable Populations, Seattle, WA.

Krupski, T., Cristofalo, M., Jenkins, L., *et al.* (2010) *Client Perspectives on the Rethinking Care Program: Report of a Telephone Survey*. Center for Healthcare Improvement for Addictions, Mental Illness and Medically Vulnerable Populations, Seattle, WA.

Lessler, D. (2010) Meeting notes for KCCP Care Management Team Meeting (Personal communication, September 10, 2010).

Linden, A., Butterworth, S.W., Prochaska, J. (2010) Motivational interviewing-based health coaching as a chronic intervention. *Journal of Evaluation in Clinical Practice*, 16, 166–174.

Rollnick, S., Miller, W.R., & Butler, C.C. (2008) *Motivational Interviewing in Health Care: Helping Patients Change Behavior*. Guilford Press, New York, NY.

West, I.I., Joesch, J.M., Atkins, D., *et al.* (2010). *Clients Assigned to the Rethinking Care Program Intervention: How Do Clients Who Started an Assessment Differ From Those Who Did Not?* Center for Healthcare Improvement for Addictions, Mental Illness and Medically Vulnerable Populations, Seattle, WA.

Chapter 20

Predictive Risk Intelligence System (PRISM): A decision-support tool for coordinating care for complex Medicaid clients

Beverly J. Court, David Mancuso, Chad Zhu, and Antoinette Krupski

Introduction

The Predictive Risk Intelligence SysteM (PRISM) is an integrated, information-rich decision support tool used by Washington State Medicaid programs. PRISM is designed to support care management interventions for high-risk, chronically ill Medicaid patients. The PRISM tool combines three key innovations: (1) identification of clients most in need of comprehensive care coordination based on risk scores developed through predictive modeling, (2) integration of information from medical, social service, behavioral health, and long-term care payment and assessment data systems, and (3) an intuitive and accessible display of client health and demographic data from administrative data sources.

This chapter will describe the main components of the PRISM tool, illustrate its capabilities and uses for comprehensive care coordination, and discuss its strengths and limitations.

Background

When Washington State's Medicaid Purchasing Administration and Aging and Disability Services Administration initiated a set of chronic care management pilots in early 2007, they contracted with a commercial vendor to provide a predictive modeling tool to use as a risk-stratification and clinical-decision support tool for nurse care managers who staffed the interventions. However, the commercial application was found to have several limitations: (1) direct access to the application was limited to a handful of program staff and not available to nurse care managers who directly worked with patients, (2) the commercial application was not recalibrated for Medicaid populations, and had a lower level of predictive accuracy than tools that were already being used by the state, and (3) the commercial application was expensive.

Comprehensive Care Coordination for Chronically Ill Adults, First Edition. Edited by Cheryl Schraeder and Paul Shelton.
© 2011 John Wiley & Sons, Inc. Published 2011 by John Wiley & Sons, Inc.

Within Washington State's Research and Data Analysis Division of the Department of Social and Health Services, a team headed by health economist David Mancuso and application architect Chad Zhu had extensive background in linking diverse state agency databases, conducting predictive modeling, and developing secure web applications. They proposed developing the PRISM tool to support care management interventions. Today the PRISM tool serves over 200 users with 28 distinct population groups, and continues to evolve to meet changing program needs.

Innovation #1: Predictive risk scores

Risk scores estimate the risk of an individual experiencing an event in the future based on their characteristics in the past. Commonly, risk scores are developed to measure expected future medical costs or an estimated probability of an event, such as an inpatient admission within a certain time interval.

A medical cost-risk score is built on an individual's expected per-member-per-month (PMPM) future expenditures divided by the average PMPM of the individual's medical coverage group. It is expressed as a ratio, with 1.0 equaling the "average" score for the group. A medical risk score of 1.5 would mean that the individual was likely to incur 50% more in future medical costs than the average member within the group. Risk scores from proprietary commercial vendors are calculated based on general commercial populations, which are less accurate and more confusing to interpret than risk scores based on a population of complex chronically ill adults.

It can be difficult for clinicians using a commercial application applied to a Medicaid population to understand how to set minimum-risk score targets for care management interventions for high-risk patients. For example, a risk score of 1.5 derived from a commercial application translates to "a Medicaid client who is expected to incur 50% higher future medical costs than the average patient enrolled in a commercial health plan." This level of risk is actually below average for disabled Medicaid populations, and targeting patients with this relatively low level of risk could result in the misallocation of limited care management resources. This is one reason why it is important to recalibrate risk scores to the population treated, assuming the population is sufficiently large, rather than using scores based on clinically different populations.

The actual calculation of a medical cost risk score is based on a risk grouping algorithm that combines groups of diagnoses and/or medications into categories that are relatively homogenous in terms of their clinical application and relationship to expected future medical service utilization. The medical risk score contained in PRISM is a combination of the Chronic Illness and Disability Payment System (CDPS) and Medicaid-Rx risk groupers developed and maintained as open source software by Rick Kronick and Todd Gilmer at the University of California, San Diego (Gilmer *et al.* 2001; Kronick *et al.* 2000). The CDPS and Medicaid-Rx software are widely used by state Medicaid programs for risk adjustment purposes, and have been shown in repeated Society of Actuaries studies (Winkelman & Mehmud 2007) to have comparable predictive accuracy to the proprietary commercial alternatives. The availability of the CDPS and Medicaid-Rx groupers was essential for the rapid, low-cost in-house development of PRISM predictive risk scores.

Risk scores and their associated clinical risk groups are used for a wide range of purposes, including (1) profiling of patients, providers, and health plans, (2) profiling of high-risk populations to inform the design of care management interventions, (3) risk stratification to support targeting of interventions to facilitate the efficient allocation of limited care management resources, (4) risk adjustment of health plan capitation payments, and (5) case mix adjustment in health outcome measurement at the population level.

While useful for organizing and quantifying expected future medical expenses, clinicians are counseled not to take the numeric value of the medical risk score itself too literally. A client with a score of 1.20 will generally be less complex than a client with a score of 7.0, but the differences between 1.2 and 1.3 are likely to be negligible from a care management perspective. The score is a place to start identifying those who have high needs.

Innovation #2: Integration of comprehensive cross-agency data

One of the major advantages of PRISM is that it contains a much broader range of health services data than is typically found in commercial predictive modeling applications. This includes service encounters from mental health and chemical dependency treatment provided through other state programs, as well as long-term care service and assessment data. Predictive risk modeling can be accomplished without this broader array of data, but the ability of the care manager to develop comprehensive care plans and effective interventions is greatly enhanced.

Service funding silos are often associated with payment and assessment information that present barriers to integrated care for complex populations. Different systems often use different means of identifying patients, with different reporting schedules. The ability to combine these different streams of data is not trivial. From a development standpoint, data integration is usually the most resource-intensive part of developing a PRISM-like application.

Innovation #3: Easy to use display of administrative information

The same diverse administrative data that enable predictive risk-modeling also serves as a rich source of clinically relevant data that can inform care management interventions. PRISM displays data on utilization, diagnoses, and filled prescriptions in a clinically meaningful and easily navigated manner. In this way, administrative data becomes a clinical tool for care managers. PRISM is built to be viewed through a secure web application, making it accessible to authorized users anywhere there is internet access. PRISM users can only access the records of clients they are authorized to view.

The first PRISM view (Figure 20.1) is a search screen that allows users to find an individual if they have all or part of a client's name, or if they know a client's Medicaid

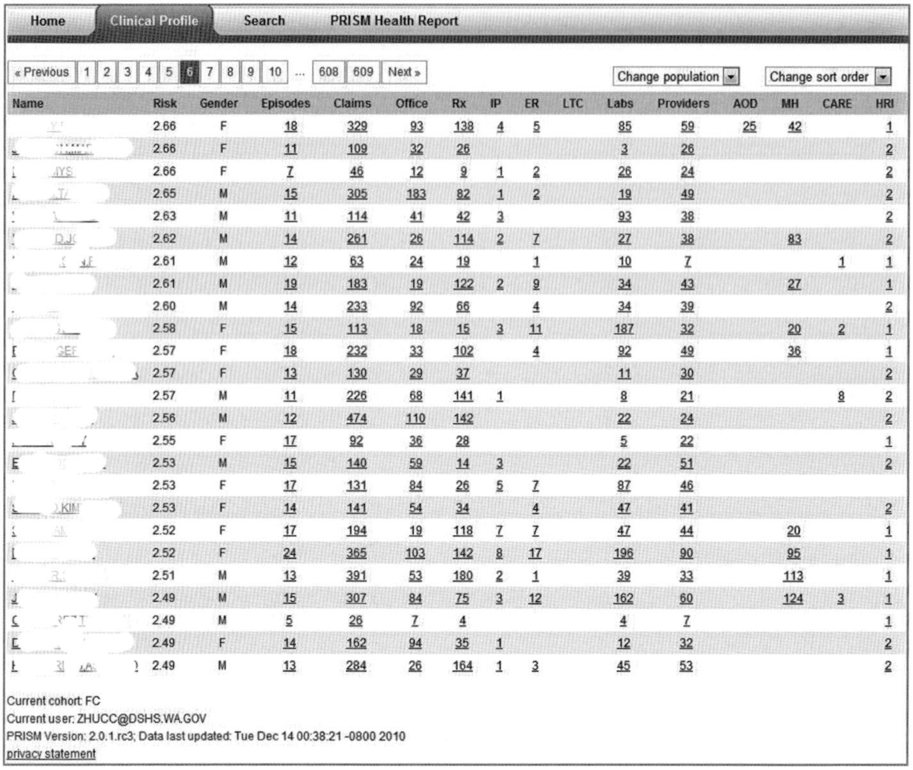

	Home	Clinical Profile	Search	PRISM Health Report		

« Previous 1 2 3 4 5 **6** 7 8 9 10 ... 608 609 Next »   Change population ▾   Change sort order ▾

Name	Risk	Gender	Episodes	Claims	Office	Rx	IP	ER	LTC	Labs	Providers	AOD	MH	CARE	HRI
	2.66	F	18	329	93	138	4	5		85	59	25	42		1
	2.66	F	11	109	32	26				3	26				2
IYS	2.66	F	7	46	12	9	1	2		26	24				2
	2.65	M	15	305	183	82	1	2		19	49				2
	2.63	M	11	114	41	42	3			93	38				2
DJ	2.62	M	14	261	26	114	2	7		27	38		83		2
	2.61	M	12	63	24	19		1		10	7			1	1
	2.61	M	19	183	19	122	2	9		34	43		27		1
	2.60	M	14	233	92	66		4		34	39				2
	2.58	F	15	113	18	15	3	11		187	32		20	2	1
GEF	2.57	F	18	232	33	102		4		92	49		36		1
	2.57	F	13	130	29	37				11	30				2
	2.57	M	11	226	68	141	1			8	21			8	2
	2.56	M	12	474	110	142				22	24				2
	2.55	F	17	92	36	28				5	22				1
E	2.53	M	15	140	59	14	3			22	51				2
	2.53	F	17	131	84	26	5	7		87	46				
KIM	2.53	F	14	141	54	34		4		47	41				2
	2.52	F	17	194	19	118	7	7		47	44		20		1
	2.52	F	24	365	103	142	8	17		196	90		95		1
	2.51	M	13	391	53	180	2	1		39	33		113		1
	2.49	M	15	307	84	75	3	12		162	60		124	3	1
	2.49	M	5	26	7	4				4	7				1
	2.49	F	14	162	94	35	1			12	32				2
	2.49	M	13	284	26	164	1	3		45	53				2

Current cohort: FC
Current user: ZHUCC@DSHS.WA.GOV
PRISM Version: 2.0.1.rc3; Data last updated: Tue Dec 14 00:38:21 -0800 2010
privacy statement

Figure 20.1 PRISM Population Screen here

ID. With one click, users can navigate to a sortable listing of each client in the population they manage.

The population screen shows each client's name, risk score, gender, and counts of key events including: (1) Episodes - key risk areas, (2) Claims – total claims, (3) Office – office visits, (4) RX – prescriptions filled, (5) IP – inpatient admissions, (6) ER – outpatient emergency room visits, (7) LTC – long term care services, (8) Lab – laboratory, (9) Providers – unique number of providers, (10) AOD – alcohol and drug treatment, (11) MH – mental health services, (12) CARE – long-term care functional assessments, and (13) HRI – health risk indicators.

Once an individual patient is chosen, the PRISM tool organizes data much as a sophisticated electronic medical record would, with summary sheets on major topics, use of graphic displays for conveying dense information, the ability to sort all fields, and the ability to drill down (connect through hyperlinks) for more detailed information.

Each summary sheet can be printed out as a .pdf document. Client-specific summary sheets all share synopses of demographics (including name, age, gender, phone, current address, whether hearing impaired, the need for interpreter services) and a risk profile (risk score, expected annual cost, primary and secondary risk conditions and diagnoses, mental health and substance use indicators), with topic-specific detail, as illustrated in Table 20.1 A pie chart illustrates the relative contribution of each risk factor to the client's

Table 20.1 Client-Specific PRISM Summaries

Summary Topics by Tab	Data
Medical Risk Factors	By disease category, reports the most recent diagnosis and/or prescription, number of claims and relative contribution to the total risk score
Hospitalizations	Admission and discharge dates, total cost, primary diagnosis, whether admission was through the emergency department, length of stay, drill-down links to hospital and attending physician contact information, and access to the complete claim
Outpatient Emergency Department Visits	Date, primary diagnosis, paid amount, classification of whether the visit was avoidable (using the New York University algorithm (Billings, *et al.* 2000), name of hospital, with drill down to hospital contact information
Prescriptions Filled	Fill date, generic drug name, drug class, quantity, days supplied, reimbursement, pharmacy, prescriber, and refill sequence
Office Visits	Date, claims line number, drug indicator, primary diagnosis, procedure, revenue code, provider (including a link to contact information), line amount, paid amount and claim type
Lab Orders Filled	Date, procedure, revenue code description, provider, paid amount, referring provider
Substance Abuse Services	Admission date, discharge date, quantity, description of service
Mental Health Services	Service date, service code, quantity, unit, description of service
Long-Term Care	Service date, service code, quantity, unit, description of service
Long-Term Care Needs Assessment	By assessment identifier, type of assessment, whether it is current or historical, assessment date and detailed assessor's notes. Sub-screens provide additional detail including activities of daily living (ADL) score, cognitive performance score, depression score, change in health status from last assessment, self-rated health status, detailed description of behavioral problems and functional limitations, fall risk, pain impacts on functioning, and identification of long-term care caseworker and primary care physician (including contact information)
Health Risk Indicators (For Clients Age 18 and Under)	Risk score; substance use disorder diagnosis subsequent to last treatment encounter, inpatient admissions in last 12 months, outpatient ER visits in last 12 months, failure to thrive diagnosis, treatment for injury diagnosis, nutrition problem diagnosis, crisis mental health encounter (past 12 months), mental health inpatient stay (past 12 months), outpatient ER with primary psychiatric diagnosis (past 12 months), child under age 6 receiving psych RX in past 12 months.
Providers	Most likely primary care providers based on an attribution model, name of billing and performing provider, last service date and number of claims with links to all visits with provider contact information
Eligibility	By year/month, patient's living arrangement, placement status, whether they are dually eligible for Medicare, their Medicaid program coverage group and the type of managed care provider or care coordination coverage they have, with links to contact information

Source: Billings, Parikh, & Mijanovich (2000)

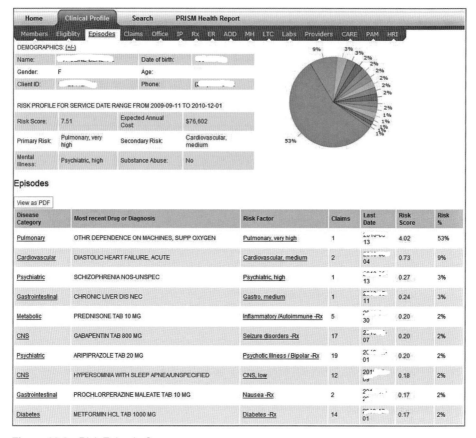

Figure 20.2   Risk Episode Summary

total risk score. Full descriptions of each risk factor are viewed by hovering the cursor over each section of the pie chart.

The summary sheet of risk factors (Figure 20.2) is usually the first stop for a clinician reviewing a client for the first time.

In this example, the primary risk factor, pulmonary, is very high, making up 53% of the patient's total risk score of 7.51. PRISM lists the most recent description of the drug or diagnosis for that risk factor, with links to all claims associated with the condition. By scanning the risk factor list, the clinician can discern which risk factors may respond to intervention. The risk factors don't substitute for professional judgment; they act as supplements. The designers of PRISM chose to not load the risk factor page with multiple alerts based on single disease protocols, because prior experience showed that too many alerts diverted attention away from what might have been the root source of the patient's dysfunction. Instead, the focus was on building an application that allowed the user's attention to scan the breath of information on a client, looking for clues as to where care management may have an impact.

As an example of the comprehensive story one can glean from a 10-minute review of the PRISM tool about a Medicaid client referred to chronic care management, consider Janet Doe (not her real name):

> Janet Doe presents as a high-risk client whose medical risk score is 7.5, which means her future medical expenditures are expected to be seven-and-a-half times that of the average non-dual SSI Medicaid client. Her highest risk factor is pulmonary – she is on portable oxygen for her COPD, and is also being treated for schizophrenia and depression, chronic liver disease, and diabetes. She has been hospitalized 4 times in the past 15 months, with 12 additional outpatient emergency department visits. The dates of her hospitalizations correspond roughly to dates when her medications would have run out.
>
> She is being regularly seen at her local community mental health agency. The caseworker at the Area Agency on Aging, a different agency, notes "The client requests in-home, long-term care services because she had fallen without help about a month ago. She fell at night and was unable to get up to call for help. She was on the floor all night until her son saw her the next morning. The client said she is alone during the day. She falls a lot due to dizziness and her legs give out on her. She also has seizures." PRISM shows she has not yet received in-home long-term care services.
>
> Her initial assessment nine months earlier by a different case worker indicates "Client is a 'frequent flier' - has had nine hospitalizations in [an] eight-month period. Is noncompliant with diet; medication management due to memory loss and MH issues. Recently assigned a nurse care manager to provide case management with medical concerns. Diagnosis includes IDDM; arthritis; schizoaffective disorder; COPD; and bipolar disorder."
>
> Though she has seen many different primary care providers, she has most often seen Dr. Johnson at the downtown federally qualified health center. She lives at home and doesn't need an interpreter.

Armed with such detailed data, an assigned nurse care-manager can locate the client, engage her in the program, and work with her to develop a care plan.

Equally important as the development of the care plan is the ability to provide invaluable summary sheets of filled medications, recent hospitalizations and other clinically relevant information tracked by PRISM to treating physicians and health care providers. The care coordinator's ability to provide the comprehensive filled-medication list (Figure 20.3), in particular, transforms the relationship between the care coordinator and the medical team. Janet Doe, for example, has had 216 prescriptions filled in the past 15 months, through her extensive interactions with primary care providers, specialists, hospital emergency departments, and behavioral health and long-term care systems. No other source draws together in one place the drug name, drug class, days supplied, dates and prescribers from all these different sources.

Uses of PRISM

The PRISM application is being used for care coordination in a wide range of populations, including children in foster care, working-age adults with high-risk physical health conditions and significant co-occurring behavioral health needs, and adults with major

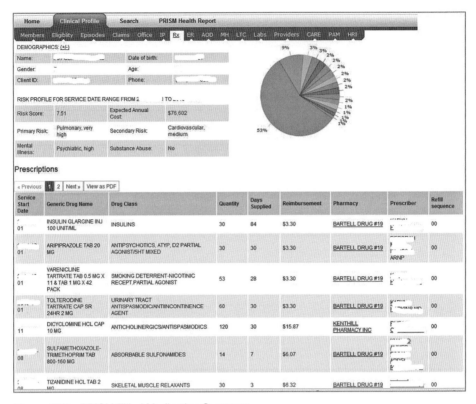

Figure 20.3   PRISM Filled Medication Summary

functional limitations and severe chronic disease conditions receiving in-home long-term care services.

Other uses are: (1) medical evidence gathering for determining eligibility for disability-related medical coverage; (2) triaging high-risk populations to more efficiently allocate scarce care management resources; for example, stratifying by recent inpatient and emergency department activity; (3) identification of child health risk indicators for high-risk children [mental health crisis, substance abuse, ED use, nutrition or feeding problems]; (4) identification of behavioral health needs (redacting information where required by state and federal law); (5) medication adherence monitoring; (6) identification of other potential barriers to care, including the patient's housing status (for example, whether they are homeless), whether they are known to be hearing impaired, and whether they have a non-English primary language; (7) access to treating and prescribing provider contact information for care coordination; (8) creation of child health summary reports for foster parents and pediatricians; and (9) a source of regularly updated contact information from the medical eligibility determination process.

The PRISM application is continuously evolving, with new risk factors, outcome measures, uses, and utilities identified by users and implemented by the PRISM application team. Areas that hold future promise include identifying "impactable" costs or sentinel events where care coordination intervention may have the most impact, for example avoiding re-hospitalization; provider profiling, especially related to medication adherence; and identifying risk factors predicting institutionalization of clients receiving community-based long-term care.

Strengths/weaknesses of PRISM

In summary, the strengths of PRISM include (1) "One-stop shopping" for information from administrative data systems to support care management decision making through a single point of entry for information about a patient's risk factors and health service utilization across medical, behavioral health and long-term care systems; (2) an intuitive user interface; (3) the ability to create and share a comprehensive profile of a client; (4) state-of-the-art prediction of prospective medical costs; and (5) data on psychosocial risk factors, including behavioral health, homelessness, and functional limitations from care coordination assessments.

Limitations include the relationship between traditional measures of medical risk and impactability is not well understood. Traditional quality measures have limited empirical data to support their relationship to health outcomes in complex populations. There is a recognized risk of creating the wrong priorities for clinical staff by focusing on standard quality of care measures to prioritize interventions in highly complex populations. Although the PRISM application is refreshed weekly, there is potential for incomplete information due to: lags in processing claims and in submitting encounter data; claims paid through separate coverage like Medicare or private insurance; services paid out-of-pocket; and redaction of chemical dependency treatment system data where written consent documentation process is not in place. Data quality issues, such as the accuracy of behavioral health diagnoses recorded by medical professionals (for example, misdiagnosis of bipolar disorder as depression). The application is not an electronic medical record, lab results and clinical notes are not currently linked into the application.

Issues for states considering in-house development of predictive modeling tools

The Washington State Department of Social and Health Services has a strong internal Research and Data Analysis Division (RDA) that includes staff with the econometric, actuarial, database, and software engineering skills necessary to calibrate commercial-grade medical risk models and implement state-of-the-art secure web applications. These staff resources are available because parts of the agency have invested in an internal health services research capability, rather than contracting research out to academic institutions or private consulting firms. Without a strong legacy of support for in-house analytic and information technology capacity, internal development of the PRISM application would have been far more challenging.

PRISM's more holistic view of the patient's health service experience was made possible by prior investment in cross-system data integration. A major challenge in this area is that different state information systems use different patient identifiers. Prior support for data integration meant that timely and well-organized multi-system service and assessment data were available for linkage to medical service data through sophisticated processes that were already well-established. The transition to a new Medicaid management information and payment system has also significantly simplified data integration within the PRISM application by providing a more unified source for medical and behavioral health fee-for-service claims and encounter data.

Several other factors created the opportunity for Washington State to develop in-house predictive risk scores and decision-support tools that have been found to be more useful and less expensive to operate than the commercial alternatives. These include implementing Medicaid service integration pilots that built team expertise in integration of medical, behavioral health, and long-term care service and assessment data; integration of research staff into program design and operations which deepened the research team's knowledge and built trust in the research team's capabilities; and the availability of open-source risk-adjustment tools maintained by UC San Diego.

Without this initial investment in analytical capacity and data and service integration, it may be difficult for Medicaid agencies to replicate all three components of the PRISM tool: (1) commercial-grade predictive modeling; (2) integration of health service utilization across medical, behavioral health and long-term care systems; and (3) a highly intuitive web-based user interface. However, this investment in internal development provides several benefits that would not be obtained through contracting with an external vendor. The application's initial design and ongoing evolution is more responsive to the agency's internal needs. There is intellectual ownership of the application, which translates into more control over the pace of development, ability to calibrate to state-specific populations, ability for rapid migration to new information systems, increased ease of extending access to agency staff, greater ability to leverage agency staff's deep program expertise, and constant interaction between the development team and system users.

Furthermore, internal development creates a professionally rewarding environment to help retain highly skilled staff in state service. This in turn creates positive spillovers in other areas. The PRISM team also provides quasi-experimental program evaluation, operational program support, and actuarial support. Project staff are also available to act as internal information technology consultants on other projects.

There are drawbacks, however, in attempting to develop such a sophisticated application internally. They include dependency on key staff to maintain the application and risk of loss of funding for internal analytical infrastructure in tough economic times. Internal analytical capacity can, perversely, be seen as a luxury in the government sector. One reason that the project team was eager to develop the PRISM application was a recognition that a closer connection to program operations might help preserve support in a difficult economic climate, in addition to making more valuable use of analytical and data resources. Commercial vendors can offer attractive packages for predictive modeling and clinical decision support applications that do not require the infrastructure investment, often with the promise of guaranteed cost-savings or other contractual incentives combined with their care coordination products.

The future

The health impacts and cost effectiveness of care management interventions that make use of the PRISM application are currently being evaluated. Access to the PRISM application is being expanded to health plan staff for Medicaid population management activities that have a broader focus than the current pilots serving high-risk aged or disabled patients. Consideration is being given to extending the use of PRISM (or developing new PRISM-like web-based, integrated predictive modeling tools) to other programs, including the cash assistance and child protective services programs.

References

Billings, J., Parikh, N., & Mijanovich, T. (2000) *Emergency Room Use: The New York Story*. The Commonwealth Fund, New York, NY.

Gilmer, T., Kronick R., Fishman P., *et al.* (2001) The Medicaid Rx model: pharmacy-based risk adjustment for public programs. *Medical Care*, 39, 1188–1202.

Kronick, R., Gilmer T., Dreyfus T., *et al.* (2000) Improving health based payment for Medicaid beneficiaries: CDPS. *Health Care Financing Review*, 21(3), 29–64.

Winkelman, R. & Mehmud, S. (2007) *A Comparative Analysis of Claims-Based Tools for Health Risk Assessment*. Society of Actuaries, Schaumburg, IL.

Chapter 21

High-risk patients in a complex health system: coordinating and managing care

Maria C. Raven

Introduction

Patients with frequent hospital admissions account for a disproportionate share of visits and costs (Kaiser Family Foundation [KKF] 2007a; Sommers & Cohen 2006). Specifically, Medicaid patients in the fee-for-service (FFS) sector comprise a minority of enrollees, yet account for the majority of Medicaid spending due to their disproportionately high use of health care services. Often this health services use is suboptimal, with patients frequenting hospital emergency departments (ED) or inpatient units, yet having no consistent source of outpatient primary care. In the face of state budget constraints and the large portion of state spending attributable to Medicaid dollars, these high-cost cases have contributed to a movement by states to shift Medicaid patients from FFS into managed care models or "high risk" case management programs. Such state initiatives create an impetus for hospitals and health care providers to better understand and control expenditures for the highest users of health services (Billings & Mijanovich 2007). In order to do so, we have conducted research with this population of high-cost, high-risk FFS Medicaid patients since 2005, developing and testing interventions with goals of improving care and reducing costs to Medicaid. A description of this work, the patients involved, the setting in which it takes place, and its implications for future health policy is what follows.

How did we get to where we are? use of evidence-based policy and management (EBPM) strategies

The New York City Health and Hospital Corporation (HHC) is New York City's public hospital system, and cares for a very diverse and geographically extensive patient base and serves many of its most vulnerable patients. Hospital to Home (H2H) is one of six current New York State Department of Health Chronic Illness Demonstration Projects designed to find and enroll FFS Medicaid patients identified as high-cost and high-risk for hospitalization in the 12 months following discharge. The H2H program model aims to

Comprehensive Care Coordination for Chronically Ill Adults, First Edition. Edited by Cheryl Schraeder and Paul Shelton.
© 2011 John Wiley & Sons, Inc. Published 2011 by John Wiley & Sons, Inc.

integrate evidence and innovation into care management for complex, high-cost patients, and to lay a foundation for further development and dissemination of best practices for this high-risk patient population.

What is EBPM?

The H2H program model was developed through pilot research with the target population, using research based within an evidence-based policy and management (EBPM) framework. What does EBPM mean? Rather than implementing a costly, large-scale intervention based on our ideas of what we thought would work, we opted to develop our intervention model in phases, and test it on a small scale before expanding. This ensured we were properly focused on the needs of the patients we'd be working with, and it also helped to determine if our intervention was feasible and could operate within the HHC environment. These efforts were supported by the United Hospital Fund and the New York Community Trust.

Identifying eligible patients: the importance of predictive modeling

Throughout these phases, eligible patients from our target population were identified using a predictive "case-finding algorithm" developed by John Billings, a professor at the New York University Wagner School for Public Policy. His work is focused on high-cost, high-risk patients. Research has shown that many patients who are high-cost one year will not remain high-cost the next, due to a phenomenon called regression to the mean. As many interventions in health care are quite costly, and there is no "new" money, it is key to assure that patients targeted for intervention are those who actually stand to benefit. The current best practice is to use predictive modeling to identify which patients are not only high-risk now, but will continue to be high-risk and high-cost in the future.

The predictive algorithm we used to identify patients has been described in detail elsewhere (Billings & Mujanovich 2007; Billings *et al.* 2006). In short, the algorithm can employ hospital or state-level administrative data to identify patients who are at high risk of subsequent readmission in the next 12 months based on their International Classification of Diseases, Ninth Revision (ICD-9) diagnoses and service utilization history (for example, ED visits, inpatient admissions, outpatient clinic visits) over the past four to five years. The algorithm assigns each patient a risk score of 0 to 100, with 100 being those patients at highest risk of subsequent readmission. A cut-off point of greater than 50 has been demonstrated to predict high probability (positive predictive value 0.7) of admission in the following 12 months (Billings & Mujanovich 2007; Billings *et al.* 2006; Raven *et al.* 2009).

Figure 21.1 illustrates how the algorithm would use five years of hospital or system-level administrative data to examine prior utilization and predict future hospital admission. Use of this methodology to identify patients for inclusion adds to our evidence-based best practices by identifying patients for whom intervention spending is most likely to offset future health care costs.

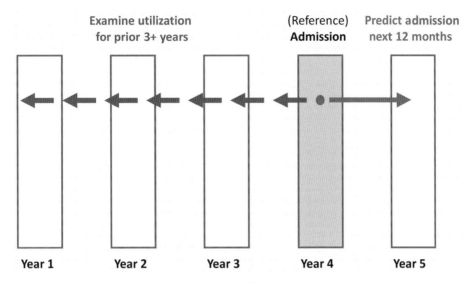

Figure 21.1   Case-Finding Risk Prediction Algorithm

Phase I: patient interviews

In 2005-06, we conducted interviews with 50 FFS Medicaid patients who were identified with predictive methodology used by our current Hospital to Home program. This process allowed us to define remediable medical and social risk factors that might be addressed by an intervention to improve health and reduce admissions and costs among the frequent hospital users identified. Through this process we were able to identify hospitalization risk factors among frequently admitted patients identified by the algorithm. This approach was paramount in informing our intervention model on ways to improve care for this patient population.

During the interviews we discovered that the majority of patients had no usual source of primary care; the ED was the single most common source cited for care. Unstable housing, substance abuse, and mental illness also emerged as strong drivers of hospitalization. The 50 interviewed patients consumed a per-person average of nearly $40,000 in Medicaid funds during the prior year, most of which were spent on hospital admissions. As a point of reference, mean New York State Medicaid payments for all Medicaid enrollees totaled $7,583 during the same year (KFF 2007b). Prior research has demonstrated that such patients will generate even higher costs in the 12 months following discharge if no intervention is undertaken to reduce health services use (Billings *et al.* 2006). This was indeed the case for our study population whose costs more than doubled in the year following study enrollment (Raven *et al.* 2009).

Phase II: pilot, small-scale, local intervention

Based on our interview data, in addition to site visits to and discussions with leadership from similar programs around the country, we developed a program model we felt would best serve the needs of the patient population, and decided to pilot it for a small number of patients to determine feasibility and effectiveness. The pilot program was structured to begin at the point of enrollment, whether at the patient's bedside in the hospital, or in a homeless shelter utilizing a flexible, patient-centered, intensive care management model with a multidisciplinary team approach. Although the program is tailored to the needs of each patient, it is designed to be responsive to local institutional patient flow, and thus readily adaptable to other settings.

Care management teams composed of social workers, community based care managers (CBCMs), and dedicated clinicians work to meet patients' needs in both health care and community settings. The model incorporates motivational interviewing, harm reduction, access to housing through our community partners utilizing a Housing First approach (Larimer *et al.* 2009), and provides cellular phones for patients when needed to better enable regular communication with program staff.

For the pilot, we enrolled 19 Medicaid FFS patients between 18 and 64 years of age who were admitted to our urban public hospital and identified by Billings' predictive case-finding algorithm as being high-cost and high-risk for future hospital readmission. All were male, a majority were substance users (17 of 19), and almost half (8 of 19) were homeless. They were evaluated to identify needs for things such as transportation to and advocacy during medical appointments, mental health and substance use treatment, and home visits. A community housing partner, Common Ground Community, initiated housing applications in-hospital for homeless patients. CBCMs facilitated appropriate discharge plans, then worked closely with the patients in the community using a harm reduction approach.

The 19 patients had a total of 64 inpatient admissions in the 12 months before the intervention versus 40 inpatient admissions in the following 12 months, which is a 37.5% reduction. A majority (11 of 15, or 73.3%) had fewer inpatient admissions in the year after the intervention compared to the prior year. Overall, ED visits also decreased, while outpatient clinic visits increased. Yearly Medicaid hospital reimbursements declined an average of $16,383 per patient. Because it was a pilot, the program was not to scale. However, subtracting our overall annualized pilot intervention costs from annual per-person Medicaid savings, the pilot resulted in over $5,000 savings to Medicaid per patient. Given these promising results, we have now expanded the model to serve more patients at additional hospitals to see if the pilot's success can be replicated.

New York State Department of Health chronic illness demonstration project: hospital to home (H2H)

Chronic Illness Demonstration Project

Building on the momentum from the pilot work, in 2007, the New York State Medicaid Office of Health Insurance Programs decided to fund seven Chronic Illness Demonstration Projects (CIDPs) across New York State. The goal of each three-year CIDP is to find and enroll FFS Medicaid patients identified as high-cost and high-risk for hospitalization in the 12 months following discharge, and to work with patients to improve their health and well-being while reducing costs to Medicaid, primarily through reductions in costly hospital admissions. The New York City HHC was awarded one of six CIDP contracts, in essence providing an opportunity to create and test the effectiveness of our program model on a much larger scale for some of the most vulnerable patients in New York City.

In April 2009, Hospital to Home was initiated by the HHC and implemented by three of its member hospitals: Bellevue Hospital Center in Manhattan, Woodhull Hospital in Brooklyn, and Elmhurst Hospital in Queens. While all a part of the same corporation, each of these facilities differs from one another in terms of layout, population served, surrounding community resources, and embedded hospital resources. However, the program model, messaging, philosophy, and staffing patterns are uniform across facilities. The experience of implementing a single program across three individual facilities has been, and will continue to be, an essential part of determining whether such a program can be implemented at multiple distinct sites (and later disseminated to other facilities) while maintaining its singular programmatic goals and policies.

Why is this important for the future of health care and Medicaid?

Currently, there is much discussion about the importance of the medical home and the formation of Accountable Care Organizations. If such models for care are to succeed for health care providers serving complex, high cost patients, strategies such as those employed by H2H will be needed. Providers will increasingly be responsible for their patients across a continuum of care that extends beyond the walls of the clinic or hospital. To be competitive, they will have to grapple with the issue of following patients outside the traditional confines of the health care system into the community, into their homes or shelters, necessitating interaction and collaboration with community-based providers, and if they exist, family members and friends. This is a notable difference from the current standard of care. Providers and policy makers in areas with high concentrations of Medicaid-insured and other potentially vulnerable populations must begin to think *now* about how to contain costs and optimize health care utilization and outcomes for such patients if they are to have a chance to succeed.

Hospital to Home addresses exactly these issues. We prioritize two key concepts: care coordination and accountability. Our program motto is "we'll meet you where you are" and we mean this both literally and figuratively. Our staff conducts much of its work not in the hospital, but in the community, aiming to surround patients with needed services and support as they move in and out of the health care system.

Health system deficiencies H2H addresses to coordinate care

As previously mentioned, our H2H enrollees are algorithmically identified FFS Medicaid patients with many health and social needs, and serious health and social stressors that interfere with their ability to interface effectively with the complex system on which their health and social well-being depend. H2H aims to help patients overcome specific inadequacies in the health system that fragment care and contribute to health care system inefficiency.

Currently, much of health care is siloed and commonly not co-located with behavioral health services (Druss & Newcomer 2007; Druss & von Esenwein 2006). Patients with mental illness have unaddressed chronic disease and preventive health needs (Raven *et al.* 2009), and organizations governing substance use services and mental illness, which often share patients with hospitals and health care systems, are distinct from one another and subject to restrictive funding streams that often make management of co-occurring disorders difficult (KFF 2007b). Perverse incentives that financially reward hospitalizations and underpay outpatient and primary care provide inadequate incentives to prioritize basic care coordination and preventive care (Larimer *et al.* 2009). Finally, a general lack of financial incentive for provision of post-discharge follow-up in the community, combined with an often precariously housed patient base, make continuity of care difficult (Druss & Newcomer 2007). As these realities are unlikely to change in the near future, we factored these challenges into our program design with the intent of eventual dissemination.

H2H rationale and program model

The essential mechanism by which we function is to specifically address these system misalignments at the individual level by engaging patients with a consistent, multidisciplinary care management team (along the lines of the Medical Home model) including a key "go-to" person (the CBCM), so that care can be managed and coordinated across multiple locations and providers. The CBCM is similar to a "patient navigator" where there is extensive literature that has demonstrated effectiveness. The main role of patient navigators is to provide basic care management, eliminate barriers to care, provide emotional support, and link the patient to appropriate community supportive agencies and resources (Dohan & Schrag 2005; Wells *et al.* 2008).

Our program philosophy is to "meet patients where they are" both literally and figuratively. As such, care team staff aims to show patients, many of whom have had negative experiences within the health care system, that improved care management and coordination via H2H can allow for a different, more positive experience, both within and outside of the health care system. This helps patients to become more engaged in and hopeful about their own care. Intervention staff focuses not only on care team-identified goals, but also patient identified goals over both the short and long term. By improving care provision via needed coordination and oversight, we anticipate that we will be able to improve health status and patient satisfaction as we demonstrated in our pilot work, while averting hospital admissions that are costly to Medicaid.

H2H staffing

Each of the three participating HHC hospitals is staffed with a social work supervisor (LCSW) who oversees a staff of CBCMs. CBCMs are required to have a minimum of a high school diploma and relevant experience working in direct patient services. CBCMs are required to build their own caseloads, which are capped at 25 patients. They are the most important single point of contact for the patients. In addition, we have a full-time housing coordinator to work with our homeless patients to obtain housing and some degree of dedicated primary care at the participating hospitals.

Once a patient is enrolled, CBCMs work with them to complete an in-depth health assessment to identify immediate, short, and long term goals to help improve health and well-being and optimize health care utilization. From this, a care plan is created. Goals range from obtaining glasses or dentures, to connecting to stable primary care, cutting down on the amount of alcohol consumed, and obtaining housing. We issue cell phones to patients who don't have other ways to keep in contact with our staff, and we use motivational interviewing techniques and take a harm-reduction approach.

The care plan and interventions needed are tailored for each patient depending on his or her unique needs and desires. Some patients obtain care within HHC, and others outside of it. Many have people who contribute to their care, including case managers at methadone programs or in shelters, psychiatrists, or family members.

Each week, the care team at each hospital, consisting of the CBCMs, social work supervisor, and participating physician, holds care management rounds. During rounds, each CBCM presents their cases which are reviewed and discussed by the team and next steps for the coming week are determined. In addition, each month we hold program-wide care management rounds that include the above mentioned staff in addition to the Housing Coordinator, site coordinators from each hospital, and program management and administration. These meetings provide the team with an opportunity to see one another and exchange ideas. Each site presents a challenging case for group discussion, and we review program updates and any administrative issues.

H2H finances

At present, H2H is not financially feasible for HHC. Ironically, because of the way the health care payment system is currently structured, we are the only CIDP participant who actually stands to *lose* revenue by fulfilling the CIDP objectives. For hospital systems, admissions (unless they occur within 30 days of discharge, a marker for poor discharge planning and follow-up which is penalized by insurers) are the largest source of revenue for hospitals. Conversely, outpatient appointments, which would be an ideal setting for care coordination and information gathering regarding social risk factors, are reimbursed at comparatively low rates. As a result, to maximize revenue, patients are booked for 15-minute appointment slots, hardly enough time to address a laundry list of health and social issues, let alone coordinate with outside agencies to improve follow-up in the community.

If HHC stands to lose money by cutting Medicaid costs, why would we participate? First, it's the right thing to do. Currently, many of the patients eligible to enroll don't receive the coordinated health and social care that could exist under health care reform, and they are suffering for it; the financial incentives to undertake the cultural and logistical changes needed to expand the locus of care simply do not exist. Secondly, when improved payments to health care providers for care coordination and accountability do come to fruition in the next few years, incentives will be more appropriately aligned. Health care provider groups, which could/should include social workers, nurses, mid-level providers, and possibly, partnerships with providers at community-based organizations, will determine what services are needed to optimize patients' health and social outcomes, and will also bear financial risk for the patients they serve. H2H allows HHC to develop and test, for more vulnerable patients not properly engaged with the system, viable strategies for the future.

How do we get patients to join H2H?

In an ideal world, patients would be eager to find and take part in an organization focused on improving care. While a small number of our eligible patients come to us via response to a mailing, most high-cost, high-risk patients eligible for our program must be found, and it takes some detective work, due largely to the fact that we must rely on whatever basic demographic data is available in the Medicaid database. This leaves us with many inaccurate addresses and phone numbers, or missing data. Once those obstacles are surmounted, upon hearing about what our program does, most patients are interested, and we have a very low refusal rate (under 10%) for participation. As few similar programs currently exist, our program is appealing to most eligible enrollees. In the coming years, however, it is likely that competition for patient participation in similar programs will increase, particularly for the newly insured either through Medicaid or state exchanges.

Many patients are distrustful of the health care system due to past experiences. How do we engage them? First, we hire staff members who want to do this work with this particular patient population, and most are hired based on experience in working with our target population. Many staff are multi-lingual and all have access through our facilities to interpreter services, both on- and off-site 24 hours a day, seven days a week. In addition, our staff undergoes rigorous training in motivational interviewing techniques, recognizing various aspects of medical and social issues they will encounter with our patient population, and our singular program philosophy. Because our motto is "we'll meet you where you are" staff are trained to listen to and elicit the patients' needs and goals, rather than impose our own standards onto them. When a CBCM first meets a patient, they are trained to attempt to fill some immediate need for that person, even if it's just a cup of coffee or an ear to help to establish rapport. CBCMs are also trained to help patients identify small, short term, achievable goals (such as establishing primary care, obtaining eyeglasses, coming to our staff offices) in addition to more challenging long term goals (including weight loss and tobacco cessation) so that small victories can be focused upon and recognized.

In order to help this process, we have a "patient necessities fund" comprised of petty cash that can be used for small purchases to fill immediate needs that would otherwise go unaddressed (such as socks, a calendar, or a coat). Because we anticipated from prior research that a significant portion of patients would be homeless, we contracted with the New York City Department of Homeless Services (DHS) to assist with outreach and enrollment of homeless eligible enrollees, and we employ a full-time Housing Coordinator skilled in outreaching to and working with the unique needs of the homeless.

Our patient alert system allows us to receive real-time e-mail notifications when eligible individuals register at any HHC outpatient clinic, ED, or are hospitalized at any HHC hospital. Because our staff can meet with patients to engage them within the hospital setting, they often have the opportunity to explore the reason for the current visit or prior visits, and to bring an immediate focus to some aspect of their health or care that our program can address. In addition, our staff has a willingness to focus on work that is not health care related. Much of their day-to-day work might consist of tasks not directly connected to the health care system, but that affect our patients' health.

How do we use technology to coordinate care and increase accountability?

In order to help coordinate care, we rely on technology a great deal. All of our staff have Blackberries that enable immediate e-mail and text services to help coordinate care on password-protected devices. We also provide our patients who do not have phones with mobile phones, and pay for their minutes. Patients must sign a contract upon receipt of the phone for tracking purposes, and staff emphasizes that H2H phones are to be used primarily for staying in touch with the program or related matters. Minute usage and potential overages are monitored by our administrative staff, and overages are viewed as an opportunity to discuss any potential issues with the patient. CBCMs train patients on how to use the phones and keep them charged, and they add relevant program numbers into the phone.

As mentioned previously, our patient alert system allows patient-services staff to receive real-time notification of a patient's presence at any acute-care facility in the HHC system. As a part of this program, we worked with HHCs Medicaid HMO to adapt their current database to work for H2H. The result is a program-specific database (distinct from the patient's electronic medical record) that our staff uses to enter all information about our enrolled patients. This database allows us to generate reports that assist with staff management and oversight regarding outreach and enrollment, proper and up-to-date documentation, our ability to follow through with initial and ongoing goals and referrals for our patients, and other issues such as billing Medicaid. Our staff also has access to the electronic medical record at their base hospital which aids in care coordination and management.

Patient vignette

Ms. W is a 43-year-old woman with morbid obesity, insulin-dependent diabetes, neuropathy and nephropathy, hepatitis C, hypertension, and asthma. She is a smoker and has a past history of IV drug use; she suffers from depression, and has had suicide attempts in the past. Prior to enrollment she was homeless in a shelter and had frequent hospital admissions for high blood-sugar and related infections, in addition to difficulty remembering to take all of her medications.

The H2H program and her care manager provided her with a cellular phone, outpatient appointment reminders, and frequent moral support. Our Housing Coordinator assisted with housing placement, and she moved into a permanent supportive housing environment where H2H arranged for a home health aide for medication assistance. Through H2H she was assigned to a primary care physician who has linked to the various subspecialists she requires. She has also been attending the monthly H2H support groups. Since enrollment, she has had only one hospitalization, although she continues to have difficulty with adequate blood-sugar control.

Dissemination and replication

By the conclusion of the project, we will have developed a user-friendly description of the intervention that includes staffing patterns and all elements of service delivery that can be disseminated to stakeholders. Lessons learned from this project have already begun to be disseminated to interested parties within and outside of HHC. Importantly, the New York State Department of Health is conducting an independent analysis of the six Chronic Illness Demonstration Projects currently being implemented across the state, and the results will help to inform the future direction of Medicaid regarding this patient population. Finally, because we are partnering with several community-based organizations in New York City, we plan to work with them to disseminate our project results as well. Replication of this project by other institutions will be facilitated by the fact that our intervention is designed to be flexible, enabling providers to tailor the intervention to individual patient needs at different hospitals or health care settings.

References

Billings, J., Dixon, J. M., Mijanovich, T., *et al.* (2006) Case finding for patients at risk of readmission to hospital: development of algorithm to identify high risk patient. *British Medical Journal*, 333, 327–332.

Billings, J., & Mijanovich, T. (2007) Improving the management of care for high-cost Medicaid patients. *Health Affairs*, 26, 1643–1654.

Dohan, D., & Schrag, D. (2005) Using navigators to improve care of underserved patients: current practices and approaches. *Cancer*, 104, 848–855.

Druss, B.G., & von Esenwein, S.A. (2006) Improving general medical care for persons with mental and addictive disorders: systematic review. *General Hospital Psychiatry*, 28, 145–153.

Druss, B., & Newcomer, J. (2007) Challenges and solutions to integrating mental and physical health care. *The Journal of Clinical Psychiatry*, 68(4), e09.

Kaiser Family Foundation. (2007a) *Medicaid, A Primer*. The Henry J. Kaiser Family Foundation, Melano Park, CA. Retrieved from http://www.kff.org/medicaid/7334-02.cfm.

Kaiser Family Foundation. (2007b) *State Health Facts*. The Henry J. Kaiser Family Foundation, Melano Park, CA. Retrieved from http://www.statehealthfacts.org/cgi-bin/healthfacts.cgi?action=profile&area=New+York&category=Health+Coverage+%26+Uninsured&subcategory=Health+Insurance+Status&topic=Total+Population.

Larimer, M.E., Malone, D.K., Garner, M.D., *et al.* (2009) Health care and public service use and costs before and after provision of hoursing for chronically homeless persons with severe alcohol problems. *Journal of the American Medical Association*, 301, 1349–1357.

Raven, M., Billings, J., Goldfrank, L., *et al.* (2009) Medicaid patients at high risk for frequent hospital admission: real-time identification and remediable risks. *Journal of Urban Health*, 86, 230–241.

Sommers, A., & Cohen, M. (2006) *Medicaid's High Cost Enrollees: How Much Do They Drive Program Spending*. The Henry J. Kaiser Family Foundation, Melano Park, CA. Retrieved from http://www.kff.org/medicaid/7490.cfm.

Wells, K., Battaglia, T., Dudley, D., *et al.* (2008) Patient navigation: state of the art or is it science? *Cancer*, 113, 1999–2010.

Chapter 22

The SoonerCare Health Management Program

Carolyn J. Reconnu and Mike Herndon

Introduction

The SoonerCare Health Management Program (HMP) is an ongoing quality improvement initiative aimed at improving the lives of Oklahomans with chronic disease as well as reducing future incidence. The SoonerCare HMP was developed in response to the Oklahoma Medicaid Reform Act of 2006. The Reform Act mandates resulted from the task force developed by the Oklahoma Legislature, whose mission was to identify $100 million in savings through efficiencies to the Medicaid system. While the task force findings overall were positive, one element of this legislation required the Oklahoma Health Care Authority (OHCA), Oklahoma's single-state agency for Medicaid administration, to create a disease management program to improve quality of care and reduce the cost of care for those with chronic conditions. This recommendation supported OHCA's stated mission to purchase state and federally funded health care in the most efficient and comprehensive manner possible, and to study and recommend strategies for optimizing the accessibility and quality of health care.

After consulting with local and national industry experts in disease management principles and programs, the OHCA used the Chronic Care Model (Wagner 1998) as a basis to create the SoonerCare HMP. A guiding principle of the Chronic Care Model is to pair an informed and activated patient with a prepared and proactive provider in order to create the best possible health outcome. The SoonerCare HMP addresses both of these key components, which optimizes sustainability. OHCA partners with a vendor, determined through competitive bid, to operate the program. Our vendor, Iowa Foundation for Medical Care (IFMC), initiated services to our SoonerCare members and providers in February 2008.

The HMP program

Nurse Case Management

The HMP program comprises two primary components: Nurse Case Management and Practice Facilitation. Nurse case management in our program emphasizes self-management principles and is provided for up to 5,000 of our highest risk members.

Comprehensive Care Coordination for Chronically Ill Adults, First Edition. Edited by Cheryl Schraeder and Paul Shelton.
© 2011 John Wiley & Sons, Inc. Published 2011 by John Wiley & Sons, Inc.

SoonerCare had approximately 500,000 members in the adult and children categories at the time the HMP was being developed, with about 20% having a chronic disease. It was estimated that 5% or less of our members spend 50% or more of our Medicaid dollars. Therefore, the determination was made to serve our top 5% highest risk members with chronic disease, or 5,000 members, through concentrated case management efforts.

These highest risk members are identified with predictive modeling software that utilizes a sophisticated approach to trend episodes of care and treatment groups to evaluate current gaps in care and future risk. The first 1,000 of these members at highest risk (Tier 1) are provided face-to-face nurse case management. The remaining 4,000 high-risk members (Tier 2) are provided telephonic nurse case management. Both tiers of members receive comprehensive health status, health literacy, behavioral health, and pharmacy assessments. At a minimum, on a monthly basis, either face-to-face or telephonically, the HMP nurses work with individual members on goals directed at their transformation to a more informed and engaged patient. This work includes a strong educational component, as well as increased access to community resources. The HMP nurses work to involve the primary care provider (PCP) in their care plan and keep them apprised of the member's progress. To date, approximately 10,000 SoonerCare members have been served by this program.

Patient example

An example of the success of the SoonerCare HMP is Robert B, age 41. Robert has type 2 diabetes, congestive heart failure, hypertension, hyperlipidemia, obesity, and non-organic psychosis. Robert accepted our offer of case management in August 2008. At that time, he qualified as a Tier 2 member to receive telephonic nurse case management. He was transferred to Tier 1 in March 2009 for more intensive and personal involvement due to his high level of need. At the time of enrollment to our program, Robert smoked ten cigarettes per day and led a sedentary lifestyle. A diabetic diet had been recommended by his physician but he did not follow the dietary guidelines because of lack of knowledge. After working with his HMP nurse case manager and with supervision of his primary care provider, Robert adopted an 1,100 calorie per day diet, lost 89 pounds in one year (going from 309 to 220 lbs) quit smoking, and started an exercise program. His hemoglobin A1C went from 7.3% to 5.2% in 16 months. He achieved decreases in his total cholesterol from 129 mg/dL to 98 mg/dL and his triglyceride levels decreased from 249 mg/dL to 127 mg/dL.

From a cost-savings perspective, impact is also realized utilizing predictive modeling profiles. After five months in the case management program, a consistent positive variance was demonstrated between Robert's forecasted cost for an upcoming year and the actual cost expenditures for that same year. This cost variance, which ranged from 1.7% to 13.6%, has been sustained over the six months of currently available data.

Practice facilitation

The other key component to the SoonerCare HMP is the necessary support to assist the primary care provider in becoming more prepared and proactive. This component is commonly known as practice facilitation. Within our program structure, the practice facilitators are specially trained nurses working as free consultants who help providers improve their office efficiency and identify methods to improve the quality of care. The SoonerCare HMP incorporated this key support for practitioners to enhance the sustainability of the program. We have found that a fundamental element is assistance in developing structured policies and procedures, formal job descriptions, and a team-centered environment. For an office to function efficiently, all team members must fully understand their roles in the various processes and procedures that comprise daily workflow. Increased definition and structure of the office environment enhances the team members' confidence in their various roles, which diminishes turnover rates and enables the team to function more effectively.

Once the foundation is in place, the practice facilitator conducts a comprehensive assessment of the practice. The practice is asked to conduct a self-assessment, while a chart data abstraction is performed by the practice facilitator. The comparative results of these two components are shared with the practice for a baseline understanding of the current trends in care gaps and patient outcomes. Attention is given to staff capabilities regarding comprehension of quality improvement principles. Office dynamics, including interpersonal communication, clinic paradigms and culture are evaluated. Educational needs and learning styles are assessed.

Clinic processes are mapped to analyze pain points in workflow. To further target improvements in chronic disease care, the practice facilitators expand process mapping to look at specific disease associated care opportunities in relation to standards of care. The facilitators evaluate any quality or process improvement initiatives in which the practice is currently participating. This is critical to determine if competing priorities and initiatives will divert the clinical staff's attention. It is possible for some clinics to participate in more than one quality improvement initiative, but it is optimal for an interface to exist between quality projects.

Once the practice facilitator formulates a strong understanding of the clinic's needs, they assist with identification and prioritization of specific process improvement interventions, whether these are general workflow issues or specifically related to care gaps and missed opportunities. Specific evidence-based interventions are considered if this need is identified.

The facilitators further support practice efforts by providing targeted education to staff regarding disease processes and process improvement principles. They work with the practice to implement regular meetings in an effort to sustain staff interest and foster continued learning related to the initiative.

Facilitators assist practices with the implementation of an electronic health management information system or patient registry. This web-based tool allows the practice to enter member data to track over time so that each member receives all the appropriate tests and treatment recommended for their chronic condition(s). The registry contains disease modules on coronary artery disease, hypertension, diabetes, heart failure, asthma, tobacco cessation, preventative care, and asthma. The facilitators assist with the electronic health management system and/or disease registry implementation by front-loading the data for all patients in the practice with a chronic disease, who were identified with predictive modeling software.

Other process improvement opportunities include utilization of standing orders to improve clinic efficiency and referral tracking. The practice learns how to run reports that highlight individual patient-care gaps in addition to reports that assist with overall population management.

Once the basic components of practice facilitation are applied, more advanced patient-centered principles are introduced. These may include development and deployment of a patient education or community resource library, implementation of behavioral health screening and instruction in motivational interviewing.

Practice facilitation services have been provided to over 75 Oklahoma-based practices to date, indirectly benefiting almost 90,000 SoonerCare members. While a comprehensive evaluation of the effectiveness is ongoing, review of data for three practices with solid adoption of the registry and related process improvement efforts notes a significant savings. The forecasted cost of the panel members was averaged and compared to the actual cost of their panel members a year later, revealing a 7.2 to 11.3% positive variance. When the average savings are distributed over the entire panel, this equates to $448,000 to $772,000 in savings for each of the three practices.

As the SoonerCare HMP was developed, a strong nurse case management component was expected by the authors of the legislation. OHCA supported this expectation but expanded the program even further to assist practitioners in their efforts to care for their patients. The initial indication is that both nurse case management and practice facilitation are effective methods to improve individual health outcomes and the quality of care delivered to patients. As the SoonerCare HMP matures, we realize there are opportunities for blending the practice facilitation and nurse case management activities more closely together. Contractual and state purchasing guidelines have kept us from a rapid cycle change in our HMP structure, but new models that would blend our two current HMP roles capture our interest as we look to future redesign options. Providers indicate that incorporating nurse case management into their practice would save them time and allow them to avoid missed care opportunities. We are working to strengthen the nurse case managers' relationships with the practices until more fundamental changes can be made.

Future directions

The SoonerCare HMP is into the third year of a five-year contract. An independent evaluator, Pacific Health Policy Group, provides an objective review of the program on a yearly basis. Evaluator feedback serves to guide program changes to better meet the needs of our high risk members and their providers.

Similarly, we work to respond to newly developed programs and initiatives, both internal and external. The SoonerCare HMP staff work collaboratively with key parties on current federal initiatives such as the Medicaid EHR (electronic health record) Incentive Program and Section 2703 (health homes) of the Patient Protection and Affordable Care Act. We also work to adapt our processes to support the newly adopted patient-centered medical home (PCMH) payment structure and development of health access networks (HAN) within the Oklahoma SoonerCare program. These developing programs provide unique opportunities for adaptation and continued growth of the SoonerCare Health Management Program.

Reference

Wagner, E.H. (1998) Chronic disease management: what will it take to improve care for chronic illness? *Effective Clinical Practice*, 1(1): 2–4.

Section 5

Practice change

Chapter 23

Introduction: practice change fellows initiatives

Eric A. Coleman and Nancy Whitelaw

Program overview

Our nation's health delivery system frequently does not meet the unique needs of older adults. Wide gaps remain between evidence-based approaches, nationally recognized best practices, and how care is currently delivered for many conditions that disproportionately affect this population. Strong leadership is needed to ensure that promising evidence-based innovations are widely adopted to improve health and functional outcomes in older adults.

The Practice Change Fellows program is designed to expand the number of health care leaders who can effectively promote high-quality care to older adults in a wide range of health and health care organizations. These leaders are essential for overcoming barriers and building the business case for geriatric care in health plans, hospitals, nursing homes, home care agencies, outpatient physician practices, and community-based organizations. Building a cadre of health care champions who possess the essential leadership skills and understanding of promising innovations in care for older adults will ensure that this country will be prepared to meet the challenges of an expanding aged population.

Fellows receive $90,000 to support their projects over the two-year program. The Fellow's home institution is expected to make a $45,000 monetary or in-kind contribution, recognizing that the Fellows' career development and project add value to their respective organizations. The Practice Change Fellows program is made possible by the generous support of The Atlantic Philanthropies and The John A. Hartford Foundation.

Intended outcomes

The short-term goal of this program is to transform health care professionals working within the broadly defined delivery system into effective agents of change. These leaders will have strong management skills and content expertise to effectuate practice improvement for older adults within their organizations and communities and across the nation. The long-term goal is to establish a vigorous network of health care practice change specialists with the capacity to influence care for this population on a national scale.

Comprehensive Care Coordination for Chronically Ill Adults, First Edition. Edited by Cheryl Schraeder and Paul Shelton.
© 2011 John Wiley & Sons, Inc. Published 2011 by John Wiley & Sons, Inc.

Program eligibility

Nurses, physicians, and social workers are eligible to apply. Applicants must hold a leadership role in a health care delivery organization, health-related institution, or community-based organization with direct responsibility for geriatric services or aging-related programs. Within this context, the Practice Change Fellows program welcomes applications from professionals working in the broadly defined field of geriatric services and aging-related programs.

Program activities

Three primary program activities promote Practice Change Fellows' leadership development. Over the two-year fellowship, these include: the completion of a project aimed at implementing a new geriatric program or service line; the execution of a customized leadership development learning contract; and active engagement at tri-annual national meetings.

Project

Through participation in this two-year program, Practice Change Fellows further refine their leadership skills through completion of a project aimed at integrating a new geriatric program or service line into their organization. Recognizing that leadership lessons are not learned in a vacuum, the project provides a vehicle for obtaining the requisite skills Fellows need to lead cultural and organizational change. In some cases, the project represents a new approach to improving care of older adults while in other cases the project focuses on how to translate established, or proven, evidence-based models into practice. The project is embedded in the daily workflow of the Fellow's responsibilities and is therefore not an "add-on." At the time the project is initiated, Fellows are expected to demonstrate insight into what would be required at their home institution to sustain the project after completion of their two-year participation in the Practice Change Fellows program. While the projects vary, many of them have focused on care coordination for the chronically ill elderly. For a list of projects see the organization's website (www.practicechangefellows.org).

Learning Contract

With the support of their home-organization supervisor, assigned program Mentor, and the mentoring Pod, Fellows create and execute a customized formal learning contract that articulates specific goals for the two-year Practice Change Fellows program and describes immediate plans for effectuating programmatic change within the home organization to support older adults. The learning contract identifies particular leadership skills Fellows plan to develop during their participation in the program, and describes how the conduct and completion of their project will contribute to development of these skills. Finally, the learning contract details opportunities for how these newly developed skills will be applied toward improving care to older adults more broadly. By the end of the two years, Fellows will be expected to articulate a vision for what they hope to accomplish in the upcoming five years and the steps necessary to achieve this vision within their home organizations.

Tri-Annual Meetings

Practice Change Fellows attend three highly interactive national meetings each year (the tri-annual meetings). Attended by Fellows, the National Advisory Board, and select national experts in practice change in the areas of geriatric care delivery and aging-related programs, the meetings are founded on the premise that every attendee is both a teacher and a learner. Fellows have the opportunity to receive input on their projects through "hands-on," case-based discussions complemented by group problem-solving activities. Fellows further gain exposure to evidence-based models of practice improvement and emerging changes in national health policy.

Fellows participate in skill-building seminars led by national experts who encourage active learning and peer-to-peer problem solving. The core six competencies addressed in these seminars include: selecting and measuring compelling outcomes for program sustainability; presenting a compelling business case; building high-performing teams; fostering cross-setting collaboration; leading cultural change; and negotiating conflict.

During each of the tri-annual meetings, Fellows receive mentoring from their assigned Mentor (a member of the National Advisory Board) and from participation in mentoring Pods. Composed of three to four Fellows and their assigned Mentors, as well as other leaders from the National Advisory Board, the Pod provides an interactive group approach to mentoring and shared learning that complements the more traditional one-to-one mentor-mentee relationship. The Pod concept offers a number of tangible benefits: it provides Fellows with a wider base of expertise and interdisciplinary perspectives, it insulates against Mentor attrition, and it allows more senior participants to model mentoring behavior to junior participants.

Between the tri-annual meetings, the Pods have regularly scheduled conference calls to further foster peer-to-peer learning and ensure that Fellows are receiving the support they need to successfully conduct their projects and develop their leadership skills.

Practice meets policy

The program recognizes that it plays a unique and important role at the interface between health care policy and health care practice. Whether through legislative or regulatory approaches, delivery system reform cannot be successful without the experience, expertise, and voice of practice leaders. Based upon successful leadership experiences, the Practice Change Fellows National Advisory Board, Fellows, and National Program Office understand how to implement a patient-centered medical home, an accountable care organization, a bundled-payment approach, and strategies to realize the potential of health information technology. For more additional information, application procedures, and timelines, and for a variety of web-related aging resources, see the Practice Change Fellows web site.

Suggested reading

The Atlantic Philanthropies web site is available at: http://www.atlanticphilanthropies.org.
The John A. Hartford Foundation web site is available at: http://www.jhartfound.org.
The Practice Change Fellows web site is available at: http://www.practicechangefellows.org.

Chapter 24

Interdisciplinary care of chronically ill adults: communities of care for people living with congestive heart failure in the rural setting

Lee Greer

Introduction

Medical management of people living with chronic illnesses in rural communities presents unique challenges for health care providers. The prevalence rates of chronic illnesses are often higher in rural counties, and treatment services indicated by evidence-based standards of care are less readily available. The considerable distances patients may need to travel to visit regional health care facilities, the limited scope of medical services often available in rural communities, the lower socioeconomic status of many rural residents, and the presence of serious co-morbid medical conditions, such as obesity and hypertension, are among the factors that place rural residents with chronic illnesses at greater risk for medical complications and adverse outcomes.

To address barriers to effective medical management of chronic illness in rural communities, North Mississippi Medical Clinics, Inc.(NMMCI), a regional network of more than 30 primary and specialty clinics, launched a pilot project designed to extend the continuum of care available to rural residents diagnosed with congestive heart failure (CHF). In this chapter, we describe the services and preliminary outcomes of our project, Communities of Care for CHF.

Background

On most surveys of general health status, residents of Mississippi rank at or very near the bottom (United Health Foundation 2009; The Commonwealth Fund 2009). In NMMCI's service area, the prevalence and age-adjusted mortality rates for most chronic illnesses exceed statistics reported for the nation, as well as the State of Mississippi (Mississippi State Department of Health 2007; University of Wisconsin Population Health Institute 2010).

Comprehensive Care Coordination for Chronically Ill Adults, First Edition. Edited by Cheryl Schraeder and Paul Shelton.
© 2011 John Wiley & Sons, Inc. Published 2011 by John Wiley & Sons, Inc.

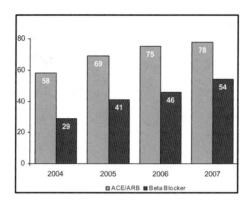

	2004	2005	2006	2007
ACE/ARB	58	69	75	78
Beta Blocker	29	41	46	54

Figure 24.1   Congestive Heart Failure, Evidence of Care

North Mississippi Health Services, the parent system of NMMCI, is one of the largest rural health systems in the United States. Approximately 61% of the residents of 24 counties in northeastern Mississippi seek high quality, cost effective health care services at one of the six hospitals and 34 clinics that comprise the health system. On average, 800 patients diagnosed with CHF are discharged annually from the health system's community hospitals, and more than 2,900 patients diagnosed with CHF are active NMMCI patients. Due to their complex medical conditions and limited opportunities to learn disease management skills, these patients are at increased risk for complications and readmission to the health system's hospitals.

One of the most formidable challenges for NMMCI's rural health care providers has been maximizing adherence to evidence-based standards of care for medical management of CHF. At the rural clinics, NMMCI's information technology system generates electronic prompts for clinicians to review patients' treatment plans for compliance with standards of care. Prior to project implementation, this technology, which was only operational at the point of care, yielded modest but inadequate gains in adherence to treatment guidelines for the use of angiotensin converting enzyme inhibitors (ACE), angiotensin II receptor blockers (ARB) and beta blockers (Figure 24.1).

Moreover, because NMMCI's rural clinics' capabilities do not afford routine access to specialized standards of care for CHF, indicated procedures, such as echocardiograms, were not always completed. In response to this issue, NMMCI clinicians reviewed the peer-reviewed literature to develop plans to expand and strengthen the continuum of care offered to patients living with CHF in rural communities.

Project plan

The Chronic Care Model (CCM) served as a template for the Communities of Care for CHF initiative (Bodenheimer *et al.* 2002a; Bodenheimer *et al.* 2002b). The project also embodied key elements of care transition models. Drawing from the exciting work of Dr. Eric Coleman, a multidisciplinary team was formed to improve transitions across NMHS' delivery system (Coleman *et al.* 2006).

Communities of Care for CHF focused on the clinic system's most medically vulnerable cohort of patients diagnosed with CHF, those aged over 65 years. Programming was implemented at 22 NMMCI clinics, and the specific aims were:

- To improve compliance with American College of Cardiology/American Heart Association standards of care for CHF (2005).
- To improve clinical outcomes of rural patients through increased adherence to indicated medications.
- To increase knowledge and improve self-care skills of patients.
- To achieve a reduction from 21% to 15% in the 30-day all-cause readmission rate for CHF patients discharged from this hospital.

To achieve these aims, existing services were intensified, and new services were added at critical junctures in the care process.

Communities of Care for CHF relied heavily on development of a more robust clinical information system capable of monitoring patients closely and generating alerts to non-adherence beyond point-of-care interactions. A registry was created containing the names and contact information for clinic patients diagnosed with CHF and was populated with data specific to the standards of care (use of ACEs, ARBs, and beta blockers; echocardiogram results; and so on). The registry was also infused with health information technology capabilities that enabled the NMMCI performance improvement data analyst to query databases to monitor adherence to specific standards of care, hospital readmissions within the past 30 days, or emergency department (ED) visits for CHF-related issues.

Effort was also directed toward designing more informative discharge summary forms to distribute to CHF patients following their clinic visits. The redesigned CHF-specific discharge summaries enabled patients to review vital sign values; changes made in prescription medications; reminders regarding diets, physical activities, and check-up visits; and other individualized recommendations.

The continuum of care for rural patients with CHF was also made more robust by introducing specialized programming at clinic sites for the highest risk patients. Each month, the CHF disease registry was queried to identify patients non-adherent to standards of care; heavy utilizers of hospital, clinic, and ED services for CHF-related issues; and/or those with high-risk health indicators, such as elevated blood pressure, or high-risk health behaviors, such as smoking. In addition, individual providers in the community were contacted for assistance in identifying vulnerable patients. These patients received invitations to attend "CHF Days" at their local clinics, and clinic staff followed up with telephone calls to urge them to attend.

For each CHF Day event, an outcomes manager, CHF nurse educator, pharmacist, and cardiology technician traveled from the health system's headquarters in Tupelo to spend the day at the rural clinics. The team reviewed clinic patients' treatment plans and offered services consistent with standards-based care, such as echocardiograms, pneumonia vaccinations, nutrition counseling, and medication reviews. The pharmacist reviewed laboratory values and current medication regimens and made recommendations for changes in medications, diet, and/or behavior.

In collaboration with the patient's primary care provider, recommendations formulated by the pharmacist and the CHF nurse educator during CHF Day events were synthesized into individualized treatment plans that were reviewed with patients during their clinic visits. As part of CHF Days, high-risk patients attended educational programs that lasted 30 to 45 minutes. Content focused on empowering patients to participate in the management of their chronic illness. Prior to leaving the clinic, high-risk patients were scheduled for check-ups with clinic physicians at three months or sooner, depending upon their medical status.

Registered nurses (RNs) employed by NurseLink, the health system's call center that performs nursing triage services, served as the CHF Care Transitions Team's outcomes and case managers. These RNs reviewed discharge records daily to identify patients diagnosed with CHF who were released from one of the health system's hospitals to their next health care delivery site: home, home with home health, or assisted living facility. Within 48 hours of discharge, an RN contacted each discharged patient to reconcile medications, begin patient education, and confirm follow-up appointments. When discrepancies were noted in medications or no follow-up appointments were scheduled, CHF Care Transitions Team members urged patients to contact their primary care providers, gently "coaching" them to manage their own health issues. Home visits were scheduled for CHF patients for whom extended services were indicated, such as patients who were unable to name their medications over the telephone.

Preliminary results

A total of 70 clinic patients participated in NMMCI's Communities of Care CHF Days pilot project and all clinic patients with CHF who were discharged from hospitals in the NMHS health system were entered into the care transitions component of the initiative. The patient registry was used to track alignment with standards-based care and to monitor clinical outcomes. To measure project impact, patient data collected during the six months preceding CHF Day events were compared with data recorded six months post participation in CHF Day events. Although all participants have not yet completed the six-month follow-up phase, preliminary results are very promising (Figure 24.2).

To summarize the data in Figure 24.2:

- 98% of the rural patients who attended a CHF Day event are currently on ACE/ARBs as part of their treatment regimens or contraindications for these interventions are now documented in their medical records compared to 86% of NMMCI clinic patients that did not participate in CHF Days; this is a statistically significant difference. Prior to introduction of the Communities of Care transition model in 2007, only 78 percent of rural clinic patients were on ACE/ARB (see Figure 24.1).

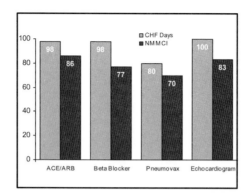

	ACE/ARB	Beta Blocker	Pneumovax	Echocardiogram
CHF Days	98	98	80	100
NMMCI	86	77	70	83

Figure 24.2   CHF Days Results

- 98% of the rural patients who attended a CHF Day event are currently on beta blockers or contraindications for this intervention are now documented in patients' medical records as compared to 77% of NMMCI patients who did not attend CHF Days, also a statistically significant finding. In 2007, only 54% of clinic patients were taking beta blockers.
- Pneumonia vaccine was administered as indicated to 80% of patients who attended a CHF Day. When compared to pneumovax administration for general CHF clinic patients (70%), the increase failed to achieve statistical significance.
- Echocardiograms were completed on 100% of patients who attended CHF Days. When compared with echocardiograms among general clinic patients with CHF (83%), a statistically significant finding was noted between the two cohorts.

No significant changes were achieved in reducing the rate of smoking among rural patients with CHF, or in reducing blood pressure readings. Forty-four percent of project participants reported histories of smoking. The number of active smokers (10%) remained constant during the project period. The Care Transitions Team attributes this finding in part to inadequate efforts to encourage smokers to quit, and failure to include access to smoking cessation services as part of the project plan.

Average blood pressure readings decreased only slightly during the pilot project. At baseline, the mean systolic blood pressure reading was 126, and the median diastolic blood pressure reading was 71. For 39 patients on whom follow-up data on blood pressure was collected and recorded six months post-CHF Day participation, both systolic and diastolic mean blood pressure decreased by just 1.8 mmHG (Figure 24.3). While primary care providers were advised to titrate medications for patients with elevated blood pressure readings, the Care Transitions Team did not monitor whether these recommendations were heeded.

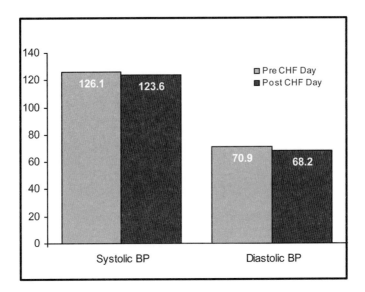

	Systolic BP	Diastolic BP
Pre CHF Day	126.1	70.9
Post CHF Day	123.6	68.2

Figure 24.3   CHF Days Hospital Utilization

Data was also collected on the hospitalization rates for patients six months post their participation in CHF Day events (Figure 24.4). In the six months prior to attending CHF Days, 20 hospitalizations were documented among the 70 project participants. Nine hospitalizations were recorded for the 41 patients who were six months post-CHF Day participation. When six-month follow-up data is available on all study participants, we will have a much better understanding of the impact of the program on rates of hospitalization. However, the number of ED visits increased to 11 post-CHF Day participation as compared to a total of six visits in the six months prior to CHF Days. None of these visits were for CHF-related issues.

On an indicator of great interest to the Centers for Medicare & Medicaid Services, the 30-day all cause system-wide hospital readmission rate for rural clinic patients with CHF decreased from 21.4% to 15.6%. Among the small sample of participants hospitalized at NMMC – Iuka, dramatic reductions were noted from 22.6% to 7.8% (Figure 24.5).

Future plans

The Communities of Care initiative piloted for people living with CHF in rural areas yielded promising results. The project design does not enable identification of the specific factors that resulted in measurable improvements, but in combination, the

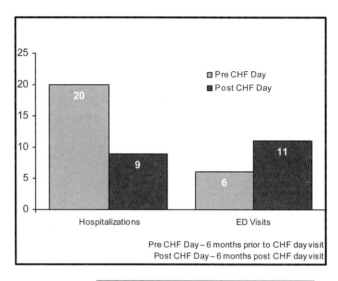

	Hospitalizations	ED Visits
Pre CHF Day	20	6
Post CHF Day	9	11

Figure 24.4 CHF Days Blood Pressure

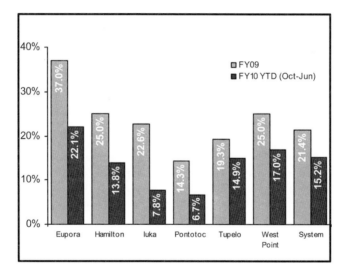

	FY09	FY10 YTD (Oct–Jun)
Eupora	37.0%	22.1%
Hamilton	25.0%	13.8%
Iuka	22.6%	7.8%
Pontotoc	14.3%	6.7%
Tupelo	19.3%	14.9%
West Point	25.0%	17.0%
System	21.4%	15.2%

Figure 24.5 CHF 30-Day Readmission Rates

following activities served to improve the general health status of rural patients living with CHF:

- Establishment of a patient registry capable of generating CHF-specific alerts and tracking standards-based care over time.
- Distributing more informative discharge summaries to educate patients and their families.
- Offering specialized programming (CHF Day events) and services (for example, medication consultations, pneumovax, echocardiograms) for the highest-risk patients.
- Creating and operating a CHF Care Transitions Team to facilitate transitions from hospitals to other care settings.

NMMCI intends to continue hosting CHF Days at rural health clinics. Lessons learned from the pilot are being used to guide development of similar programming tailored to address the medical needs of rural residents living with asthma and diabetes.

References

American College of Cardiology/American Heart Association. (2005) ACC/AHA 2005 guideline update for diagnosis and management of chronic heart failure in the adult. *Circulation*, 112, e154–e235.

Bodenheimer, T., Wagner, E.H., & Grumbach, K. (2002a) Improving primary care for patients with chronic illness. *Journal of the American Medical Association*, 288, 1775–1779.

Bodenheimer, T., Wagner, E.H., & Grumbach, K. (2002b) Improving primary care for patients with chronic illness: the chronic care model, part 2. *Journal of the American Medical Association*, 288, 1909–1914.

Coleman, E.A., Parry, C., Chalmers, S., *et al.* (2006) The care transitions intervention: results of a randomized controlled trial. *Archives of Internal Medicine*, 166, 1822–1828.

The Commonwealth Fund. (2009) *The Commonwealth Fund State Report Card.* The Commonwealth Fund, New York, NY. Retrieved from http://www.commonwealthfund.org/Maps-and-Data/State-Scorecard-2009.aspx.

Mississippi State Department of Health. (2007) *County Health Profiles.* Mississippi State Department of Health, Jackson, MS. Retrieved from http://www.msdh.state.ms.us/msdhsite/_static/31,0,211.html.

United Health Foundation. (2009) *America's Health Rankings.* United Health Foundation, Minnetonka, MN. Retrieved from http://www.americashealthrankings.org/yearcompare/2008/2009/MS.aspx.

University of Wisconsin Population Health Institute. (2010) *County Health Rankings.* University of Wisconsin Population Health Institute, Madison, WI. Retrieved from http://www.counthealthrankings.org/mississippi.

Chapter 25

Collaborative care treatment of late-life depression: development of a depression support service

Eran D. Metzger

Introduction

This chapter describes the implementation of a collaborative care model of depression treatment for long-term care residents of the Hebrew Rehabilitation Center, a chronic care hospital in Boston, Massachusetts. Experience gained from the project, which was supported in part by a grant from the Practice Change Fellows Program, led to both improved depression care at the parent organization and to dissemination of the model at local and statewide levels.

Background

At the time of inception of the project, Hebrew Rehabilitation Center (HRC), the flagship facility of Hebrew SeniorLife (HSL), was a 700-bed chronic care hospital providing long term care (LTC), sub-acute skilled nursing care, and long-term acute care. The LTC population had an average age of 88 years and was 78% female; 98% of residents were Medicaid recipients and 20% were Russian immigrants. Data available from computerized medical records and the Minimum Data Set (MDS) for 2007 indicated that approximately 51% had symptoms of depression and 20% were on antidepressant medications. Approximately 14% were dependent for all activities of daily living; 58% of patients had a diagnosis of dementia, with 87% of these in the moderate to severe stage. Thus, the HRC population represented a highly vulnerable cohort characterized by a high prevalence of depression, dementia, and frailty.

As is the case in other LTC institutions, much of the first-line treatment of depression at HRC was being managed by primary care geriatricians. Two staff psychiatrists and a psychologist were available for consultation, however they were also responsible for consultation at five other affiliated sites including two outpatient clinics, a 300-member continuing care retirement community, and sub-acute and medical acute care units at HRC. The imminent opening of two additional Hebrew SeniorLife sites, a 311-member

Comprehensive Care Coordination for Chronically Ill Adults, First Edition. Edited by Cheryl Schraeder and Paul Shelton.
© 2011 John Wiley & Sons, Inc. Published 2011 by John Wiley & Sons, Inc.

continuing care retirement community and a primary care practice site in low-income housing, was about to expand the total patient population to approximately 2,000. The psychiatrists' efforts were frequently concentrated on the acute and sub-acute units; consequently, follow-up for LTC patients after the initial consultation was inconsistent. Primary care physicians' ability to provide focused and up-to-date mental health care was limited by caseload and fiscal productivity constraints. With regard to allied staff, unit nurses and social workers had many competing tasks, limiting their abilities to monitor patients' mood and provide feedback to the primary care provider. Finally, there was no program in place to provide psychiatric education to the medical staff, to ensure compliance with psychiatry practice guidelines, or to track an individual patient's response to treatment.

The high rate of depression symptomatology at HRC is consistent with national figures. While the prevalence of depression in community-dwelling elderly is comparable to that of other age groups (Byers *et al.* 2010), it increases with presence of medical illness and need for long-term care. Approximately 10% of primary care patients and 15% to 20% of LTC residents have major depression, the most severe form of depressive illness (Parmelee *et al.* 1992). Beyond its direct effects on quality of life, depression is a risk factor for increased mortality and disability. Suicide is closely linked with depression, and the rate for white males 85 years and older is six times that of the general population (Conwell *et al.* 2000). Depression independently predicts mortality in cardiac patients (Bush *et al.* 2001) and increases the use of health care resources (Luber *et al.* 2001).

Although there has been progress in screening for depression in primary care, there remain obstacles to appropriate diagnosis, treatment, and follow-up. These obstacles include time constraints, misconceptions among primary care providers and patients about the nature of depression, and lack of resources for monitoring patients' compliance and response to treatment. Programs focusing only on increasing screening for depression or on educating primary care providers have yielded disappointing results (Schade *et al.* 1998; Ziffra & Friedman 2006). Consequently, The U.S. Preventative Services Task Force added to its previous recommendations the stipulation that depression screening should be offered in primary care settings "that have systems in place to assure accurate diagnosis, effective treatment and follow-up" (Palmer & Coyne 2003; U.S. Preventative Services Task Force 2002).

Program design

The goal of the program was to create the HRC Depression Support Service, which would provide the HRC primary care geriatricians the resources and support they needed to effectively treat depression without increased dependence on consultations by psychiatrists. An environmental scan of previously developed programs for collaborative care of depression identified reviews of a number of models which had been rigorously studied and shown to be effective (Gilbody *et al.* 2006; Oxman *et al.* 2003). A review of four "third generation" models by Oxman and colleagues highlights the important role played by the depression *care manager* (Oxman *et al.* 2003). Similar to care coordination in programs for other medical conditions (such as congestive heart failure, diabetes mellitus), the depression care manager maintains frequent contact with the patient, provides patient education, and gives feedback to the primary care physician or nurse practitioner. While the HRC program borrowed from several of these models, the program was modeled most closely after Seattle-based Improving Mood - Promoting Access to Collaborative Treatment (IMPACT). Designed for implementation in the primary care office setting, IMPACT has been shown in a large randomized controlled trial to be effective across diverse practice settings and to be cost-effective (Unutzer *et al.* 2002; Katon *et al.* 2005). The HRC Depression Support Service was tailored to meet the needs of the long-term care environment while maintaining fidelity to the IMPACT design.

Staffing structure

As mentioned above, the key innovation adopted from IMPACT and other collaborative care programs was the depression care manager. At HRC, the position of the psychologist on staff was expanded to allow her to assume this role. Her responsibilities include: (1) Intake assessment after a consultation request is received by the primary care provider; (2) Provides patient psychoeducation, elicits patient preferences with regard to medication and psychotherapy' and formulates a treatment plan; (3) Initiation of short-term psychotherapy when clinically appropriate; (4) Weekly follow-up sessions with the patient for monitoring treatment adherence, response to treatment, and for continuing psychotherapy; (5) Documenting treatment response; (6) Weekly supervision with the psychiatrist to review cases being followed; and (7) Communication back to the geriatrician including response to treatment and recommendations for medication changes.

Two features of the model deserve emphasis. First, as illustrated in the collaborative care schema (Figure 25.1), the primary care geriatricians continue to be the clinicians responsible for prescribing and continuing the antidepressant medication, with ongoing support and feedback from the Depression Support Service. Second is the importance of the depression care manager's role in providing psychoeducation and eliciting patient preferences at the outset of treatment. Both activities, which may be overlooked in primary care practices not utilizing a depression care manager, have been shown to affect positively patient adherence and outcome (Gum *et al.* 2006; Proctor *et al.* 2008; Raue *et al.* 2009; Clever *et al.* 2006).

Resources

A collection of resources, often referred to as the depression "toolkit," was assembled for use in the HRC Depression Support Service.

Depression screening

During the initial rollout of the Depression Support Service, all of the HRC residents were being assessed for depression via the MDS, administered by nursing staff quarterly. While there was reason to believe that the MDS depression rating scale was not the optimal instrument for identifying depression (Anderson *et al.* 2003), staffing constraints did not permit administering to all residents one of the preferred screening instruments such as the Geriatric Depression Scale or the Patient Health Questionnaire (PHQ) (Snowden *et al.*

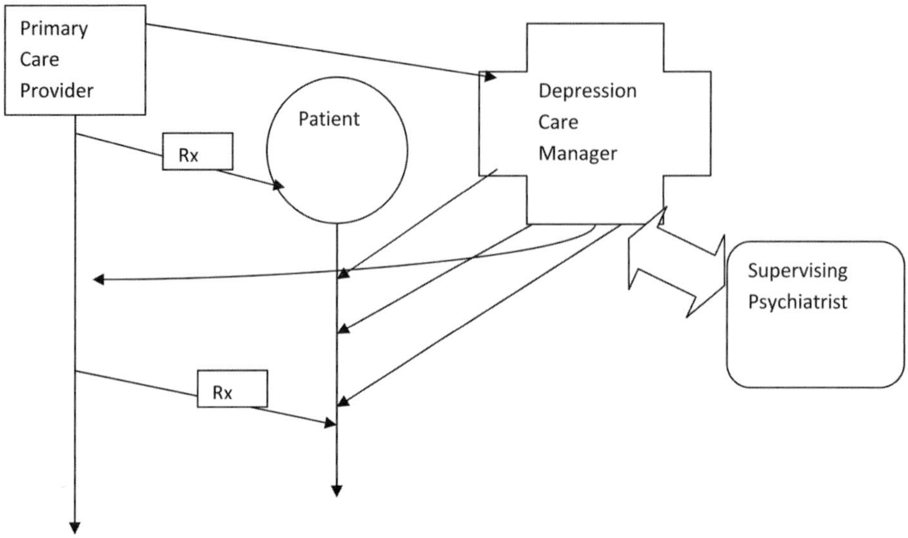

Figure 25.1   Flowchart for the Collaborative Care Model. The primary care provider makes a referral to the depression care manager who begins to meet with the patient regularly. The depression care manager receives supervision from the psychiatrist and provides feedback to the primary care provider, who retains the responsibility for prescribing antidepressant medication.

2009). This issue was resolved with incorporation of the PHQ-9 in the recently released MDS 3.0 (Saliba & Buchanan 2008).

Clinician education modules

Three 30-minute presentations were created and presented to the medical staff during regularly scheduled medical staff meetings. Topics covered included: barriers to identifying depression, updates on late-life depression psychopharmacology, and an introduction to the collaborative care model. Minutes of these meetings were distributed to all of the medical staff with information on how to access the education modules.

Quick reference for antidepressant medications (Table 25.1)

A double-sided laminated guide was provided to each of the geriatricians and posted on each of the nursing units. The reference was adapted and updated from a similar resource developed by the MacArthur Foundation (MacArthur Initiative on Depression and Primary Care).

Psychotherapy

Most depression toolkits include references and forms for initiating and continuing short-term psychotherapy. After relatively brief training, depression care managers without advance degrees can provide effective Problem Solving Therapy or Behavior Activation

Table 25.1 Quick Reference for Antidepressants

Antidepressant	Therapeutic Dose Range (mg/day)	Initial Suggested Dose	Titration Schedule	Advantages	Disadvantages
Serotonin Reuptake Inhibitors (SSRIs)					
Citalopram (Celexa)	10–40	10 mg daily with food.	If no response after 3 wks, increase by 10 mg increments every 2 wks	Shown to be helpful for anxiety (all SSRIs). Low risk of CP450 interactions.	Use with caution if h/o hyponatremia or GI bleed (all SSRIs).
Escitalopram (Lexapro)	5–20	5 mg daily with food.	Increase by 5 mg increments	No advantages over citalopram.	No generic—EXPENSIVE.
Fluoxetine (Prozac)	10–80	10 mg daily for 6 wks.	If no response after 6 wks, increase by 10 mg increments every 4 wks	Helpful for OCD. Long half-life good for poor compliers.	Inhibits cP450 2D6 (e.g. metoprolol, codeine, risperidone, trazadone). Higher incidence of insomnia.
Paroxetine (Paxil)	10–40	10 mg daily with food or HS if found to be sedating.	If no response after 3 wks, increase by 10 mg increments every 2 wks	Can be mildly sedating and helpful for sleep.	Most anticholinergic of SSRIs. Inhibits cP450 2D6. Withdrawal syndrome.
Sertraline (Zoloft)	25–200	25 mg daily with food.	If no response after 3 wks, increase by 25 mg increments every 2 wks	Low risk of cP450 interactions.	
Norepinephrine and Dopamine Reuptake Inhibitor					
Bupropion SR (Wellbutrin)	100–300	100 mg daily.	If no response after 3 wks, increase to 100 mg b.i.d. then increase to 150 mg b.i.d.	May be activating. No risk of GI bleed or hyponatremia. May be better in Parkinson's.	B.i.d. dosing (using SR). May lower seizure threshold. May cause insomnia.

(Continued)

Table 25.1 (*Continued*)

Antidepressant	Therapeutic Dose Range (mg/day)	Initial Suggested Dose	Titration Schedule	Advantages	Disadvantages
Serotonin and Norepinephrine Antagonist					
Mirtazapine (Remeron)	15–45	7.5 mg q HS.	If no response after 3 wks, increase by 7.5 mg increments every 2 wks thereafter.	May stimulate appetite. Sedating. Less sedation at higher dose.	Too sedating for some pts.
Serotonin and Norepinephrine Reuptake Inhibitors					
Duloxetine (Cymbalta)	20–60	20 mg daily.	After 1 wk, increase to 20 mg bid. If no response after 3 wks, increase to 30 mg bid.	Also indicated for neuropathic pain.	No generic—EXPENSIVE.
Venlafaxine (Effexor, Effexor XR)	37.5–225	37.5 mg daily with food.	If no response after 3 wks, increase to 37.5 mg bid. Increase by 37.5 mg increments every 2 wks thereafter.	Also indicated for anxiety disorders. Available as XR for once daily dosing, but this is not generic.	May increase blood pressure.
Norepinephrine Reuptake Inhibitors					
Amitriptyline, Desipramine, Doxepin, Imipramine, Nortriptyline	Depends on individual medication.	Depends on individual medication.	Depends on individual medication.	Effective for neuropathic pain. Serum drug levels guide dosing. Inexpensive.	Anticholinergic. Can exacerbate cardiac conduction problems. Lethal in overdose.
Monoamine Oxidase Inhibitors					
Phenelzine, Tranyl-cypromine, Selegiline	Depends on individual medication.	Depends on individual medication.	Depends on individual medication.	Effective for some refractory cases. Selegiline available as transdermal patch.	Dietary restrictions, risk of hypertensive crisis from tyramine or other medications. Postural hypotension common.

Modified from The MacArthur Initiative on Depression & Primary Care at Dartmouth & Duke Depression Management Tool Kit, pp. 32-34. Used with permission.

Therapy (Arean *et al.* 2008). Because the first depression care manager in the HRC Depression Support Service was a PhD psychologist with experience in short-term therapy, she did not undergo re-training in one of these modalities. With expansion of the program (see below), the next depression care manager, a nurse practitioner without specialized training in psychiatry, underwent live IMPACT training at the University of Washington.

Communication form (Table 25.2)

This form was completed by the depression care manager and the psychiatrist during supervisory sessions and was the primary form of communication between the Depression Support Service and the primary care team. The form was reviewed with other clinical documents (for example laboratory results, consultation reports) by the primary care team during routine rounds. The primary care team had the option of contacting the depression care manager or psychiatrist directly with additional questions.

Depression care manager tracking form (Figure 25.2)

The depression care manager initiated a tracking form for each resident entered into the Depression Support Service. The form assisted the care manager and supervising psychiatrist in tracking the primary care team's response to the care manager's recommendations and tracking the resident's response to treatment.

Measurement

Process and outcome measures were identified to quantify the results of this pilot phase of the Depression Support Service. Process measures were selected to measure the geriatricians' acceptance of the new program and included attendance at the education modules, orders entered requesting the Depression Support Service, and change in orders requesting traditional psychiatric consultation for depression. Outcome measures included changes in residents' scores on the MDS Depression Rating Scale, clinicians' completion of a knowledge and attitude survey on late-life depression, and physician productivity as measured by billing before and after the rollout of the Depression Support Service. For the purposes of this pilot phase, the nursing units caring for residents with end-stage dementia were excluded from measurement, limiting the study population to 6 geriatricians and 252 residents.

The HRC experience, facilitators and barriers

Rollout

The Depression Support Service was introduced to the medical staff with the first education module at a regularly scheduled meeting. The physician-in-chief's championing of the new service and willingness to include the education modules on the agendas of the mandatory medical staff meetings were strong facilitators of the rollout process. Attendance for the medical staff meetings at which the education modules were presented averaged 60%,

Table 25.2 Depression Support Service Communication Form

Date:_____ | Patient Label

Week_____ of Treatment

1. Diagnostic Impression:

_____

_____

_____

2.   Treatment

Antidepressant / dosage	Therapy(s)
	☐ Cognitive Behavioral
	☐ Supportive
	☐ Brief Dynamic
	☐ Other

3. Patient Response to Treatment and Recommendations for Primary Care Physician

_____

_____

_____

Depression Care Manager:_____

Psychiatry:_____

comparable to usual attendance. Completion of the knowledge and attitude survey by the geriatricians was 100%.

Referrals to the depression support service

During the initial 12-month pilot phase, the Depression Support Service received 72 referrals. An order for the new service was added to the menu of the recently adopted

Initial Needs Assessment						Patient Label

Diagnosis(es): _____					Y	N	
_____ _____	Y	N	Creative Arts therapy				
Medication			Recreation therapy				Date:
Psychotherapy			Family therapy				

Treatment Tracker

Week #	1	2	3	4	5	6	Comments
Psychotherapy							
Medication dose change							
Team Meeting							
Creative Arts							
Recreational							
Family							
Status							

(left label: Treatment)

Week #	7	8	9	10	11	12	Comments
Psychotherapy							
Medication dose change							
Team Meeting							
Creative Arts							
Recreational							
Family							
Status							

(left label: Treatment)

Status Codes: I=improved W= worse U=unchanged H=hospitalized T = treatment terminated

Figure 25.2 Depression Care Manager Tracking Form

electronic order entry system, which facilitated clinicians' access to the service. Referrals for consultation from the psychiatrist for depression showed a corresponding decrease for these units, declining from 96 over the course of the previous year to 18 during the support service pilot phase. Review of the requests for traditional psychiatric consultation revealed that a number were because of family request or extenuating circumstances (for example, history of bipolar disorder).

Effect on depression

MDS Depression Rating Scale scores were calculated for all residents on the units studied for the quarter prior to the rollout of the Depression Support Service and the quarter one year into service implementation. For the six units combined, there was a trend toward improvement of depression scores. There was significant improvement in depression scores on one of the units.

Impact on the geriatricians

Medical staff participation in the depression knowledge survey was 100% for both the pre- and post-tests. Mean scores on the primary care provider survey items of *knowledge* of depression and on *confidence* in treating depression did not change significantly during the project period, however the sample size was insufficient to rule out a type II error. A qualitative review of the surveys indicated that: (1) primary care providers believed it was their responsibility to manage depression (100% response); (2) primary care providers had accurate beliefs about how antidepressants work (72%); and (3) providers felt at least "mostly" confident about treating depression (100%). High pre-implementation scores indicated a high baseline level of knowledge about geriatric depression, and the lack of change in the scores indicated a ceiling effect. The primary care physicians in this project were all board certified in geriatrics, which may in part account for their high baseline knowledge of geriatric depression. Being members of a closed medical staff with frequent contact with the psychiatrists may also have contributed to their knowledge and confidence in depression management.

Provider productivity was measured by Medicare Resource Value Units (RVUs) before and after implementation of the Depression Support Service. Total RVUs for the six clinicians decreased from 782 to 637 between the two time periods, but was not statistically significant. This trend toward a decrease in RVUs for the physicians participating in the project was unexpected. However, coincident with the implementation of the Depression Support Service the hospital implemented both a new electronic medical record and a new voice recognition software system for dictating progress notes. Subjective reports from the physicians were that the introduction of both these technologies had significant short-term impact on their productivity. As described previously, more sophisticated studies of collaborative care programs like IMPACT have demonstrated cost effectiveness.

Dissemination: A statewide project

Researchers at Masspro, a healthcare performance improvement organization which serves as the federal subcontractor for the Quality Improvement Organization within Massachusetts, sought ways to decrease the prescription of medications considered to be potentially inappropriate for older patients. Improving the diagnosis and treatment of late-life depression can decrease prescribing of anti-anxiety and antipsychotic medications known to be associated with increased morbidity and mortality in older patients. Masspro has teamed up with HRC staff involved with the HRC Depression Support Service in order to disseminate this model to community health centers across the state. In addition to live presentations, the team has produced 10 informational webinars describing in detail the collaborative care approach to treating late-life depression.

Future directions: An expanding role for collaborative care depression treatment in the HSL system

As described at the outset of this chapter, the HSL system of medical care and housing has continued to grow. Accompanying this growth has been an increased demand for psychiatric services, making the Depression Support Service more relevant than ever. The positive HRC pilot results, in combination with the results of larger studies described previously, have led to acceptance of the model by both hospital administration and the department of medicine and a commitment to expand the service. Financial support from both HSL and a technical implementation package awarded by the Centers for Disease Control and Prevention, the Carter Center, and the University of Washington allowed for a medical nurse practitioner to attend an IMPACT training and begin depression care manager work at HSL's community elder housing sites. As illustrated by the following case, expansion into the outpatient arena has brought new challenges.

Case study

Ms. R an 82-year-old widowed woman, and has resided at the HSL senior housing, Center Communities of Brookline, for three years. She was insured by a Medicare Advantage HMO and became one of the first clients of the HSL outpatient Depression Support Service when her primary care physician referred her for depressed affect, social isolation, and insomnia. She was visited by the nurse practitioner depression care manager and was determined to be an appropriate referral for collaborative care treatment of her depression. Her initial PHQ-9 score was 11/27, consistent with mild depression. A chief psychosocial precipitant to the depression was Ms. R's husband having been diagnosed with Alzheimer's disease. Starting with the first visit, Ms. R began a course of Problem Solving Psychotherapy and a low dose of antidepressant medication. Ms. R began to report subjective benefit from the visits and her PHQ 9 score dropped to 9 after two visits.

Prior to the third visit, Ms. R called the depression care manger to inform her that she would be reducing her visits to monthly. On questioning, Ms. R confessed that the reason behind the change was the HMO mandated $25 co-pay per session, which was prohibitive on her fixed income. Discussions ensued in the business office about the legality and sustainability of waiving co-payments in these instances, with the conclusion that the co-payments would need to be enforced. At follow-up one month later, Ms. R had not completed her prescribed Problem Solving homework for the session and had neglected to refill her antidepressant medication prescription. Her PHQ 9 score had increased to 12. The depression care manager called Ms. R's primary care geriatrician to share her concerns about worsening depression.

In seeking to expand the Depression Support Service, HSL has had to address issues faced by many organizations which seek to sustain a successful collaborative care service after completion of a grant (Bachman *et al.* 2006; Belnap *et al.* 2006). The most frequently encountered issue is funding for the care manager position. HSL's initial care managers were a PhD psychologist and a nurse practitioner. Advantages of utilizing an advance practice clinician in this role included: (1) prior psychiatric training; (2)

ability to at least partially support the position by billing for psychotherapy services when appropriate. Disadvantages of filling additional depression care manager positions with advance practice staff include: (1) lack of availability of advance practice clinicians with geriatrics expertise or interest; (2) higher cost of advance practice clinicians' salaries; and (3) as illustrated by the case above, monetary constraints placed on the patient when the depression care manager bills insurance to help support the position.

Future directions: Support of collaborative care for late-life depression on a national level

Depressive illness is a major public health concern and has been identified by the World Health Organization as one of the leading causes of disability (Pan American Health Organization). In the United States alone, direct and indirect costs of depression are estimated at $83 billion (Greenberg *et al.* 2003). In patients with physical illness, co-morbid depression increases healthcare service utilization by as much as 50% (Luber *et al.* 2001). As the portion of the elderly population continues to increase, the number of geropsychiatric specialists will not keep pace (Bartels 2003). Although collaborative care programs have been proven both clinically efficacious and cost effective for the health care systems responsible for medical and psychiatric care, significant barriers remain which have prevented more widespread dissemination. As described above, foremost among these barriers has been finding funding for the depression care manager position, a key component of the collaborative care model. Recent developments offer hope that coalitions on a statewide level may provide means for overcoming these barriers.

Depression Improvement Across Minnesota, Offering a New Direction (DIAMOND) is a project involving a unique collaboration between medical groups, commercial health plans, and the Minnesota Department of Human Services (Institute for Clinical Systems Improvement 2008). Also based on the IMPACT model of collaborative care treatment of depression, the program utilizes depression care managers and a depression toolkit as described in this chapter. Unique to the DIAMOND program is a new payment system whereby health plans pay a "care management fee" to participating medical groups to cover the expenses of the depression care manager and supervising psychiatrist. Forty-five clinics have been enrolled to date with another 40 scheduled to be enrolled by the end of 2010. DIAMOND's results, which are currently being studied under an NIMH grant, may encourage similar collaborations in other states.

Collaborations between medical groups and payers are also occurring in many states to support the development of the Patient-Centered Medical Home model of primary care. The Medical Home model, a hallmark of which is coordination of care, is ideally suited to support collaborative care treatment of depression. The Patient-Centered Primary Care Collaborative (PCPCC), a national coalition which includes employers, primary care societies, national health plans, and patient groups, lists 17 states with one or more Patient-Centered Medical Home pilots underway (PCPCC 2008). Recognizing the value of such statewide collaboration, the Departments of Health and Human Services and the Centers for Medicare & Medicaid Services (CMS) announced in June 2010 that they would support up to six state demonstration projects of Multi-Payer Advanced Primary Care (MPAPC) practices (CMS 2009).

Barriers to implementation of effective depression treatment for elders can also be addressed by national health care policy which supports the dissemination of this successful intervention. As highlighted by the Institute of Medicine (IOM) report, "Retooling for an Aging America," fee-for-service Medicare, in which the majority of Medicare recipients are enrolled, discourages adoption of collaborative care models because: (1) Statutorily established benefit categories do not cover reimbursement for many of the services provided by the collaborative care model; and (2) Nurses and social workers, ideally suited for the roll of depression care managers, do not qualify for reimbursement (IOM 2008).

Summary

This chapter describes the introduction of a program for coordinated care of depression in the long-term care setting using a collaborative care model adapted from IMPACT. The program's successful pilot has led to institutional support of the expansion of the program to other practice sites in the organization as well as to support from the state's Medicare Quality Improvement contractor to disseminate the model to community health centers across the state. Barriers to adoption of the collaborative care model are chiefly around funding for the depression care manager and supervising psychiatrist roles. Research is currently underway to determine if promising statewide collaborations between medical practices and payers will overcome these barriers and lead to nationwide implementation of this effective means for treating depression.

References

Anderson, R.L., Buckwalter, K.C., Buchanan, R.J., *et al.* (2003) Validity and reliability of the Minimum Data Set Depression Rating Scale (MDSDRS) for older adults in nursing homes. *Age and Ageing*, 32, 435–438.

Arean, P., Hegel, M., Vannoy, S., *et al.* (2008) The effectiveness of problem solving therapy for older primary care patients with depression: results from the IMPACT project. *The Gerontologist*, 48, 311–323.

Bachman, J., Pincus, H.A., Houtsinger, J.K., *et al.* (2006) Funding mechanisms for depression care management: opportunities and challenges. *General Hospital Psychiatry*, 28, 278–288.

Bartels, S.J. (2003) Improving the system of care for older adults with mental illness in the United States. Findings and recommendations for the President's New Freedom Commission on Mental Health. *American Journal of Geriatric Psychiatry*, 11, 486–496.

Belnap, B.H., Kuebler, J., Upshur, C., *et al.* (2006) Challenges of implementing depression care management in the primary care setting. *Administration and Policy in Mental Health and Mental Health Services Research*, 33(1), 65–75.

Bush, D.E., Ziegeistein, R.C., Tayback, M., *et al.* (2001) Even minimal symptoms of depression increase mortality risk after acute myocardial infarction. *American Journal of Cardiology*, 88, 337–341.

Byers, A.L., Yaffe, K., Covinsky, K.E., *et al.* (2010) High occurrence of mood and anxiety disorders among older adults: The National Comorbidity Survey replication. *Archives of General Psychiatry*, 67, 489–496.

Centers for Medicare & Medicaid Services. (2009) *Multi-payer Advanced Primary Care Practice (MAPCP) Demonstration Fact Sheet.* Retrieved from http://www.cms.hhs.gov/DemoProjectsEvalRpts/MD/itemdetail.asp?itemID=CMS1230016.

Clever, S.L., Ford, D.E., Rubenstein, L.V., *et al.* (2006) Primary care patients' involvement in decision-making is associated with improvement in depression. *Medical Care,* 44, 398–405.

Conwell, Y., Lyness, J.M., & Duberstein, P. (2000) Completed suicide among older patients in primary care practices: a controlled study. *Journal of the American Geriatrics Society,* 48(1): 23–29.

Gilbody, S., Bower, P., Fletcher, J., *et al.* (2006). Collaborative care for depression: a cumulative meta-analysis and review of longer-term outcomes. *Archives of Internal Medicine,* 166, 2314–2320.

Greenberg, P.E., Kessler, R.C., Birnbaum, H.G., *et al.* (2003) The economic burden of depression in the United States: how did it change between 1990 and 2000? *Journal of Clinical Psychiatry,* 64, 1465–1475.

Gum, A.M., Arean, P.A., Hunkeler, E., *et al.* (2006) Depression treatment preferences in older primary care patients. *The Gerontologist,* 46(1), 14–22.

Institute for Clinical Systems Improvement. (2008) *Depression Improvement Across Minnesota, Offering a New Direction.* Institute for Clinical Systems Improvement, Minneapolis, MN. Retrieved from http://www.icis.org/health_care_redesign/diamond_35953/.

Institute of Medicine on the Future of Health Care Workforce for Older Americans. (2008) *Retooling for an Aging America: Building the Health Care Workforce.* National Academies Press, Washington, DC.

Katon, W.J., Schoenbaum, M., Fan, M., *et al.* (2005) Cost-effectiveness of improving primary care treatment of late-life depression. *Archives of General Psychiatry,* 62, 1313–1320.

Luber, M.P., Meyers, B.S., Williams-Russo, P.G., *et al.* (2001) Depression and service utilization in elderly primary care patients. *American Journal of Geriatric Psychiatry,* 9, 562–571.

MacArthur Initiative on Depression and Primary Care. Resources for Clinicians. Retrieved from http://www.depression-primarycare.org/clinicians/toolkits.

Oxman, T.E., Dietrich, A.J., & Schulberg, H.C. (2003) The depression care manager and mental health specialist as collaborators within primary care. *American Journal of Geriatric Psychiatry,* 11, 507–516.

Palmer, S.C., & Coyne, J.C. (2003) Screening for depression in medical care: pitfalls, alternatives, and revised priorities. *Journal of Psychosomatic Research,* 54, 279–287.

Pan American Health Organization. *144th Session of the Executive Committee, Pan American Health Organization, World Health Organization.* Retrieved from www.http://new.paho.org.

Parmelee, P.A., Katz, I.R., & Lawton, M.P. (1992) Incidence of depression in long-term care settings. *Journal of Gerontology: Medical Sciences,* 47, M189–196.

Patient-Centered Primary Care Collaborative. (2008) *Patient Centered Medical Home: Building Evidence and Momentum.* Retrieved from http://www.pcpcc.net/content/pcpcc_pilot_report.pdf.

Proctor, E.K., Hasche, L., Morrow-Howell, N., *et al.* (2008) Perceptions about competing psychosocial problems and treatment priorities among older adults with depression. *Psychiatric Services,* 59, 670–675.

Raue, P.J., Schulberg, H.C., Heo, M., *et al.* (2009) Patient's depression treatment preferences and initiation, adherence, and outcome: a randomized primary care study. *Psychiatric Services,* 60, 337–343.

Saliba, D., & Buchanan, J. (2008) *Development and Validation of a Revised Nursing Home Assessment Tool: MDS 3.0.* Retrieved from http://www.cms.hhs.gov/NursingHomeQualityInits/Downloads/MDS30FinalReport.pdf.

Schade, C.P., Jones, E.R., & Wittlin, B.J. (1998) A ten-year review of the validity and clinical utility of depression screening. *Psychiatric Services*, 49, 55–61.

Snowden, M.B., Steinman, L., Frederick, J., *et al.* (2009) Screening for depression in older adults: recommended instruments and consideration for community-based practice. *Clinical Geriatrics*, 17(9), 26–31.

U.S. Preventative Services Task Force. (2002) Screening for depression: recommendations and rationale. *Annals of Internal Medicine*, 136, 760–764.

Unutzer, J., Daton, W., Callahan, C.M., *et al.* (2002) Collaborative care management of late-life depression in the primary care setting: a randomized control trial. *Journal of the American Management Association*, 288, 2836–2846.

Ziffra, M.S., & Friedman, R.S. (2006) To screen or not to screen: is that the question? Improving the outcomes of depression in primary care. *Journal of Clinical Outcomes Management*, 13, 562–571.

Chapter 26

Geriatric Telemedicine: supporting interdisciplinary care

Daniel A. Reece

Introduction

Although most communities have inadequate access to geriatric medical specialists, the problem is particularly acute in rural communities. Many of these communities have a high percentage of older adults. Older adults who would benefit from a comprehensive geriatric assessment are likely to be experiencing physical and mental limitations that make traveling for medical services especially burdensome.

Geriatric interdisciplinary teams have been found to be effective in delivering high quality, evidence-based care, with positive outcomes on patients' functioning and quality of life (Stock *et al.* 2008). These teams provide comprehensive, coordinated care in partnership with patients, caregivers, and other service organizations. The team addresses a broad range of factors that can affect patients' health, including social and emotional issues. Teams often comprise a geriatric physician, an advanced practice geriatric nurse, a pharmacist, and a social worker. Other professionals might participate on an ad hoc basis (for example, physical therapists, dieticians, and chaplains) (Stock *et al.* 2004). Rural communities may have some components of an interdisciplinary team, but usually do not have a geriatrician.

Telemedicine solutions

Telemedicine is the use of medical information exchanged from one site to another via electronic communications to improve patients' health status (American Telemedicine Association [ATA]). There are multiple categories of telemedicine services, including specialist provider to provider consultations; patient assessments via live interactive audio and video; and asynchronous store & forward (such as radiology reads and remote patient monitoring). The standard terminology refers to the patient's location as the "Originating Site" and the provider's location as the "Distant Site."

Telemedicine is now provided in all 50 states and is expected to comprise 15% of all health care by 2015 (ATA). Live interactive audio-video conferencing has been demonstrated to be effective in providing a variety of clinical services, including

Comprehensive Care Coordination for Chronically Ill Adults, First Edition. Edited by Cheryl Schraeder and Paul Shelton.
© 2011 John Wiley & Sons, Inc. Published 2011 by John Wiley & Sons, Inc.

neurology stroke assessments, dermatology, and psychiatry. Primary care can also be provided via telemedicine, such as in Ohio and Texas, where prison populations are served from remote university medical centers. The ATA has organized national expert panels to devise standards and guidelines for the provision of telemedicine services (ATA 2008).

Although elderly patients often comprise a significant portion of the patients in telemedicine studies, there have not been many studies specially examining the efficacy of tele-geriatric assessments. The available evidence suggests that tele-geriatric assessment can be both effective and well received by elderly patients (Jones *et al.* 2001; Brignell *et al.* 2007).

Project description

The Geriatric Telemedicine Assessment Service used telemedicine technology and processes to extend geriatric services based at the PeaceHealth Gerontology Institute's Senior Health and Wellness Center (SHWC) in Eugene, Oregon, to patients at Ketchikan General Hospital (KGH), located in Ketchikan, Alaska. The service model is based on the SHWC's outpatient assessment service. The Geriatric Telemedicine Assessment Service pilot program with KGH demonstrated the clinical viability of telemedicine as a means of extending geriatric expertise to patients who would otherwise not have access to geriatricians. KGH was selected for the pilot based on several factors: (1) KGH and the SHWC are both part of the same health system; (2) KGH and the SHWC share the same electronic medical record; (3) KGH administrators and clinicians expressed a need for and a strong interest in the service; and (4) Ketchikan, Alaska meets Centers for Medicare & Medicaid Services (CMS) criteria for telemedicine reimbursement.

Systemic support

Early in the project, PeaceHealth telemedicine supporters across clinical service lines joined with the Telemedicine Alliance of Oregon (TOA) to work collaboratively in advocating for telemedicine. For example, TAO was instrumental in passage of state legislation requiring commercial insurers to cover telemedicine services. TAO also supported a successful $20 million FCC grant to develop statewide access to broadband networks. This led to the creation of the Oregon Health Network. PeaceHealth also made use of resources from the American Telemedicine Alliance and the Northwest Regional Telehealth Resource Center. The organizations provided critical information about technology, reimbursement and best practice standards.

Project implementation

There were multiple implementation components, some of which were pursued concurrently, and some that needed to occur sequentially. During the initial site visit to KGH, project developers identified the target patient population, organized the key individuals required for implementation, and assessed the existing technology resources. Later steps involved licensing and privileging the telemedicine geriatrician, practicing telemedicine consultations, resolving reimbursement issues, and designing the telemedicine workflow process.

Target patient population

Initially, patients were referred by KGH's skilled nursing facility (SNF). The SHWC geriatrician had particular expertise in the assessment of gait and fall risk, which are issues of concern in the SNF population; moreover, project developers believed these types of referrals would be optimal for testing the telemedicine process. Patients were referred based on changes in their physical or mental functioning, with the aim of exploring community placement. Subsequent referrals came from a state-operated assisted living facility (ALF) and the KGH home health agency.

Key stakeholders

It was critical for KGH to have a physician champion. Fortunately, the KGH medical director, a highly respected practicing primary care physician, was prepared to serve this role. Other stakeholders included the director of quality improvement, the vice president for ambulatory services, the ambulatory services manager, the director of medical staff services (credentialing), the patient accounts manager (billing), the SNF unit manager, the health information manager (medical records), the admissions supervisor, a financial analyst, and the KGH information technology manager. The KGH social worker emerged as one of the key champions of the service and was the individual who was most involved in hands-on project implementation.

Key participants at the SHWC included the Gerontology Institute's executive director, the director of clinical services and quality, the geriatrician, and the outpatient consultation coordinator (medical office assistant). The geriatrician joined the executive director on the second KGH site visit, during which he met with administrators and physicians and viewed the connectivity between and KGH and the SHWC. This experience reinforced his confidence that a high-quality service could be provided.

Licensing and privileging

Prior to delivering patient care, the SHWC geriatrician needed to be licensed in the State of Alaska and credentialed for medical staff privileges at KGH. The licensing process for the geriatrician was the same as for any other provider. The KGH privileging process was largely the same, but included exceptions based on the more limited scope of practice (for example, telemedicine providers do not have call responsibilities). The state licensing and hospital credentialing processes required more than six months to complete. CMS has proposed changing its credentialing requirements to allow originating sites to accept as proxy the credentialing, privileging, and peer review processes in the distant organization.

Technology resources

The Geriatric Telemedicine Service used PeaceHealth's existing Polycom videoconferencing system, which provided a high-speed link to all PeaceHealth entities in Oregon,

Washington, and Alaska. Each videoconference site had a camera, monitor, and remote control used to manipulate both the local camera and the camera in the remote location. The resolution was excellent, with a wide camera range and significant zoom capability. The geriatrician had access to a second computer monitor, placed next to the videoconference monitor, which was used to view the patient's electronic medical record during the videoconference. The SHWC used a desktop device that combined the monitor and a small, embedded camera.

The KGH videoconferencing room was deemed adequate, although not ideal, for patient assessments. However, the videoconferencing rooms were in high demand and the schedule limited times that consultations could be booked. This prompted KGH to purchase a mobile Polycom telemedicine unit that could be scheduled independently and used in multiple locations.

Shortly before the geriatric telemedicine service was proposed, PeaceHealth had initiated two other types of telemedicine services. First, a USDA grant funded the development of a tele-interpretive service that included several mobile units. Second, a pilot telepediatric service was developed linking the Sacred Heart Medical Center's emergency department in Eugene, Oregon, with pediatric intensivists at Oregon Health Science University in Portland. These projects enabled our Information Technology staff to become familiar with telemedicine products and connectivity issues. We also learned about telemedicine service delivery processes.

Reimbursement issues

The project team conducted an exhaustive assessment related to Medicare and Medicaid billing. CMS policy restricts telemedicine services to patients who reside in either a Health Provider Shortage Area (HPSA) or a U.S. Census-defined Micro Statistical Area (MSA). HPSA designation is based on the number of primary care physicians per 1,000 residents. Surprisingly, Ketchikan did not meet HPSA criteria; although some specialist services were scarce, the community had slightly more primary care physicians than the HPSA standards allowed. Fortunately, Ketchikan did have MSA designation. There were no Medicare Advantage plans offered in the KGH service area.

Mock consultations

Mock consultations were conducted to test the technology, the processes, and the patient and provider experience. The first mock consultation used a staff volunteer as the patient. The second mock consultation used a senior volunteer as the patient. These practice sessions helped test the physical environment, confirmed which examinations could be performed, pinpointed the ideal positioning of the patient and provider relative to the camera and monitor, enabled the provider to practice using the remote control, and finalized the process for orienting and interacting with patients.

Standard process flow

Based on the mock consultations, the team developed a standard work process flow diagram (Figure 26.1).

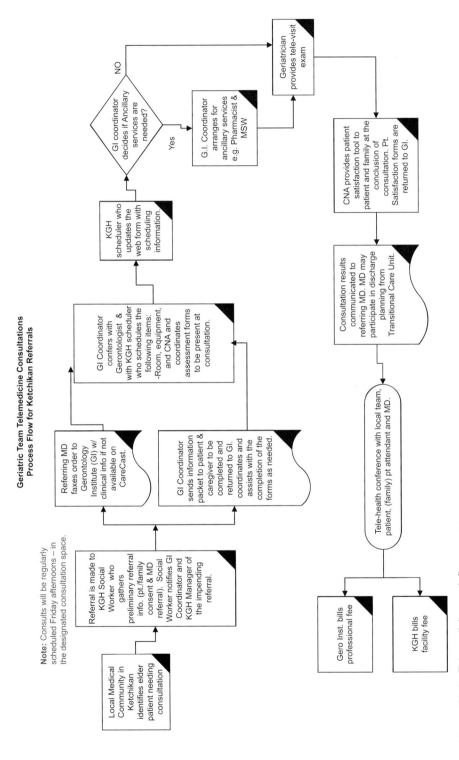

**Geriatric Team Telemedicine Consultations
Process Flow for Ketchikan Referrals**

Note: Consults will be regularly scheduled Friday afternoons – in the designated consultation space.

Local Medical Community in Ketchikan identifies elder patient needing consultation

Referral is made to KGH Social Worker who gathers preliminary referral info. (pt./family consent & MD referral). Social Worker notifies GI Coordinator and KGH Manager of the impending referral.

Referring MD faxes order to Gerontology Institute (GI) w/ clinical info if not available on CareCast.

GI Coordinator sends information packet to patient & caregiver to be completed and returned to GI. coordinates and assists with the completion of the forms as needed.

GI Coordinator confers with Gerontologist & with KGH scheduler who schedules the following items: -Room, equipment, and CNA and coordinates assessment forms to be present at consultation.

KGH scheduler who updates the web form with scheduling information.

GI coordinator decides if Ancillary services are needed?

G.I. Coordinator arranges for ancillary services e.g. Pharmacist & MSW

Geriatrician provides tele-visit exam

CNA provides patient satisfaction tool to patient and family at the conclusion of consultation. Pt. Satisfaction forms are returned to GI.

Consultation results communicated to referring MD. MD may participate in discharge planning from Transitional Care Unit.

Tele-health conference with local team, patient, (family) pt attendant and MD.

Gero Inst. bills professional fee

KGH bills facility fee

Figure 26.1 Telemedicine work flow process.

411

The diagram illustrates the roles of staff at KGH and at the SHWC. Project developers revised the flow diagram several times to add details and reflect ongoing process efficiency enhancements. Process and role refinements were made in various areas, including confirming referral orders and preauthorization, scheduling visits, registering patients, and assembling patient's medical information and histories. All patients were asked to have a family member, friend or caregiver participate in both the assessment visit and follow-up visit. A Medical Office Assistant (MOA) was assigned to room patients and their caregivers; the MOA was not required to be in the examination room at all times during the visit, but could be called in as needed. The team later developed promotional materials and user forms to support the process.

The billing processes were clarified, with KGH billing the facility fee and the SHWC billing the professional fee. Electronic billing systems and paper forms were modified to note the required telemedicine qualifier.

Results

As of this writing, the Geriatric Telemedicine Consultation Service has served 17 patients, ranging from 70 to 95 years of age. The reasons for referral mirrored outpatient assessments in Oregon, including changes in physical functions, changes in mental functioning, and exacerbation of problem behaviors. Geriatrician assessments were also similar (such as diagnoses, medication interventions, behavioral interventions, caregiver recommendations, and social service referrals).

The geriatrician experience

The geriatrician reported that, using telemedicine, he was able to complete all of the assessments he would normally complete in an office visit (including mobility and mental status examinations). The camera could be moved into the hallway to observe gait, and the resolution was sufficient to allow him to observe the clock-drawing test. As with conventional outpatient assessments, the assessment process primarily entailed review of medical records, observing patients and interviewing patients, family members and caregivers. The geriatrician believed that the telemedicine interview process was as effective as an in-office interview; he believed having a side-by-side view of the patient with the electronic medical record is critical for optimizing visit efficiency and thoroughness.

Patients and caregivers experience

Patients or their accompanying caregivers were asked to complete a brief survey following the visit. They were very positive about their telemedicine experience and were more than willing to do it again, if necessary. Patients became comfortable with the telemedicine process after a few minutes of interaction with the distant telemedicine coordinator in Oregon and prior to the geriatrician entering the interview. One patient commented that the process did not seem unusual because, "I talk back to my television all the time."

Several patients commented that they were pleased to have access to geriatric specialty care without being required to leave their community.

Referral sources

Feedback from the caregiver teams at both the KGH SNF and the ALF was very positive. The geriatric assessments facilitated discharge planning at the SNF and helped staff manage behavior at the ALF. Direct interaction between the geriatrician and these local care teams was found to be most valuable.

Financial results

Professional fee and facility fee reimbursement has mirrored payments received for office visit assessments. However, these are now split between the originating and distant sites. The originating site does not benefit from the professional fee and the distant site does not benefit from the facility fee. The distant site does incur costs beyond that of the geriatrician (for example, the coordinator's time, which is not covered directly by a facility fee). Telemedicine assessments continue to be more time consuming for the geriatrician than office visit assessments. More time is spent gathering and reviewing medical records. There are opportunities to further refine the process, saving time and cost. The originating site facility fee does not entirely cover the cost. The likely cost benefits for the originating site's skilled care unit have not yet been quantified. Geriatric assessments have contributed to more effective care plans, reduced medications and, in some cases, progress towards discharge.

Lessons learned

- Partnerships with referring communities should begin with confirmation that caregivers and the local medical community strongly believe in the need for geriatric specialty care. Local health care leadership needs to explicitly support the service. Most importantly, a local physician should serve as the "champion" of the service; in this case, the KGH medical director was invaluable in facilitating implementation.
- If the referring organization does not have other existing telemedicine services, they should be given clear, written technology requirements, including the American Telemedicine Association's program standards.
- Geriatric provider organizations should develop internal partnerships to advance telemedicine services across clinical service lines. The infrastructure for geriatric telemedicine cannot be developed and sustained independently of other programs (see replication discussion below).
- A telemedicine visit should not be considered "special." In most respects, a telemedicine visit is the same as any other office visit. By de-mystifying the telemedicine service, program developers will increase patient and clinician comfort, as well as clinical effectiveness.

- Work process flow, including specific roles and responsibilities, should be explicitly agreed upon and clearly mapped.
- The devil is in the details. Every aspect of the standard visit (for example, registration, medical records, and billing) should be reviewed and adjusted if necessary to accommodate care provision via telemedicine.
- Consider the telemedicine experience from the patient's point of view. The nuances inherent in telemedicine interactions should be acknowledged and addressed. For example, patients and caregivers require a brief orientation to the process before the consultation begins, and should be informed about who is in the room at the provider (distance) location. Clinicians should practice providing telemedicine care to ensure that they are comfortable working with the technology and that they know how their actions will be viewed by patients. For example, clinicians should make regular eye contact with the camera and reduce the viewing angle between the camera and monitor; otherwise, the provider appears to be looking down at the patient's lap.
- The technology infrastructure should be reliable, fast, and clear, while the end-user technology should be simple to operate. Ideally, telemedicine should be supported with high-speed fiber-optic connectivity. It is vital to avoid network disruptions, slow response times, and poor audio-visual quality. Although maintaining network quality can be complicated and available IT expertise is essential, using the technology (such as accessing the network and operating the camera) should be straightforward and intuitive.
- Clinicians can conduct comprehensive geriatric assessments using telemedicine. Geriatric assessments largely do not require clinicians to touch patients. Although peripheral telemedicine devices can allow providers to do physical examinations (such as listening to chest and lung sounds), these devices are costly and generally are not necessary.
- Elderly patients acclimate to telemedicine relatively quickly. Moreover, providers and staff also quickly become accustomed to telemedicine interactions. The experience is not that different from other types of telecommunications we use in our daily lives.
- The ultimate value of geriatric consultations is based on the degree to which the clinician's findings and recommendations can be shared with the care team and integrated into the care plan. To the extent possible, telemedicine geriatric consultations should be incorporated into the local care planning process and the geriatricians should be considered part of the local care team. For example, the Geriatric Telemedicine Consultation Service strived to include a representative of the care team in each visit, especially during the second visit when recommendations are shared. The physical setting of the local telemedicine visit (originating site) should allow for participation of family members and the patient's local care team.
- Although telemedicine can improve access to geriatric services and extend the reach of geriatric providers, it does not necessarily enhance the capacity of geriatric providers. There continues to be a serious national shortage of geriatricians and telemedicine services can only be developed where there is capacity. Most health care systems will be challenged to stretch a limited number of geriatric providers across the continuum of care.

Policy implications

Geriatric telemedicine will be encouraged or limited to the degree that CMS polices allow for reimbursement. Medicare currently only pays for telemedicine services provided to patients who reside in either a HPSA or a federally designated MSA. HPSA designation is based on the ratio of primary care providers to residents in a given area. However, this is frequently not the most relevant access issue, as telemedicine is often most applicable to medical specialties with little or no presence in a community. Furthermore, the CMS policy requiring HPSA or MSA designation for telemedicine reimbursement erroneously implies that access to medical services is primarily a rural issue. There are significant needs and opportunities to employ telemedicine in urban areas as well (for example, hospitals and SNFs could benefit from geriatricians regularly rounding on patients via telemedicine). CMS policy implies that telemedicine is inherently inferior to traditional face-to-face visits. Although there are some limitations to the services that can be provided during a telemedicine visit, there is no evidence that the care is substandard. On the contrary, patients and providers report that telemedicine visits are beneficial and appreciated, especially given the vastly greater convenience for patients who would otherwise be required to travel to receive specialty care.

It is encouraging that CMS is broadening coverage for telemedicine, albeit incrementally. In 2008, CMS expanded the list of services that could be provided via telemedicine and allowed reimbursement for telemedicine services provided in nursing facilities. There could be significant patient benefit in telemedicine home visits, especially when accompanied by telemedicine home monitoring.

In March of 2011, CMS is expected to issue new regulations allowing originating site organizations to accept the credentialing, privileging, and peer review processes of providers at the distant site. This would address one of the most significant barriers to broadening access to telemedicine services.

Recent increases in funding for health care technology adoption is very encouraging. The 2009 economic stimulus package passed by Congress provides substantial funding for the further development of health information networks that will provide the backbone for telemedicine services. It also includes funding for telemedicine demonstration projects. These resources will facilitate the adoption of telemedicine and improve access to specialty care for patients with a broad array of care needs.

References

American Telemedicine Association. *Telemedicine Defined*. American Telemedicine Association, Washington, DC. Available at: http://www.americantelemed.org/i4a/pages/index.cfm?pageID=3333

American Telemedicine Association. (2008) *Telemedicine Standards and Guidelines*. American Telemedicine Association, Washington, DC. Available at: http://www.americantelemed.org/i4a/pages/index.cfm?pageID=3311.

Brignell, M., Wooton, R., & Gray, L. (2007) The application of telemedicine to geriatric medicine. *Age and Aging*, 36, 369–374.

Jones, B.N., Johnston, D., Reboussin, B., *et al.* (2001) Reliability of telepsychiatry assessments: subjective versus observational ratings. *Journal of Geriatric Psychiatry and Neurology*, 14, 66–71.

Stock, R., Reece, D., & Cesario, L. (2004) Developing a comprehensive interdisciplinary senior healthcare practice. *Journal of the American Geriatrics Society*, 52, 2128–2133.

Stock, R., Mahoney, E.R., Reece, D., *et al.* (2008) Developing a senior healthcare practice using the chronic care model: effect on physical function and health-related quality of life. *Journal of the American Geriatrics Society*, 56, 1342–1348.

Chapter 27

Integrated Patient-Centered Care: the I-PiCC pilot

Karyn Rizzo

I-PiCC pilot overview

As 25% of Medicare recipients are utilizing 85% of Medicare dollars, it is imperative that the needs of this subgroup of geriatric patients be scrutinized and targeted for new and innovative ways to approach care delivery, care coordination, and disease education. Currently, 13% of the overall population in the United States is 65 years of age and older and account for approximately 36% of health care expenditures. The percentage of geriatric patients is rapidly expanding as is national health care expenditures (Machlin 2009). Changes in health care reimbursement have moved funds away from the primary care physician (PCP) to the specialty physician, which has contributed to a model of fragmented care. This shift in funds, along with other administrative burdens, has led to a shortage of PCPs and an even greater scarcity of geriatric-trained clinicians. This trend puts the vulnerable geriatric patient at great risk.

Care coordination and patient education need to be aligned at the PCP level. Education provided in the acute care setting is not easily absorbed during times of transition and heightened anxiety for hospitalized elders. Patients with multiple chronic illness and polypharmacy issues are best served by an interdisciplinary team with greater continuity of care throughout their aging process. Physicians should focus on the patient's medical condition(s) and rely on other members of the health care team to ensure the patient's needs are met. Registered nurses (RNs) are a perfect adjunct to assist with disease education and lifestyle modification. Pharmacists can provide a significant contribution to chronically ill elderly patients in terms of drug interactions, dosage recommendations and spotting potential polypharmacy reactions. Social service workers have a unique set of skills that are ideal when strategizing behavior change and facing "geriatric syndromes" challenges (such as sleep issues, pain, incontinence, eating problems, confusion, falls and skin breakdown).

Research shows that if primary care practices restructure how they operate, being more accessible, promoting prevention, proactively supporting patients with chronic illness, and engaging patients in self-management, they provide better care more efficiently (National Committee on Quality Assurance [NCQA] 2009). The name

Comprehensive Care Coordination for Chronically Ill Adults, First Edition. Edited by Cheryl Schraeder and Paul Shelton.
© 2011 John Wiley & Sons, Inc. Published 2011 by John Wiley & Sons, Inc.

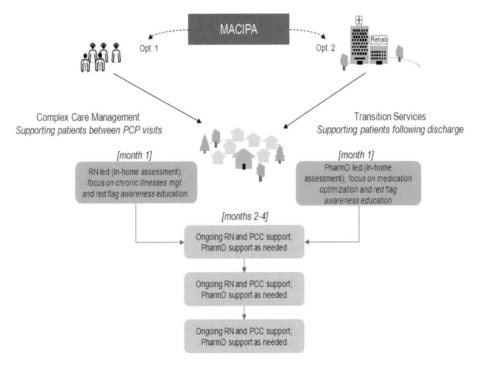

Figure 27.1   IPiCC Process Flow

attributed to this conceptualization of primary care is the "Patient-Centered Medical Home" (PCMH).

Integrated Patient-Centered Care (I-PiCC) was a pilot project designed to extend the reach and impact of the PCP and support the more complex geriatric clients in the community. I-PiCC supported the PCP practice by providing structured and scheduled in-home visits between scheduled office visits and upon hospital discharge by an interdisciplinary team consisting of an advanced practice nurse (APN), RN, pharmacist, social worker, and non-clinical support staff. These visits focused on risk reduction, medication optimization and ongoing health education. This cadre of services not only helps patients but helps to extend the PCP practice and move it closer to the PCMH model. Figure 27.1 provides a schematic representation of the I-PiCC program.

Areas of focus

The target population of the I-PiCC pilot was high-risk, high-cost elderly individuals living in the community with multiple co-morbid conditions who would benefit from greater PCP integration and involvement. Focusing on aged patients in their homes allows a clinician to see the many challenges this population must overcome in order to maintain independence and successfully age in place.

Many factors contributed in choosing in-home visits to address care coordination and chronic disease education as opposed to an office-based or hospital-based model:

- "Geriatric syndromes" are best observed in a person's home, not in the PCP's office or in a hospital.
- Lifestyle impact on health becomes more apparent in the home environment (such as food choices, smoking, alcohol consumption, financial resources, and caregiving challenges).
- Over-the-counter medications that many people "forget" to tell their PCPs about are not necessarily harmless, and often contribute to polypharmacy challenges. They are also frequently omitted from a patient's medication profile.
- Adults learn better when they are not at a point of transition/anxiety (hospital admission/discharge or in their PCP's office) and when information is repeated many times, especially if it is unfamiliar.
- To assist our seniors and keep them on-track to successful aging, clinicians need to meet them "where they are most comfortable" and in control – in their homes.

Program-planning involved contributions from every team member. The following principles and considerations were integrated into program operations:

- Historically, the population we were targeting is generally considered to be made up of "passive participants" in the health care system.
- The intervention needed to be structured to ensure maximum engagement of the participants and motivate them to pursue lasting behavior change after the pilot was completed. Our strategy was to coach our patients so we coined the phrase "Cue, Don't Do." An interdisciplinary team was imperative to meet the wide variety of needs the target population had.
- Geriatrics is a specialty. Specific education and training in geriatrics prior to starting the project was an absolute necessity to ensure all team members had a minimal level of competency.
- The program focus was on coaching, engaging, and motivating our patients, not providing skilled hands-on care that could be provided by home health personnel.
- Care plans are passive so we decided to use a more "pro-active" tool to engage participants. The I-PiCC team opted to implement a Co-Plan. This tool was more patient-centered and identified interventions and actions that the patients could do to change their health, in addition to the contributions of team members.
- Transitions of care needed to be specifically addressed because they are particularly difficult for the geriatric patient (Coleman & Boult 2003).
- A non-clinical teammate was chosen to address non-clinical "care coordination" participant needs.
- The duration of the intervention would be four months (16 weeks). This time frame was similar to successful transition projects administered by Naylor and colleagues. This length of time was also determined to be the minimum amount of time necessary to observe behavior change (Naylor 1990).

- The model's interventions needed to be easily replicated with specific measurable outcomes, as well as successful clinical outcomes, be cost effective, and demonstrate a return on investment.
- The model had to "wrap around" existing primary care practices to expand into their patient's homes and perhaps offer solutions to the PCP crises.

Patient selection

Our target population was geriatric patients, 65 years of age and older, taking five or more medications a day with two or more co-morbid conditions, and with cognition that allowed them to be coached (or a caregiver willing to accept the coaching on behalf of the patients). In addition, they were identified by the practice manager as being a "high cost" managed care member. We looked to target those individuals who were seriously ill but not actively or imminently dying. A total of 78 individuals were identified by the physician practice management team in accordance with project guidelines; seven were screened who did not meet criteria, 31 declined to participate and four were identified as end stage and were referred to hospice. Forty individuals enrolled in the program; 32 completed the entire four month intervention, and eight completed at least two but not all four months due to death or subsequent placement in long term care.

Prior to entry all participants completed the SF-12 (V2), an instrument used to measure self-perception of health (Ware *et al*. 1996) in a face-to-face interview with project staff. The SF-12 measures eight domains of health and provides two scores, one for physical health and one for mental health (Ware *et al*. 1998). Based on a score in the 30-39 range, 90% of patients were identified as "moderately disabled," indicating they were seriously ill but not terminal.

I-PiCC components

I-PiCC offered an interdisciplinary team that provided structured and scheduled in-home visits and ongoing telephonic support between regular PCP office visits. The program's initial focus during the first month was to conduct a thorough nurse-driven geriatric assessment in order to aid in targeting potential areas of knowledge deficit or personal risk, and medication reconciliation and optimization by the pharmacist. The intervention then focused on the assessment results and participant's specific health care needs.

The clinical team

A geriatric clinical nurse specialist (GCNS) lead the team and the project. The GCNS's role was to oversee the project, ensure adhearance to operational guidelines, collect data, and provide initial plus ongoing education to other team members. No direct patient care was provided by the GCNS. The GCNS held weekly clinical reviews of each patient with team members. An RN was the patient's health coach and ultimately responsible for the team's interventions and action plans. As "Co-Plan" implementer, the RN provided on-going health coaching and plan reassessment. The RN assessed the patient's readiness to learn, make change, and continue to monitor motivation for change throughout the project. The RN also conducted in-home visits once or twice a month per patient. In addition, the RN had numerous telephonic encounters driven by patient need to reinforce educational content and discuss potential risk factors for hospital readmission.

A pharmacist conducted an initial in-home assessment focusing on medication reconciliation and patient education. The reconciliation process was taken one step further by running potential drug interactions, screening for medications on the Beers lists, and offering recommendations for optimization of medications to the patient's PCP. The pharmacist worked with each patient to develop a pillbox system to meet their needs and reduce errors in filling their pillboxes, assisted with specialty packaging from their pharmacy if indicated, and guided patients in the disposal of expired or unused medication. They made follow-up visits if there was ongoing knowledge deficit or whenever a participant was admitted to the hospital and returned home with medication changes. Additionally, a social worker assisted patients in overcoming behaviors that unfavorably impacted their health, and assisted with identification of community resources when needed.

When a patient required care coordination, we utilized a personal care coordinator (PCC) to address the patient's care coordination needs. The PCC was a non-licensed support person who assisted the patients, their caregivers, and the clinical staff. They supplemented the clinical team by assisting with making follow-up appointments with physicians, leaving appointment reminders, and identifying community resources to support aging in place (e.g., homemakers, home repairs, transportation etc). The PCC filled a vital role that supported wellness, personal well being and an overall decrease in health care spending.

Acknowledging geriatrics as a specialty, a 16-hour orientation was developed that focused on common geriatric syndromes and chronic diseases, behavioral change theory, coaching, medication optimization and reconciliation, and orientation to home care/community care.

The patient Co-Plan

Care plans have been used by many disciplines within the health care system to prioritize goals of care and interventions. It is generally not given to the patient and the degree of patient input is highly variable, even within identical settings. Our purpose of modifying the traditional care plan was three-fold: (1) clinician's negative perceptions of care plans – the team overwhelmingly felt that care plans were a significant amount of upfront work and did little to help the clinician or patient; (2) the change in wording made it "ok" for patients, caregivers, clinicians, and non-clinicians to contribute to the document; and (3) use of the term "Co-Plan" instead of care plan was decided so that it was clear to the participant that this was not a passive process and their actions would be required to meet the goals that they set.

The traditional care plan has three components: problems, interventions, and goals. The interventions section of a traditional care plan captures the clinical team's actions. I-PiCC chose to make the interventions applicable to both clinicians and patients. The goals are usually health care team goals, not patient goals, so the clinicians were mindful that Co-Plan goals were the individual patients'.

In the health care system clinicians struggle with the patient's "health care wants" and "health care needs". Reconciling wants and needs is not an easy negotiation and clinicians, due to time constraints and numerous other factors, frequently default to addressing the patient's "needs" by placing the most critical at the top of the list. If a patient does not share the team's assessment of his/her needs, or feels that his/her "wants" are ignored, unwittingly this may create a situation that fosters an unengaged patient. Sometimes these individuals may be given the ominous title of "non-compliant." In our model there could never be a non-compliant patient. The goals were determined by the patient in a marriage of wants and needs. The action items were set by the patient. The deliverables from the health care team were clearly stated so the patient knew what to expect "next". Co-Plans were updated at every point of contact (phone or in person) by each team member, as well as by patient or caregiver request. When a Co-Plan was updated the patient was provided with a copy of the revisions within 24 hours.

Behavior change approach

Our overall goal was to coach and empower the patients, positioning them with skills to better manage their health and future health care experiences. We acknowledged that this would require a significant behavior change for many patients. There are numerous theories that address behavioral change. We chose to use motivational interviewing and the Transtheoretical Model (TTM) of change. The TTM assesses an individual's readiness to act on a new behavior and provides strategies to guide the individual through the stages of change to a point of action and sustainability (maintenance). A person can move forward in the process and continue to progress (to the right of the diagram) or regress (movement to the left; Prochaska & Velicer 1997; 1998).

We embedded the TTM assessment within the nursing assessment and scored patients' readiness for change in each area where a knowledge deficit was detected. When the clinical team assembled the Co-Plan goals with the patient they considered their readiness to change when developing a plan. For example, a patient was considering smoking cessation. They may be in the contemplative stage with no near future plan to stop. Providing them with a stop date is unlikely to result in a behavior change. Asking the patient permission to provide information on quitting options at the next visit might have

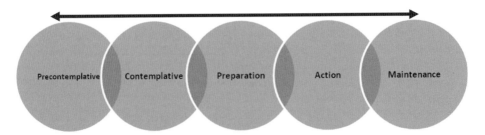

Figure 27.2   The Transtheoretical Model of Change

a greater chance of success. The TTM takes into account that behavior change is a linear process and flows both forwards and backwards. The clinician may not be able to bring the patient to the point of smoking cessation, but there is some success if she/he moved from not considering cessation to a willingness to consider it in the near future.

Behavior change takes time and to ensure sustainability we would recommend an intervention period from four to six months. By using the TTM model clinicians were able to measure the smaller more incremental steps of progress instead of an "all or none" approach" to behavior change. Research using the TTM model indicates that in any given sample of 100 participants, 25 will make and maintain change, 25 will make no change, and 50 will make steps toward progress but may require more time or resources to achieve additional behavior change (Prochaska & Velicer 1997; 1998). We acknowledged up front that 12 weeks may not be enough time to see significant behavior change, but by staging the patients we were able to share with them their incremental progress and frame it as a starting point for future chances of success.

Project challenges

One of the many challenges we experienced was to train an interdisciplinary team to find the right balance of "cueing" (patient coaching) versus "doing" (care coordination). The TTM provided us with a means to assess readiness for change, the SF-12 scores provided insight on the patient's perception of their health, and the Co-Plan guided us to their priorities. This information helped the team in identifying what a patient was willing or unwilling to address, but it did not address if the patient was able. When staff were frustrated and not succeeding in helping to motivate behavior change, it was frequently because the patients were willing but not able. A program adaptation was necessary to address the varying level of limitations that occurred due to normal aging or impact of their illnesses.

An additional challenge was to implement a model to support PCP's who were struggling with managing their complex geriatric patients. While our program was designed to "stand alone," an additional benefit was that these services, when coupled with the existing PCP practice, enabled the PCP and their staff to partially meet three of the nine standards required to achieve PCMH accreditation through the NCQA. The benefit, beyond clinical implications, is that PCMH accreditation may provide additional financial

Table 27.1 Willing and Able

	Willing	**Unwilling**
Able	If patient is willing and able, plan is to **coach** and support	Is patient is unwilling but able, plan is to **coach** and continue to assess readiness to change. Continue to model the desirable behavior.
Unable	If patient is willing but unable, **care coordination** should be implemented with a plan for ongoing support	If patient is unwilling and unable, **care coordination** should be implemented with a plan for ongoing support

Note: This chart was used by the clinical team to guide them regarding when coaching might be of benefit and when they would need to be more active in preventing decline in health.

incentives for the PCP practice. Medicare is in the process of funding several national PCMH pilots and looking to realign reimbursement for those practices that better manage their patients using the PCMH approach. A delivery model that is in alignment with future Medicare reimbursement changes has a greater chance of replication and implementation than a model that requires a full overhaul of the existing Medicare reimbursement process (NCQA 2009).

Patient education materials

Healthwise for Life: A Self-Care Guide for People Age 50 or Better (Metter & Kemper 2003) was selected as the educational tool used by clinicians for self-management. The manual provides a wide variety of information on prevention, chronic disease, myths on aging, first aid, as well as information on different types of insurance plans. It is printed in a large font size to facilitate ease in reading for the geriatric patient, and is easily understood while providing a comprehensive overview of most challenges faced by the aged population. Each patient was provided a manual and instructed on its use.

Our focus was on patient education; content was used to prepare patients to ask specific questions about their health issues and concerns with their physician at regular visits. All project staff were trained to use the manual in a consistent manner. Project staff referred to the manual when providing either in-home or telephonic support. When appropriate, patients were given "reading assignments" from the book in preparation for the team member's visit or phone call. Patient feedback on the manual was overwhelmingly positive and was a resource that could continue to be utilized post-project.

I-PiCC results

Patient characteristics

The average age of the 40 enrolled patients was 81 (range 69 to 93 years); 38% were male. These patients averaged eight chronic illnesses, were taking 12.5 medications daily, were cognitively intact and able to be coached, or else had mild impairment and their caregivers were willing to be the recipients of disease education. All patients lived in the community, either in their own homes, senior housing, or an assisted living facility. English was a second language for 15% of patients. All 40 patients had experienced a hospitalization, emergency room (ER) visit, or had above average health care expenditures in the past year.

Intervention intensity

Each patient averaged four in-home visits and nine telephone calls from RNs during the four-month intervention period that focused on disease coaching, care coordination, and preparation for physician appointments. Each patient also averaged 25 telephone calls from the PCC to reinforce goals of care, appointment reminders and care coordination activities. The intervention team made 93 referrals to non-skilled community resources and 79 referrals and coordination calls to specialty physicians.

Lessons learned

The overall project evaluation indicated that the intervention had a positive impact on improving care and a positive impact on some utilization outcomes. During the project, 5% of patients had ER visits compared to the national average of 20% for elderly individuals (Machlin 2009). We believe that this difference was due to several factors: participants were coached to see their PCPs with greater frequency (95% of patients saw their PCP at least once during the study period); each person was coached to be aware of their "red flags" and to contact their PCP office at the first signs of any of these changes; and frequent telephone calls from the PCC to those patients identified at greatest risk for hospitalization.

The hospitalization rate was 35%, well above the national average of 18% (Hall *et al.* 2010). However, the 30-day hospital readmission rate was only 7.5% compared to the national rate of approximately 18%. We believe the pharmacist in-home visits, that included reconciling and optimizing medications, was one of the main reasons for this reduction in readmissions. Additionally, patients were coached to return to their PCP within seven days of discharge, and this also may have contributed to the program's success.

Care coordination is not usually reimbursed within the existing health care system, yet it is vital for allowing the elderly person to age in place in the community where cost of care is much less expensive. Research indicates and supports that, overwhelmingly, people want to remain in their homes as they age and not be placed in residential facilities. Assistance with care coordination helps to compensate for the decline and losses (personal, professional, functional, sensory and financial) that occur with aging. In our model, we chose to address this need with a PCC who was non-licensed and non-clinical. Lack of clinical expertise posed no threats to patient safety and we found that the care coordination role was one that was teachable.

We considered care management/complex care management as a vital part of the program that was accomplished by the clinical team. We broadly defined care management as a holistic view of all things that impacted the participants' health. When assembling the participants Co-Plan, care management strategies were employed. We revisited the person's "global health needs" during weekly clinical review, and it was the focus of the team leader (GCNS) to keep a vision of the patient's care management needs. The RN addressed these needs on an ongoing basis in addition to coaching and providing disease education. The PCC supplemented these needs in addressing care coordination items. Clinicians delegated tasks, pre- or post-visits, and calls. These encounters were tracked and showed a significant investment in time to support each patient.

The role of the PCC was significant and contributed to the program's success in supporting aging, frail, community-based elders. The PCMH model looks to hold PCP practices accountable for patient care coordination as part of the services provided to meet PCMH standards. Our concern with this standard is that NCQA blends care management with care coordination so we continue with a delivery model of compensating over-qualified staff to do the task. Continuing to define care coordination and distinguishing it from care management is needed in order to drive payment reform in the right direction.

Focusing on participant empowerment we were able to provide personal, patient-centered, patient-driven care. Coaching was often time consuming and frustrating for the clinical team but the long-term benefits to the patient were clearly visible. It is vital that all team members be skilled in coaching and motivational interviewing because they are important skills needed by clinicians to facilitate health care system change.

I-PiCC case study

Mr. T is a 70-year-old man. Past medical history includes chronic renal insufficiency, benign prostate hypertrophy with urinary frequency, insomnia, hypertension, coronary artery disease, hypothyroid and major depression disorder. He lives in subsidized housing and is the primary caregiver for his 96-year-old mother. He is on a fixed income and is challenged with being able to purchase food and medications. His TMM category of "contemplative" suggested that he was ready to make changes in his life to improve his health.

Mr. T identified the following concerns: depression, financial limitation, poor sleep, urinary frequency, and placement of his mother in a long term care facility due to her declining health. During the assessment Mr. T shared that he had stopped his Levothyroxine, Qualaquin, Zolpidem, and aspirin due to either side effects and/or cost. In addition, he was taking Advil-PM as a sleep aid.

Patient Co-Plan

- My strengths and resources are:
  - I have friends to help me.
  - I can walk to everything I need in my neighborhood.
  - My memory is good.
- I will support my goals by doing the following:
  - Make an appointment with my PCP.
  - Take my medications as directed.
  - Go to an appointment with a mental health professional.
  - Work on a healthier bed time routine.
- My team will support my goals by:
  - Looking into medication funding resources.
  - Identifying a mental health worker within the MACIPA system.
  - Optimizing my medications with my PCP.
  - Setting up a medication system for me to follow.
  - Provide education on my medications.
  - Order a commode.
- These are the goals I want to accomplish by the end of this program:
  - I want to be able to get a good night's sleep.
  - I want to walk more.

- ○ I want to get help for caring for my mother.
- ○ I want to feel less sad and lonely.
- My goals for the next 30 days are:
  - ○ I will use my pill box and take all my pills.
  - ○ I will take a walk after dinner two times this week.
  - ○ I will go to my appointment with my mental health worker.

Intervention services

Mr. T received the following services during his four-month participation in the I-PiCC program:

- Four in-home RN visits focusing on lifestyle modification and chronic disease education.
- One in-home pharmacy visit.
- 22 telephone sessions to reinforce his co-plan, disease education, lifestyle modification, and medication education (calls placed by all members of the team).
- 18 calls were made to the patient or on the patient's behalf for care coordination.
- The pharmacist identified a mail order pharmacy that would provide medications with a significant cost savings and assisted Mr. T. in initiating the process.
- A medication box was put in place with a system to reduce errors.
- A Mental Health consult was obtained and Mr. T. started on an antidepressant with good effects.
- Mr. T. was able to initiate a daily increase in exercise with an afternoon or evening walk to assist with health and promote sleep.
- A social worker worked with him and helped him complete a SNAP(Supplemental Nutrition Assistance Program) application to provide assistance with meals and income supplementation.
- Mr. T. was placed in an insurance-provided high-risk case manager program to continue to receive ongoing support after I-PiCC ended.
- Mr. T. received assistance in selecting a nursing home for his mother that was within walking distance of where he lived.
- A sleep hygiene program was implemented to improve insomnia.
- A commode was purchased and placed at his bedside for nighttime urinary frequency.

Summary

The cost of the I-PiCC intervention per enrollee was approximately $1,000. The model provided elderly individuals with the knowledge to manage their ongoing health concerns using an interdisciplinary team approach to geriatric care. Clinicians expressed increased job satisfaction as they felt their interventions and encounters were more meaningful and patient centered. Follow-up calls made by the PCC after the intervention ended indicated long term sustainable changes for the majority of participants. They valued the resources provided, indicated improved relationships with their PCPs' practice, and felt more knowledgeable about the health care system. This type of interdisciplinary intervention has potential for future care coordination efforts with at risk Medicare patient populations.

References

Coleman, E.B., & Boult, C.E. (2003) Improving the quality of transitional care for persons with complex care needs: positional statement of the American Geriatrics Society health care systems committee. *Journal of the American Geriatrics Society*, 556–557.

Hall, M.J., DeFrances, C.J., Williams, S.N., *et al.* (2010) *National Hospital Discharge Survey: 2007 Summary*. National Health Statistics Reports Number 29. National Center for Health Statistics, Hyattsville, MD.

Machlin, S.R. (2009) *Trends in Healthcare Expenditures for the Elderly Age 65 and Over: 2006 versus 1996. Statistical Brief #256*. Agency for Healthcare Research and Quality, Rockville, MD.

Metter, M., & Kemper, D.W. (2003) *Healthwise for Life: A Self-Care Guide for People Age 50 or Better*. Healthwise Publications, Boise, ID.

National Committee on Quality Assurance. (2009) *Physician Practice Connections – Patient-Centered Medical Home (PPC-PCMH)*. National Committee on Quality Assurance, Washington, DC. Retrieved from http://www.ncqa.org/tabid/631/default.aspx.

Naylor M. (1990) Comprehensive discharge planning for hospitalized elderly: a pilot study. *Nursing Research*, 39, 156–160.

Prochaska, J.O., & Velicer, W.F. (1997) The transtheoretical model of health behavior change. *American Journal of Health Promotion*, 12(1), 38–48.

Prochaska, J.O., & Velicer, W.F. (1998) The transtheoretical model of health behavior change. *Homeostasis in Health and Disease*, 38(5–6), 216–233.

Ware, Jr., J., Kosinksi, M., & Keller, S. (1996) A 12-item short form health survey: construction of scales and preliminary tests of validity and reliability. *Medical Care*, 34, 220–233.

Ware, Jr., J., Kosinksi, M., & Keller, S. (1998) *SF-12: How to Score the SF-12 Physical and Mental Health Summary Scales*, 3rd edn. Quality Metric, Lincoln, RI.

Section 6
Medicare managed care

Chapter 28

Longitudinal care management: High risk care management

Chandra L. Torgerson and Lynda Hedstrom

Introduction

Although the United States spends more per capita on health care than any other country, 50% of Americans do not receive recommended preventive care, 30% do not receive needed care for acute medical conditions, and 40% go without necessary care for chronic conditions. As a group, Medicare beneficiaries have complex health care needs: 82% have at least one chronic condition; 20% have multiple chronic illnesses, accounting for two thirds of all Medicare spending; beneficiaries with multiple chronic illnesses account for 76% of all hospital admissions, and 70% of seniors do not receive recommended geriatric interventions (Centers for Disease Control and the Merck Company Foundation 2007).

Successful business models will depend on improving the ability to manage the risks of all segments of the population while improving quality (Bodenheimer 2003). Providers of Medicare Advantage Plans, such as United Healthcare Medicare & Retirement, have the infrastructure, interest and experience to coordinate care through targeted interventions and programs that are based on individual needs.

In the United Healthcare Medicare & Retirement High Risk Care Management Program, nursing (RN) care managers provide identified individuals with longitudinal telephonic case management. Longitudinal case management includes specific nursing interventions delivered over time while creating long-term relationships with members. Care managers work with the member to meet the member's goals and perceived needs, address their symptoms and provide condition management. Interventions focus on long-term care planning, member education, coordination of services and a schedule of focused follow-up.

Data from this experimental study design, using multivariant testing, indicate a 25% reduction in hospital admissions for the targeted population. Participants are predominantly dually eligible Special Needs Plan members. The results suggest that a predictable set of clinical nursing interventions can be identified, tracked, studied, and tied directly to improved outcomes for individuals in care coordination programs.

Comprehensive Care Coordination for Chronically Ill Adults, First Edition. Edited by Cheryl Schraeder and Paul Shelton.
© 2011 John Wiley & Sons, Inc. Published 2011 by John Wiley & Sons, Inc.

Background

United Healthcare is committed to improving the lives of the more than 9 million Medicare members served through a variety of services and benefits offered through the health plans. United Healthcare has a rich history of clinical program deployment, including a focus on frail, at-risk populations. Evercare, United Healthcare's flagship Special Needs Plan, was one of the first Centers for Medicare & Medicaid Services (CMS) demonstration projects for at-risk populations. This care model identifies frail elders living permanently in a nursing facility and provides a unique collection of services and benefits to the members residing there. In the Evercare model, assigned Nurse Practitioners provide ongoing services, including geriatric care, chronic condition management, appropriate prevention and wellness services, and advanced care planning. Nurse Practitioners have the ability to identify early changes in patient condition and bring care to the individual at the facility. This minimizes unnecessary transfers and hospitalizations, and improves quality of care resulting in greater member and family satisfaction (Kane *et al.* 2002; Kane *et al.* 2003; Kane *et al.* 2004).

In 2006, United Healthcare's commitment to serving the frail and at-risk populations extended to those populations living in the community setting. The Dually Eligible Individual Special Needs Plans formalized a creative care coordination program to address the needs of this population. Outcomes of interest include ensuring access to care, improvement in quality, communication with the primary care physician, and reduction in cost.

Highlighting United Healthcare's long-held value for the role of nursing in serving geriatric and frail populations, this clinical model was designed as a nurse-delivered telephonic care management model serving the frailest elders living in the community. The basic premise of the model is that nursing interventions can make a difference for dually eligible individuals, including those with multiple chronic conditions and a high need for community or caregiver support (Bodenheimer *et al.* 2002). These individuals could benefit from a long-term care management program using targeted interventions to address the needs of the individual comprehensively, rather than a short-term, face-to-face, or telephonic program. Identified individuals agree to participate and are assigned a care manager. They maintain continuous enrollment until they die or disenroll from the health plan. The target population includes individuals enrolled in United Healthcare's Dual and Chronic Special Needs Plans with high CMS hierarchical condition category (HCC) scores (HCC scores of 4.27 or greater; Institute for Health Policy Solutions 2005). Referrals can be made into the program and individuals are then assessed for inclusion. A study was designed to determine what specific nursing interventions were effective in reducing unnecessary admissions to the hospital.

Rationale

Analysis conducted by the UnitedHealth Group Center for Health Reform and Modernization estimates that the United States will spend $5 trillion on health care for the dually eligible population over the next 10 years. This dually eligible population has many challenges. Demographics show that these individuals typically earn less than

$20,000 per year, do not have a high school education, and many live in rural areas. These specific demographics lead to challenges in accessing and affording health care. Limited resources may also affect the individual's ability to follow through with the needed care, unless extra support is offered. Nurse driven care coordination models can provide that support.

Intervention

The philosophical approach is to begin first "where the individual is" on enrollment into the program, where the individual's basic needs and concerns are assessed and addressed (Lorig & Holman 2003). For example, it is unrealistic to consider disease management or self care if the individual doesn't have enough to eat. Once basic needs and significant areas of concern are addressed, the care manager can begin to work with the member on chronic condition management and education. Helping the individual achieve a working relationship with their primary care provider is a valuable strategy. Individuals learn to plan their visits with their provider and learn how to talk with their physician about their concerns. Care managers will work directly with the primary care physician or nurse, if needed, to ensure the member's needs are met. Management of care transitions and advanced care planning are priorities.

The following interventions have demonstrated a statistical difference in reducing hospital admissions. These are implemented and used in a standardized approach by all care managers with the members they serve.

Frequent touch

A decision-support tool based on certain criteria directs the nurse to the next touch point for an individual member. The criteria uses information gathered at each call to guide the process. The RN may call back the next day, in a week, or follow the standard protocol of 30 days.

Self management: change in condition

As individuals gain understanding of their chronic conditions and gain competency in managing their medications, an educational tool is introduced. This tool informs them of signs and symptoms that may indicate changes in their condition. The care manager works with the member and the tool to provide an action plan. The plan offers strategies in symptom management, such as dietary changes, taking prescribed medication, calling the physician or seeking care immediately in the emergency room. Care managers review this plan regularly with their assigned members.

Co-management with behavioral health specialists

Anxiety and depression have been shown to interfere with effective self-management of chronic conditions. This needs to be identified by the care manager and effective treatment initiated. When a care manager identifies an individual who may be demonstrating signs or symptoms of anxiety or depression, a consult with the individual's primary physician is recommended. A behavioral health specialist is engaged if the member consents and co-management begins.

Advanced care planning using the five wishes document

During the assessment process individuals without advanced care directives are identi-fied. The Five Wishes document is used to guide conversation with the individual. The care manager encourages the individual to discuss these wishes with their family and/or caregivers and make decisions if they so choose. Advanced Care Planning is an ongoing conversation which is included regularly in care management activities.

Care manager specific feedback on adherence to specified interventions

Individual care manager feedback is an important piece of ensuring that standard in-terventions are deployed for measurement. Activity reports inform the care manager regarding the outcomes they are responsible for, productivity standards and case loads. Care managers get information updated daily, weekly, and monthly regarding the individ-ual, touches, member hospitalizations, and assessments/care plan completion. In addition, calls are recorded and reviewed with Supervisors to assess the quality of interactions and adherence to the priority interventions. Regular feedback on performance is shared with all care managers to improve their competency and professional development.

An unanticipated secondary impact: Staff performance

The whole process of identifying and testing effective nursing interventions in this struc-tured way resulted in improved staff satisfaction and performance. This outcome had not been anticipated. Each intervention tested involved detailed recipes for implementation; with each member contact, care managers are required to follow a standardized process. Each care manager has to perform and document certain designated interventions in the same way. This degree of standardization allowed for consistency and thoroughness in documentation. It allowed consistent tracking of activities with data that could be trusted and acted upon. Care managers and supervisors alike can see what occurs between the member and their care manager. Productivity and application of the interventions are readily apparent.

In addition to standardization and consistency, the recipes allowed for better overall task management. Staff that had previously experienced difficulty in structuring their day became more efficient within a matter of days or weeks. Performance scores soared, increasing 30% or more on average. These performance measures are monitored weekly for each care manager and have not regressed over time.

One other development in the care manager team was a new appreciation for data or evidence to drive daily activities. Care managers were initially blinded from seeing which interventions were working until the results of the study were validated. The care managers couldn't wait for the results. They became thoroughly engaged in the testing process and strived to obtain the best possible outcomes. They suggested new ideas for testing and process improvements and were eager to implement the results. This created an environment of continuous quality improvement and innovation within the team and a desire to practice based on what the evidence shows. This has also kept adherence to the proven interventions high – at 98% or greater. Staff retention remains greater than 90%.

Case studies

The cases and names have been altered and are not reflective of any single individual.

Case study #1

Dawn, the High Risk Case Manager, was assigned to Mary on June 2, 2009. The initial assessment and conversation included findings on several debilitating conditions.

Mary's diabetes was being treated with daily Insulin of 60 units each morning, and she is to use sliding scale insulin based on her blood sugar levels throughout the day. A significant complication to her diabetes is the diagnosis of heart failure. Mary has been hospitalized repeatedly – four times in the last year. She is also morbidly obese and wheelchair bound.

Mary is dependent on others to bring her food; neighbors and a daughter stop by regularly. Unfortunately, the food they bring rarely adheres to her dietary requirements for diabetes and heart disease. From a practical perspective of managing in her home, Mary's wheelchair would not fit through the bathroom door, forcing her to use a bedside commode. Mary was not able to get to her physician appointments, as local transportation could not accommodate her size and weight. The only medical treatment she received was in the local emergency room when she was transported by ambulance.

Dawn immediately identified several interventions to help Mary improve her health and quality of life. Dawn found a transportation provider who could accommodate Mary's size and wheelchair, allowing her to get to and from her physician appointments. Mary is a very motivated individual and began to see her doctors and specialists on a regular basis. Dawn talked to Mary about basic needs and nutrition. By using Mary's Medicaid benefits, she arranged for Mary to receive two meals a day delivered to her home that met her dietary requirements. Next, Dawn worked with the PCP office staff to find a personal care aide for assistance with ADLs. The aide was also able to help prepare meals in compliance with Mary's dietary requirements. After lots of research by the care manager, a local charity arranged to have new doors put into Mary's bathroom. A short series of visits from a home health physical therapist helped Mary to manage in the bathroom safely when she was alone.

During Dawn's frequent follow up calls it became apparent that Mary was losing weight and feeling better. Over the course of a few months Mary was able to stop taking her daytime sliding scale insulin and reduced her morning insulin from 60 to 35 units. Her spirits began to lift and Dawn could tell a difference with every phone call.

After 18 months of care management, Mary's progress was remarkable. Through support by Dawn's prioritized and strategic case management interventions, Mary lost

185 pounds. She has a new wheelchair and no longer requires special bariatric transportation. She lost two shoe sizes and now has diabetic shoes. Her goal is to start walking again. She is compliant with her diet and doctor visits, and she is very proud of the steps she has taken to be healthier. Mary believes the nurse made the difference. Working together with Dawn through the comprehensive High Risk Care Management program gave her the resources and encouragement to begin living a healthier life.

Case study #2

Rosina, the High Risk Care Manager, has been working with Mark since January 2010. Mark is 71 years old with a history of colon cancer and a subsequent colostomy. Mark had been instructed in the hospital and was trying to manage alone but he just couldn't get the colostomy bags to fit. At a scheduled monthly call, Rosina found that Mark's sister, the primary caregiver, was frustrated because she could not get the necessary supplies for his colostomy. She had questions regarding the supplies that were needed and was unsure whether or not these supplies were covered under Mark's insurance. Several calls to the insurance customer service line had left her with more questions than answers, and she had given up. She was also fearful of hurting Mark and she needed some basic instruction.

Rosina worked to find the right home health care provider to provide the necessary instructions, supplies, and support for Mark and his sister. Once Mark and his sister felt proficient, Rosina worked with the durable medical equipment company to regularly ship the needed supplies to their home. When Rosina called the primary care physician office to get the orders for the right supplies, the physician acknowledged the efforts of the care manager and appreciated the intervention in a very difficult situation. Mark is managing very well.

Rosina demonstrated that as a care manager she was a ready resource for them. Rosina continues with her regular contact and support for Mark and his caregiver.

Key learnings in high risk care management

Many lessons have been learned over the past three years in the High Risk Care Management program.

1. Telephonic care management works to improve individuals' lives and the return on the investment can be quantified. Care management telephonic interventions can be standardized and delivered to reduce costs and improve individual outcomes.
2. Targeting the right population with the focused interventions was critical to the success of the High Risk Care Management program.
3. Care managers gain buy-in from members when time is taken to address the member's concerns and basic needs first.
4. A longitudinal approach in the development of the relationship with the member helps to make changes to health status over time.
5. Frequent interaction between the individual, the caregiver, the primary care physician, and the care manager can make profound improvements in the individual's health and reduce costs overall.

6. Sharing data on the standardized interventions and productivity with care managers helped them take responsibility for their performance and motivated them to do well.
7. The ability to describe and test what nurses do, and the improvements those activities make, led to greater job satisfaction, higher staff retention, and the ability to measure the impact of nursing interventions in real dollars.
8. Management oversight is important to ensure standard intervention protocols are being followed. This can be done in a way that is not burdensome to the care manager or supervisor and allows for continued improvement in practice and the program.

Summary

A targeted telephonic longitudinal care management program can improve the lives of individuals, reduce costs, and demonstrate improved financial outcome to the business. Access to a care manager who works with members over time can be instrumental for frail, at-risk populations in providing improved health and outcomes in complex situations.

Acknowledgments

The authors acknowledge the partnership of many excellent clinicians, their leaders, and statisticians who contributed to this work that has demonstrated business value and most importantly contributes to improved care for the individuals and their families.

References

Bodenheimer, T. (2003) Interventions to improve chronic illness care: evaluating their effectiveness. *Disease Management*, 6, 63–71.

Bodenheimer, T., Wagner, E.H., & Grumbach, K. (2002) Improving primary care for patients with chronic illness. *Journal of the American Medical Association*, 288, 1775–1779.

Centers for Disease Control and the Merck Company Foundation. (2007) *The State of Ageing and Health in America 2007*. The Merck Company Foundation, Whitehouse Station, NJ. Available at: http://www.cdc.gov/aging/pdf/saha_2007.pdf.

Institute for Health Policy Solutions. (2005) *Risk Adjustment Methods and Their Relevance to "Pay-or-Play."* Institute for Health Policy Solutions, Washington, DC. Available at: http://www. ihps.org/pubs/2005_Apr_IHPS_SB2_ESup_Risk_Adj.pdf.

Kane, R.L., Flood, S., Keckhafer, G., *et al.* (2002) Nursing home residents covered by Medicare risk contracts: early findings from the Evercare evaluation model. *Journal of the American Geriatrics Society*, 50, 719–727.

Kane, R.L., Flood, S., Bershadsky, B., *et al.* (2003) The effect of Evercare on hospital use. *Journal of the American Geriatrics Society*, 51, 1427–1434.

Kane, R.L., Flood, S., Bershadsky, B., *et al.* (2004) Effect of an innovative Medicare managed care program on the quality of care for nursing home residents. *The Gerontologist*, 44, 95–103.

Lorig, K.L., & Holman, H.R. (2003) Self-management: history, definition, outcomes, and mechanisms. *Annals of Behavioral Medicine*, 26(1), 1–7.

International care coordination

Chapter 29

The experiences in the Republic of Korea

Weon-seob Yoo and Joo-bong Park Oh

Background information

Demographics

With 49 million people, the Republic of Korea (hereafter Korea) is going through the most rapid change in demographics as well as an epidemiological transition. Life expectancy at birth increased from 65.7 years in 1980 to 80.1 years in 2008, and the total fertility rate dropped from 2.83 to 1.19 during the same period (Ministry of Health and Welfare [MHW] 2009). As a result of this increase in life expectancy, along with having the world's lowest total fertility rate, Korea is expected to become an aged society in 18 years, since it became an aging society in 2000, and is expected to become a super-aged society in an additional 8 years (by 2026). The United Nations defines an "aging society" as a country where 7% or more of the population is 65 years or older, and a "super-aged society" as one with 20% or more 65 years of age or older. For the United States it took 72 and 16 years, respectively, to progress to an aged society and then to a super-aged society, and 24 and 12 years, respectively, for Japan. (See Table 29.1 for selected Korea demographics and health indicators.)

Health care system

Korea has implemented and maintained two national health security schemes for its 49 million citizens since 1977. One is the National Health Insurance program (NHI), a compulsory social insurance program which covers 96.3% of the whole population and the other is the Medical Aid program (MA), a public assistance program for the underprivileged of whom about 90% receive livelihood assistance.

The National Health Insurance Corporation (NHIC) is responsible for operating the NHI, while local governments are responsible for the MA. The Health Insurance Review Agency (HIRA) reviews all of the providers' claims, except those claims not covered by the NHI or the MA, while the Ministry of Health and Welfare supervises the NHIC, the local government, and the HIRA (Kwon 2009).

In 2008, Korea spent 6.5% of its GDP on health care (Organisation for Economic Co-operation and Development [OECD] 2010). Of the total health care budget,

Comprehensive Care Coordination for Chronically Ill Adults, First Edition. Edited by Cheryl Schraeder and Paul Shelton.
© 2011 John Wiley & Sons, Inc. Published 2011 by John Wiley & Sons, Inc.

Table 29.1   Selected Demographics and Health Indicators, 2008

Population	
Population (millions)	48.6
Aged 65 and older (percent)	10.3
Life expectancy at birth (years)	
Female	83.3
Male	76.5
Infant mortality rate (per 1,000 live births), 2006	4.1
Total fertility rate	1.19
GDP per capita (P.P.P.$)	27,658
GDP given to health (percent)	6.5
Doctor consultations per capita	13

Source: OECD (2010)

government sources and social insurance accounted for 55.5%, while the remaining 44.5% had to be paid privately (Jeong 2010). Though the health care spending of Korea, as a share of GDP, is the third lowest among the OECD nations, its growth rate was the fastest over the past decade due to the rapid aging of the population and the expanding of NHI benefits (Jones 2010).

Health care services are delivered mainly by the private sector; 90% of physicians work in private clinics and hospitals, and 96% of hospitals and clinics are privately owned, which accounts for 90% of beds (Jones 2010). Providers are reimbursed mainly by a fee-for-service scheme supplemented by a diagnosis-related group (DRG) in some inpatient care. There is no formal gate-keeper, and clinics and hospitals perform similar functions, resulting in a limited role of primary care, and competition rather than coordination among physicians in clinics and hospitals is prevalent (Kwon 2009).

Current programs for care coordination

There are three nation-wide care coordination programs for people with chronic conditions in the public sector. One is for NHIC's beneficiaries with targeted chronic diseases, another is for MA's beneficiaries who heavily use medical services, and the third is for residents who voluntarily enrolled in local public community health centers (PCHCs). Through community-based intervention, all of these programs are trying to achieve common goals of reducing cost, ensuring quality services, and improving clients' health outcomes.

Case management of NHIC

When NHIC experienced a financial deficit in 1997, various efforts aiming at fiscal sustainability and cost containment were made. In 2002, NHIC introduced the Case Management Program for Chronic Diseases (CMPCD) as a demonstration project from August 2002 to December 2003. During that period, 15 teams composed of two case managers were deployed to 15 local NHIC offices with support from professionals in medicine, nursing, and social welfare from 13 local universities. By the end of the CMPCD, target population priority, an education program for the CMPCD's case managers, five disease-specific needs assessment tools, care plans based on comprehensive need assessment, a case management process, and an information system supporting the case managers' routine work had been developed with active participation of the case managers (Kim *et al.* 2008).

Target population

At first, CMPCD targeted five major chronic diseases: essential hypertension (HTN), type 2 diabetes mellitus (type 2 DM), congestive heart failure (CHF), stroke, and children's asthma based on the burden of each disease and the availability of effective intervention. Using NHIC's nationwide claim data, NHIC identified those people with one of these five target diseases, and classified them into an under-utilizing or an over-utilizing group, according to their total number of consultations and treatment days.

However, there have been some unexpected problems with identifying and selecting two target populations. Clients with CHF were rare and it was difficult to meet them within the community. For children's asthma, the disease code in the claims data was frequently found to be incorrect. As a result, CHF and children's asthma were excluded from the target diseases to increase the efficiency of the CMPCD since 2004. Arthritis was newly included as another target disease in 2007 (Kim *et al.* 2008).

In 2010, NHIC has reformed to link its biennial Health Screening Program (HSP) and CMPCD. The CMPCD is now targeting those people who are newly identified to have HTN or type 2 DM through HSP within the past six months. The NHIC is expecting it can provide CMPCD services for about 50,000 new clients through NHIC's 494 lay workers each year.

Case manager

In 2002, the NHIC recruited 31 registered nurses (RNs) with at least three years of clinical experience in clinics or hospitals as case managers and had developed education and training programs for their own case managers (Table 29.2). As the Korean government has been trying to reduce the NHIC's workforce to lower its operating costs since 2002, the NHIC has not been able to recruit additional RNs required when the CMPCD expanded to a nationwide service in 2004. The NHIC then decided to use lay workers (staffs of the NHIC) for the CMPCD. Before the lay workers started their new job as a case manager, they received a one-week education program and a month of field training supervised by a skilled RN case manager.

To improve the expertise of the case manager, the NHIC introduced a two-level certificate for its own case managers and has been providing training courses for the first grade (advanced level) and the second grade (skilled level) case managers since 2006. The two certification courses have been operated by the NHIC and commissioned to an external institute, the Nursing College of Seoul National University. The training course of the second grade is a three-week, 95-hour course covering 40 subjects, and the first grade is a two-week, 56-hour course covering 20 subjects that is required to successfully implement and manage the CMPCD (Shin 2009).

Table 29.2 Training Course for the NHIC's Certified Case Managers

	Case Manager	
	1st grade **(advanced level)**	**2nd grade** **(skilled level)**
Training Course	2 weeks (56 hours) 20 subjects	3 weeks (95 hours) 40 subjects
Candidates/trainees	Certified 2nd grade Case managers who have worked at least 2 years in the case management service	NHIC staff who have worked for at least 3 months in the case management service
Number of 2006		108
newly 2007		40
certified 2008	22	40
case 2009	22	40
managers 2010	–	45
Total	44	273

Source: Modified from Shin (2009)

Process

Every six months, case managers of a local office receive a list of the target population residing in each designated area and send a letter to potential clients introducing the CMPCD and informing them how to utilize the service. After they have received consent from the clients, case managers provide a 12-week service consisting of at least four home-visits and two telephone calls. The first home-visit is for needs assessment and the last one is for identifying the effectiveness of the services. Telephone calls are made to monitor and support clients during the intervention phase.

Through a face-to-face interview, case managers assess the client's needs using a questionnaire, 'needs assessment tool' developed by the NHIC. The questionnaire covers seven categories: socioeconomic information, medical information, utilization of health care services, knowledge about their specific disease, self-management, health-related behavior, and social support. An individualized care plan and goals of each action plan are developed based on the data collected during the first visit and entered into the NHIC's information system (see Table 29.3).

With an individualized comprehensive care plan, case managers can identify diverse needs and concentrate their efforts on higher priority needs. However, the care management program has a limited role because there is no obligation or financial incentive for physicians to cooperate with the case manager and the NHIC's CMPCD does not include any kind of formal cooperation with physicians who provide care for the clients.

Recently, with the change of the target population, focusing on the newly identified patients with HTN or type 2 DM and patients with low compliance, there has been efforts made to modify the intensity and method of interventions depending on the level of motivation of the clients.

Table 29.3   Process of NHIC's Case Management Program

Process	Activities
Phase 1 Selecting clients	Select a client based on preset criteria Send an information letter Make an appointment by telephone
Phase 2 Assessing needs and planning interventions	1st visit Undertake needs assessment using the needs assessment tool Select problems by preset standard Establish care plans with client
Phase 3 Doing interventions	2nd visit-1st phone call 3rd visit-2nd phone call Provide interventions concerning the problem list
Phase 4 Evaluating the effectiveness of Case Management services	4th visit Identify changes of the client using the same needs assessment tool Evaluate the achievement of goals of services

Source: Modified from So (2008)

Results

A total of 171,919 clients utilized the CMPCD service through 2008 and clients' satisfaction was very high (84.9 on a 100 point scale). There have been many studies reporting the short-term effect of the NHIC's CMPCD, including the improvement of blood pressure or blood sugar control, daily life practices, physical activities, medication adherence, functional status, and caregiver burden (Shin *et al.* 2003; Kim *et al.* 2004; So *et al.* 2008). However, there is no evidence supporting the long-term effects of the services and their impact on cost containment has not been identified.

Case management of medical aid

In May 2003, the Case Management for the Medical Aid Beneficiaries (CMMAB) was introduced by MHW in 28 districts of Korea as a demonstration project to support self-management and health service utilization of clients and to reduce costs. Through a gradual expansion, in 2006 all 232 districts in Korea provided CMMAB to those people who need help for effective self-care and a guide to complex health care services, and have a tendency to use medical services heavily.

The Medical Aid program is composed of individuals with higher needs for health care than NHIC. For example, the ratio of the elderly in MA is approximately four times that of the NHIC, and the registered disabled and people with a rare and incurable disease, like chronic renal failure, are much more concentrated in MA.

Unlike the NHIC's CMPCD which focuses on a specific disease, CMMAB focuses on an individual, and most have multiple chronic conditions. In addition, case managers may limit access to medical service for clients if they receive permission from the local Medical Aid committee, based on the Medical Aid Act. If a client receives this penalty, the MA benefit will be stopped until the end of the year, and the client must pay all of the cost without the support of the MA benefit.

The Medical Aid Case Management Center (MACMC), supervised by the MHW, was established in 2007. Its main functions are planning and evaluating CMMAB, providing a training program and technical support for case managers and updating practice guidelines.

Target population

The CMMAB targeted those people newly entitled to MA benefits and those who are more likely to heavily use medical services; people whose medication is prescribed beyond 365 days a year for the same disease, who have a tendency to visit two or more clinics (or hospitals) frequently for the same disease, and those who are on long-term inpatient care for more than 31 days. In 2010, CMMAB added hospitals and long-term care facilities as another subject of CMMAB intervention where long-term hospitalizations are occurring more frequently than others.

The MA target population, and the list of clients, is identified using claims data from the HIRA, which is updated periodically. Of the 247,878 CMMAB recipients in 2009, 51,747 (20.6%) were re-enrolled clients who had received the CMMAB service the previous year (MACMC 2010).

Case manager

At first, the MHW recruited 28 case managers from licensed RNs and social workers, but has narrowed employment criteria only to RNs with three or more years of clinical experience.

With stepwise expansion of the CMMAB, the number of MA case managers also increased. At the end of 2009, there were 463 case managers, deployed in the local government at a ratio of one case manager per 2,500 MA beneficiaries. In 2010, a skilled case manager has been placed in the regional administrative authority to supervise and support CMMAB within local areas. A case manager is supposed to provide services to 320 clients per year (MHW 2010b).

The MACMC provides two three-day training courses several times a year for the case managers. One is for the new case manager, and the other is for the experienced. Case managers must complete at least one course per year. In addition, there are other intermittent education programs operated at the regional or local level. Currently, there is no certification or license program for the MA case manager.

Process

Based on the claims data, the HIRA identifies and selects the list of clients for each local area and provides it to local case managers on a quarterly schedule. Priority is given to newly enrolled MA beneficiaries, heavy users of outpatient services, and patients on long-term hospitalization.

According to the client's previous pattern of service utilization, case managers classify their clients into four subgroups: a high-risk group, an unmet-need group, a temporary-management group, and a newly enrolled group. The high-risk group is in danger of abusing or misusing medications and medical services, as they are likely to visit medical institutions more frequently than other clients and get duplicated prescriptions. The unmet-need group is likely to under-use medical services given the client's needs of diagnosed disease. The temporary-management group consists of clients who are not identified by HIRA but only by a case manager. The newly enrolled group is composed of the people who enrolled in MA for the first time and need basic information about MA.

The intensity of provided services depends on group assignment. More than two home-visits and four phone calls are provided for the high-risk group, more than one home-visit and two phone calls for the unmet-need group, one or two home-visits or phone calls for the temporary-management group, and one or two phone calls and a mailing of informational pamphlets for the newly enrolled group.

Needs assessment information is collected in a face-to-face interview during home-visits using the structured needs assessment tool and computerized information already available to the local authorities, the NHIC, and the HIRA. The needs assessment tool, developed and periodically being revised by the MACMC, covers seven categories: demographic information, knowledge about MA, pattern and quantity of medical service utilization, health status, self-care, social support, and residential environment.

Based on the comprehensive needs assessment, a care plan for each client and goals for action plans are made. Before they terminate services, case managers evaluate the services by re-measuring the client's needs using the same need assessment tool.

Results

In 2009, of the total 1.7 million MA beneficiaries, 247,878 clients (14.7%) were provided services by 463 case managers. Approximately 32% of beneficiaries receiving services were initially classified in the high-risk group as well as the temporary-management group, 19% were in the newly enrolled group and 10% were in the unmet-need group. Satisfaction with the services provided was high (80.4 on a 100 point scale), and it is estimated that approximately $23 million was saved due to the nation-wide CMMAB (MACMC 2010). The improvement of health related quality of life, self-care, and changes in service utilization were significantly greater in the high-risk group than the unmet-need group (Ahn 2010).

Case management of community health center

The Individual Home Visiting Health Care (IHVHC) is the representative service of Public Community Health Centers (PCHC) and it is provided by 253 PCHCs nationwide. Its prototype began in 1990, but a full-scale IHVHS with a greater expansion of workforce and a more systematic approach began in 2007.

Target population

The IHVHC provides services for low-income populations with priority given to pregnant women, infants, immigrants, the disabled, and the elderly. In 2009, of 1.5 million clients, 930,403 (77.7%) had one or more chronic conditions in need of care. Unlike CMPCD or CMMAB, the clients are identified and enrolled by self-registration, referral from CMPCD or CMMAB, or by lay people.

Case manager

A multidisciplinary team provides its services based on an individual care plan. There are 2,700 IHVHC staff and RN case managers that play a core role with other PCHC staff, including physical therapists, dietitians, dental hygienists, and social workers. There are two training courses for RN case managers. One is for new case managers and the other is for the already skilled.

   The RN case managers assess the client's needs and create a care plan using a comprehensive needs assessment tool and a computerized information system. They can provide home nursing services, which is not possible in the CMPCD or the CMMAB.

Process

Case managers implement needs assessment during the initial home visit. Based on the results, clients are classified into three subgroups: an intensive care group, a routine care group, and a well-controlled group.

   According to an individual care and action plan, case managers provide or coordinate services for a year. They adjust the number of their home visits depending on group classification: for the intensive care group, at least once a month; for the routine care group, at least once every three months; and for the well-controlled group, at least once a year. Clients may use the IHVHC service up to two years if they are in need of the services. The PCHC's information system is an integral tool that assists case managers in doing their job and keeping up with vital information on their clients.

Results

A total of 1.5 million clients used the IHVHC services in 2009; routine group clients accounted for 76.7% of the service use; well-controlled clients 22.3%, and the intensive group 1%. Almost all clients (97.1%) responded that they were satisfied with the IHVHS services (MHW 2010a). According to a recent study, the benefit-cost ratio of IHVHS was 9.16 and the benefit of arthritis management was the largest among disease management programs (Kim *et al.* 2010).

Summary and future challenges

Financial instability of the health security system, and the quickly aging population with the epidemiologic transition to chronic diseases have triggered the development of individualized intensive interventions such as CMPCD, CMMAB, and IHVHC. Since 2002, education programs and training courses for case managers have developed, and knowledge, information, and an evidence-base of case management has accumulated. Though there is some evidence that current programs are effective or efficient, still there are questions to be answered. For example, the effectiveness or efficiency of current programs has to be confirmed by well-designed studies. Furthermore, the education programs or training courses for case managers should be evaluated in terms of how they meet their needs. Involving primary care physicians who could significantly change or have an effect on clients' knowledge, attitude, behavior, and medication is another critical issue to be examined.

As Korea has been experiencing a rapid aging of the population, people with chronic conditions are increasing at a rapid pace. It is difficult to expect optimized care within a fragmented and complex health care delivery system. Coordination of care is helpful and effective for these people with chronic diseases, especially those with multiple chronic conditions that need continuous attention and care. And it may provide opportunities to strengthen primary care and improve efficiency of our fragmented health system. With efforts to reform the current health care delivery system, care coordination could be a means of ensuring good care and reducing costs.

References

Ahn, Y., Kim, E., & Ko, I. (2010) The effects of tele-care case management services for medical aid beneficiaries. *Journal of Korean Academy of Community Health Nursing*, 21, 351–361 [in Korean].

Jeong, H. (2010) *2008 National Health Accounts and Total Health Expenditure in Korea*. Ministry of Health and Welfare, Seoul, Korea [in Korean].

Jones, R.J. (2010) *Health-care Reform in Korea*. Economics Department Working Papers, No. 797, Organisation for Economic Co-operation and Development, Paris, France.

Kim, E., Choi, J., Kim, C., *et al.* (2004) Effects of community-based case management program on functional Status and caregiver burden of stroke patients. *Journal of Korean Community Nursing*, 15(1), 18–28 [in Korean].

Kim, E., Kim, Y., Kim, C., *et al.* (2008) *Community-based Case Management for the Chronically Ill Patients*. Hyunmoonsa, Seoul, Korea [in Korean].

Kim, J., Lee, T., Lee, J., *et al.* (2010) A cost benefit analysis of individual home visiting health care. *Journal of Korean Academy of Community Health Nursing*, 21, 362–373 [in Korean].

Kwon, S. (2009) Thirty years of national health insurance in South Korea: lessons for achieving universal health care coverage. *Health Policy and Planning*, 24(1), 63–71.

Medical Aid Case Management Center. (2010) *Annual Report 2009*. Medical Aid Case Management Center, Seoul, Korea [in Korean].

Ministry of Health and Welfare. (2009) *Annual Report 2008*. Ministry of Health and Welfare, Seoul, Korea [in Korean].

Ministry of Health and Welfare. (2010a) *Improving Family's Health Guide 2010*. Ministry of Health and Welfare, Seoul, Korea [in Korean].

Ministry of Health and Welfare. (2010b). *Medical Aid Guide 2010*. Ministry of Health and Welfare, Seoul, Korea [in Korean].

Organisation for Economic Co-operation and Development. (2010) *OECD Health Data 2010.* Organisation for Economic Co-operation and Development, Paris, France.

Shin, E., Kim, C., Yoo, W., *et al.* (2003). The effect of case management program for diabetic patients in Korean community. *The Journal of Korean Community Nursing*, 14(4), 1–9 [in Korean].

Shin, S. (2009) Evaluating a community-based case management program for people with diabetes in Korea. PhD thesis, La Trobe University.

So, A., Kim, Y., Kim, E., *et al.* (2008). Effects of community-based case management program for clients with hypertension. *Journal of Korean Academy of Nursing*, 38, 822–830 [in Korean].

Index

Comprehensive Care Coordination for Chronically Ill Adults, First Edition. Edited by Cheryl Schraeder and Paul Shelton.
© 2011 John Wiley & Sons, Inc. Published 2011 by John Wiley & Sons, Inc.

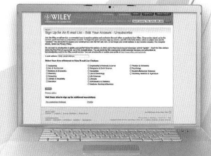